UTILIZING COMMUNITY RESOURCES
An overview of human services

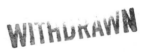

UTILIZING COMMUNITY RESOURCES
An overview of human services

William Crimando

T. F. Riggar

S^t_L

St. Lucie Press
Delray Beach, Florida

Direct all inquiries to:
    St. Lucie Press, Inc.
    100 E. Linton Blvd., Suite 403B
    Delray Beach, Florida, 33483.
    Phone: (407) 274-9906
    Fax: (407) 274-9927

S^t_L

St. Lucie Press
Delray Beach, Florida

To Liz and Mark, my life and my joy

To S. W. R., without whom nothing is possible

Contributors

Jill E. Adams, J.D. is assistant professor of Law, Southern Illinois University School of Law. She received her Juris Doctor from the University of New Mexico.

Clora Mae Baker, Ph.D. is assistant professor in Vocational Education Studies, Southern Illinois University at Carbondale. She received her doctorate in Curriculum, Instruction, and Professional Development from Ohio State University in 1989.

John J. Benshoff, Ph.D. is assistant professor of Rehabilitation Administration and Services at the Rehabilitation Institute, Southern Illinois University at Carbondale. He received his doctorate from the University of Northern Colorado in 1985. He is a charter fellow of the American College of Addiction Treatment Administrators.

Wanda D. Bracy, M.S.W. is associate professor and chairperson of the Department of Social Work, Northeastern Illinois University in Chicago. She received her M.A. degree in Sociology from Roosevelt University in 1975, and her M.S.W. from the University of Illinois at Chicago in 1985. Professor Bracy's specialty is in the areas of social welfare policy and evaluation research.

William Crimando, Ph.D., CRC is professor and coordinator of Rehabilitation Administration and Services of the Rehabilitation Institute, Southern Illinois University at Carbondale. He received his doctorate in Counseling from Michigan State University, and is the author or co-author of five books and over 40 articles.

Brian C. Cronk, M.A. is a research assistant at Chestnut Health System's Lighthouse Training Institute. He has a master's degree from Bradley University and will receive a Ph.D. in experimental psychology from the University of Wisconsin-Milwaukee.

Paula K. Davis, Ph.D. is lecturer in the Rehabilitation Institute, Southern Illinois University at Carbondale, where she received her degree in 1989 in Special Education. She has published several papers on the topic of community living skills, and has made numerous presentations at the state and national level.

Norma J. Ewing, Ph.D. is chair of the Special Education Department at Southern Illinois University at Carbondale. She is the author of numerous articles, chapters, and books. Currently, she is pursuing research on African-Americans in higher education.

Mark D. Godley, Ph.D. is director of Research and Development at Chestnut Health Systems, Bloomington, Illinois where he conducts evaluation studies of state and federal substance abuse demonstration projects. He has presented and published more than 30 papers on substance abuse.

Susan Harrington Godley, Rh.D., CRC is a consultant specializing in human service planning, development, and evaluation. She received her doctorate in 1982 from the Rehabilitation Institute, Southern Illinois University at Carbondale. She is the author or co-author of numerous rehabilitation, mental health, and program evaluation publications.

Cheryl Hanley-Maxwell, Ph.D. is an assistant professor of Special Education in the Department of Rehabilitation Psychology and Special Education at the University of Wisconsin-Madison. She received her doctorate in Education from the University of Illinois, and is the author or co-author of over 22 publications.

Debra A. Harley, M.A., CRC is project coordinator for the Off-Campus Transition Specialist Program at Southern Illinois University at Carbondale. She received her master's degree from South Carolina State College and is enrolled in the doctoral program in Special Education at SIU-C.

James T. Herbert, Ph.D., CRC is assistant professor and coordinator of the Rehabilitation Counseling Program at The Pennsylvania State University. He received his doctorate from the University of Wisconsin-Madison in Rehabilitation Psychology. Although his published work concerns the field of rehabilitation counseling, an ongoing research theme and professional interest is job placement of persons with disabilities.

Beverley E. Holland, Rh.D., R.N. is assistant professor at the School of Nursing at University of Louisville, Louisville, Kentucky. She received her doctorate in Rehabilitation from Southern Illinois University-Carbondale.

Timothy R. Janikowski, Ph.D., CRC is assistant professor of Rehabilitation Counseling at the Rehabilitation Institute, Southern Illinois University at Carbondale. He received his doctorate in Rehabilitation Psychology in 1988 from the University of Wisconsin-Madison. His professional experience includes job placement of persons who have sustained industrial injuries.

Richard Kern worked as a reporter for five years and in public relations work for two years. He is now a graduate student in rehabilitation at Southern Illinois University at Carbondale.

Robert F. Kilbury, M.S. is the executive director of the Southern Illinois Center for Independent Living in Carbondale, Illinois. He is a doctoral candidate in Rehabilitation at the Rehabilitation Institute, Southern Illinois University and earned his master's degree in Counseling Psychology from the University of Central Arkansas.

Bradley W. Kuhlman, Ph.D. is a pain rehabilitation counselor at St. Cloud Hospital's Pain Management Clinic in St. Cloud, Minnesota. He has a master's degree in Rehabilitation Counseling from St. Cloud State University and a Ph.D. in Rehabilitation Psychology from the University of Iowa.

Eugene Landrum, M.D. is a practicing psychiatrist and the Medical Director of Chestnut Health System's Lighthouse Training Institute, where he conducts evaluation studies of substance abuse demonstration projects and policy studies on AIDS, medical care, and substance abuse.

Dennis R. Maki, Ph.D., NCC, CRC received his doctorate in Rehabilitation Counseling Psychology from the University of Wisconsin-Madison, and coordinates Graduate Rehabilitation Counselor Education Programs at the University of Iowa. Named Rehabilitation Educator of the Year in 1985 by the National Council on Rehabilitation Education, Dr. Maki is a past president of American Rehabilitation Counseling Association and has been co-editor for special issues of the *Journal of Applied Rehabilitation Counseling.*

Ralph E. Matkin, Rh.D. is an associate professor in the Department of Educational Psychology and Administration at California State University, Long Beach. He is also adjunct research psychologist in the School of Medicine at the University of California, Los Angeles, and the data manager for the Rehabilitation Medicine Service-Brentwood Division, West Los Angeles VA Medical Center. Dr. Matkin has been a private consultant since 1978.

Robert Lee Matkin, M.P.F.M., is a budget officer for the Anti-terrorism Assistance Program within the United States Department of State. He received his master's degree in Public Financial Management from The American University, Washington, DC. He has worked for the United States government in federal budgeting since 1977, including eight years in the Housing and Urban Development Budget Office.

V. Robert May III, Rh.D. is senior partner and clinical rehabilitation evaluator at May Rehab and Therapy Services in Richmond Virginia. He received his doctorate from the Rehabilitation Institute, Southern Illinois University at Carbondale. He is also executive director of the National Association of Disability Evaluating Professionals (NADEP).

Vicente N. Noble, Ph.D. is a professor of Educational Psychology and coordinator of the Marriage, Family, Child Counseling graduate training program at California State University, Long Beach. He received his doctorate from the Claremont Graduate School in 1973 and has conducted studies in multicultural psychology and families.

Julie Kate O'Brien, Ph.D. is a human resource development specialist with the Region V Rehabilitation Continuing Education Program, Rehabilitation Institute, at Southern Illinois University-Carbondale. She has 12 years employment experience in rehabilitation facilities. She earned her doctorate from Colorado State University in career and guidance counseling of persons with disabilities.

Lenore Patton, M.A. is co-founder of the Alice Paul House Domestic Violence Shelter and Rape Crisis Center in Indiana, Pennsylvania. She has served as executive director of the program since 1981.

Frank D. Puckett, Rh.D. is coordinator of Clinical Services, Center for Rehabilitation Science and Biomedical Engineering, Louisiana Tech University. He earned his doctorate in rehabilitation from Southern Illinois University at Carbondale and is project manager for regional training programs in rehabilitation technology.

T. F. Riggar, Ed.D. is a professor in the Rehabilitation Administration and Services division of the Rehabilitation Institute, Southern Illinois University at Carbondale. Dr. Riggar is a graduate of the University of Northern Colorado and is the author or co-author of 12 books and over 50 articles.

M. J. Schmidt, M.A. is program director for Outpatient Services, ReMed Recovery Care Centers, Conshohocken, Pennsylvania. She received her degree in Rehabilitation Administration and Services, Southern Illinois University at Carbondale. The author or co-author of books and articles on sexual harassment and human resource management, she has consulted in the area of case management practices.

Nancy L. Schade is the program director of the Client Assistance Program, South Dakota Advocacy Services in Pierre. She received her B.S. in psychology from South Dakota State University.

Karen M. Sowers-Hoag, Ph.D. is assistant professor of Social Work at Florida International University in North Miami. She received her doctorate in social work from Florida State University in 1986, and has authored over 20 articles, most related to child and family services.

Barbara J. Stotlar, M.E. is the program director at the Southern Illinois Center for Independent Living in Carbondale, Illinois. She received her master's degree in Educational Psychology from Southern Illinois University at Carbondale.

Edna Mora Szymanski, Ph.D. is an assistant professor of Rehabilitation Psychology and Special Education at the University of Wisconsin-Madison. She received her doctorate from the University of Texas, and is the author or co-author of over 29 publications.

Joseph D. Teaff, Ed.D. is professor and director of the Office of Leisure Research, Department of Recreation, Southern Illinois University at Carbondale. He received his doctorate from Columbia University, and is the author or co-author of five books and over 30 articles and book chapters.

Bruce Thyer, Ph.D. is professor of Social Work at the University of Georgia in Athens. He received his Ph.D. in social work and psychology from the University of Michigan in 1982. Dr. Thyer is Editor of *Research on Social Work Practice* (Sage) and has authored over 100 articles in the fields of social work and behavior analysis and therapy.

Garry A. Toerber, Ph.D. is manager of Health and Medical Services in the Department of Social Services in Denver, Colorado. He received his doctorate from the University of Iowa in 1971. He has been Colorado State Medicaid Director for over 12 years.

Donald E. Vaughn, Ph.D., CPA graduated from the University of Texas-Austin in 1961. He is currently professor of Finance, College of Business and Administration, Southern Illinois University at Carbondale. He has published over 25 articles, authored or co-authored eight books, and has contributed to other books.

Susan M. Viranyi is a master's degree candidate in Rehabilitation Administration and Services, Rehabilitation Institute, Southern Illinois University at Carbondale. She is a graduate assistant in Administration, and works as a vocational specialist coordinating work experience programs for participants at the Evaluation and Developmental Center, Carbondale.

John S. Washburn, Ed.D. is professor and chair of the Department of Vocational Education Studies, Southern Illinois University at Carbondale. He received his doctorate in Educational Administration from the University of Illinois in 1977.

Richard R. Wolfe, Ph.D. is professor in Rehabilitation Counseling, University of Northern Colorado, Greeley, Colorado. Dr. Wolfe is a graduate of the University of Pittsburgh, and the Project Director of several RSA funded grants.

Henry D. Wong, Rh.D. is an assistant professor in the School of Medicine, Division of Rehabilitation Counseling, at the University of North Carolina in Chapel Hill. He received his doctorate in 1990 from the Rehabilitation Institute, Southern Illinois University at Carbondale.

Wendy York is an attorney who graduated from the University of New Mexico in 1982. She is a visiting professor at Ohio Northern University School of Law.

Table of Contents

I. Introduction

Overview

T. F. Riggar, Ed.D.

This book is intended to provide human service professionals with information to assist and guide their clients. To do this, the most prominent and beneficial human service agencies are examined. In helping clients, it is often necessary for the professional social worker, or counselor of whatever type, to look outside her or his particular organization and enlist the expertise of professionals in other specialties. When a client is accepted for service by a particular agency, and by a specific counselor, the responsibility for the whole individual is also being accepted. Help for specific problems and enhancement of the client's interaction with the community and society at large is required. With an individual who is disabled in some way—be it physical, mental, or environmental—the services of one agency are usually too limited in structure and scope to remediate all of the client's handicaps. To intervene with such an individual means that the counselor must enlist the aid of others to deal with problems outside the boundaries of the organization. For a counselor to refer, transfer, or coordinate with one or more other agencies, it is essential to be reasonably conversant with what the assisting agency can offer the client.

The intent herein is to supply information which will assist counselors to help themselves and their clients. Despite the knowledge any counselor maintains, it is usually beyond the range of any one specialty area to encompass all of the areas in which an individual may need assistance. For example, a social worker, a vocational rehabilitation counselor, or a mental health counselor may each be proficient in their respective areas, but one client may need the services of all three professionals. Unless the initial contact counselor is conversant with the range of professional activities of other counselors and their supporting agencies, it will be difficult for the client to obtain appropriate outside services.

Lack of knowledge of what can be obtained, and where it can be obtained, results in clients being rendered services which do not exactly fulfill their needs. It is incumbent upon service providers to know the "what, where, how, and why" of a broad range of community services. Only in this way may the helper confidently assist the client in gaining that which is needed. In essence, much of what is contained here will allow an individual to be "plugged in" to existing community human services. Making a client aware of what exists in the area fosters a future independence. If the same or a similar problem arises, the client will know where to go, who to see, and what to get. This development of the population in general means that human service agencies, and their workers, may more effectively assist people. It also means that the population regularly frequents the organizations which provide necessary activities.

The principles of case management require that each counselor assist each client to the maximum. How much help the client receives will often depend upon how much the assigned professional is capable of assisting. Because the total individual is the target, the case must reflect efforts toward remediating all problems and disabilities. It does no good, for instance, to get a person a job (vocational rehabilitation) if they are confused, disoriented, and disturbed (mental health), and at the same time hungry and without a place to stay (social services). Such a case is not unique. Too often the counselor initially interviewing a client will immediately note that the person needs help in many areas. Aside from their own specialties, how do counselors go about finding out who can help? What outside agencies will assist? Who in these agencies handles these specific matters? What will the other organizations and agencies really do? To what extent? How often?

The answers to these and other questions form the intent of this book. It is hoped that a human services professional following this guide will gain, over time, increased knowledge of the community and its resources. This information will be put to good use in helping individuals help themselves. Although this book contains detailed data about a variety of agencies and organizations, it does not, and cannot, provide information concerning the local addresses and individual referrals throughout the country. The responsibility for finding local community contacts rests with each professional. The location, development, and nurturance of community contacts is an important part of any counselor's job. Wide-ranging and versatile contacts expand the abilities and services which a worker may bring to bear for a client.

The information provided herein addresses the areas of responsibilities of the agencies in detail. When referring a client to another organization, it is far better to refer to a known fellow professional than to an entity. This means that although a counselor may know that certain services can be provided, actually making sure clients receive them is another matter. When transferring some of the responsibility for the total individual to another counselor, certain aspects must be considered. Among these are: (a) the ability of the client to carry through on the suggestion, and (b) the manner in which the referral is made.

The ability, desire, or necessity of a client to follow through on a suggested referral is usually determined by the initial counselor. Depending upon the type of disability manifested, and the needs and capacities of the clients, a judgment may be made as to how well individuals can help themselves. Clearly, if they are unable to really do what is required, the assigned counselor will have to make the necessary arrangements and expend extra effort to assist the clients.

Perhaps the most important part in using community human services from the counselor's perspective, is possessing knowledge of services and personnel of other agencies. As noted, it is far better to refer to a person than to an "organization." A crucial ingredient in referring an individual to another agency is to clear the obstacles usually inherent in bureaucratic systems. Even though this book will enable any counselor to determine what is potentially available and where certain items and services are most easily obtainable, it does not put the counselor in touch with those who will, in fact, provide the outside assistance.

The resultant effectiveness of this outside assistance is often dependent upon two factors. These aspects are expectations and cooperation. The expectations of both counselor and client concerning ancillary services are often dependent upon the knowledge the counselor has of the assisting agency. These expectations are imparted to the client in the form of advisements, suggestions, or comments about what the assisting agency may do for the individual. The second aspect, that of cooperation, relates to the interaction between the initial or sponsoring counselor and the cooperating counselor from the other agency. Cooperation is enhanced when both professionals are aware of the orientation and requirements of the other. When an unreasonable request for services is made, it is evident that the requesting individual is unfamiliar with the services of an agency.

With both factors, expectations and cooperation, the most important determinant of whether or not the client will receive appropriate services is the knowledge held by each counselor concerning other organizations. For all counselors, from all agencies, information about what exists by way of potential human services must be made available. The intent here is to make available that much needed information in a form which can be easily assimilated and used in everyday practice. Basically, this is a reference book which can be used by the practicing counselor on a daily basis. Most chapters have a similar format. For each agency or organization, the section is divided into three parts. These parts include: History/Legislation, Purpose/Intent, and Client Services.

The History/Legislation section outlines the historical background of the agency. Particular emphasis is placed on the legislation that has, and is currently, influencing the direction and goals of the organization. Additionally, the authority by which the service operates and, where appropriate, funding sources are examined. Agency personnel, particularly type and training, are delineated, as well as any special organizational certifications, licensing, or accreditation.

Purpose/Intent refers to the rationale for the agency. Most particularly why the agency's existence has continued over the years is examined. What the organization strives to do for citizens and how it intends to do so are detailed. This section of each chapter discusses utilization criteria. Particularly important for a counselor is the determination of how, potentially, a specific agency or organization may assist clients. Any preestablished special case management needs are detailed with data concerning their utilization by counselors.

Client Services are those particular ways in which the agency and its counselors attempt to aid clients. So that counselors from other organizations will have a clear picture of what the specific agency can offer, potential services are described and explained in some detail. Additionally, typical referral questions may be presented which will assist counselors in proper presentation of client interests to a potential agency.

All three components of each chapter are important. In the first instance, knowledge of historical background tends to show how the organization has evolved over time. The evolution which takes place in any bureaucratic system is influenced by such things as administrative changes, legislative mandates, and citizen demands. To know what they do, it is sometimes necessary to know what and how they have performed in the past. Known past activities are clear indicators as to how current and future activities will be conducted. Purpose/Intent are those paths which the agency and its counselors tread on the way toward reaching goals. Because of the ever-increasing diversification among agencies, it is necessary to know what particular segment of a population is purported to be represented. In respect to the target group, what the agency intends to do with this population describes the intended purpose. Lastly, the precise services that are sponsored are examined. As noted, there is considerable diversification and proliferation of human services agencies. Because of this, an overlap exists concerning both populations and possible services. However, for each service which may be provided, there is usually one agency whose history and intent focus directly toward that activity. All three components of each chapter, and hence the agencies concerned, contain crucial information to enable a counselor to assist a client, develop realistic expectations, and effectively cooperate with the counselors.

The book itself can be used in a number of ways. As a handy reference, the counselor may investigate the subject in which the client has either expressed an interest, or is deemed to require. In this way, the book provides extensive information concerning service agencies which exist in every locale. If a particular service seems appropriate, the book may also be of use. When it is known that a client needs or requires assistance of a certain nature, the material can be used to indicate what agency has that item as a primary responsibility or priority. As an overall source of information, the contents are suitable for use in classes which seek to instruct in what types of human services exist in every community, and as a follow-up or adjunct to case management courses. In this way, counselors, who may have some in-depth knowledge about one or two establishments, can learn and prepare to use similar information concerning dozens of other organizations. Such increased knowledge not only increases professional expertise, but means that clients will be more effectively and efficiently served.

Case Management Implications

William Crimando, Ph.D.

A "community resource" can be defined as any service vendor— public or private, fee-charging or not–available within a specific geographic area that potentially can be used to aid our clients, ourselves, or our organizations. They range from comprehensive rehabilitation hospitals and social service agencies, to neighborhood advocacy and service organizations, to a variety of educational, legal, and employment agencies, and to a host of small vendors such as physicians, counselors, pain management clinics, and churches. However broad, this definition is important. It implies critical aspects of community resources:

- They must be capable of providing a needed service or commodity;
- They must be willing to enter into a relationship in which those services and commodities can be purchased or otherwise secured;
- They must be located in a place that is geographically accessible; and
- They must have attainable (to us or our clients) eligibility requirements.

Therefore, "community" and "resource" are terms relative to the needs and abilities of our clients. A "community" could be a city block large or the entire nation, if the particular agency's services or commodities are readily available and accessible. Seider (1966) suggests that communities are not limited by geographic boundaries, and are composed of inter-connected social systems and institutions. Further, if we serve a caseload of indigent families, from our perspective a neighborhood grocer who is willing to give away day-old baked goods and produce is a resource, while a college placement office that only serves students may not be.

There are two types of community resources: single service and multiple service agencies. As their names imply, single service agencies provide services of a single type, be it vocational, educational, social, or health. Examples include physicians, legal clinics, financial counselors, and transportation vendors (e.g., cab companies and bus lines). Multiple service agencies can provide services from two or more types. Examples are community colleges, which often provide vocational and psychological guidance as well as educational services; comprehensive rehabilitation facilities from which job training, independent living skills, vocational exploration and placement services could be secured; and Public Aid, which serves a variety of physical, financial, and emotional needs.

Potentially, single-service agencies have these advantages for the case manager: (a) they usually do what they do very well; (b) they have specifically-trained personnel; and (c) their personnel can stay up-to-date in their skills. Multiple-service agencies, on the other hand, offer the advantage of being able to see a client's needs from multiple perspectives. They also obviate developing separate and possibly duplicate formal service agreements with multiple single-service vendors.

Identifying and Selecting Community Resources

The importance of a systematic method of identifying and selecting community resources cannot be overstated. Vandergoot and Jacobsen (1979) state:

A basic problem for many counselors is having enough time and resources to meet service expectations. Large caseloads and varied service needs often force counselors to decide on service priorities which exclude the needs of some clients. . . .Involving various persons and community agencies . . . could improve services and decrease counselor activity . . . [so] counselors would have more time to devote to other needs. (p. 159)

They add to these advantages (a) increased openness and public awareness, (b) elimination of duplicative service efforts, and, especially for counselors in federal programs, (c) satisfaction of congressional expectations.

These procedures have been described in previous materials (cf., Abramson, 1983; McCollum, Swenson, & Hooge, 1979; Rossi, 1982; Vandergoot & Jacobsen, 1979; Weissman, Epstein, Savage, 1983).

NEEDS ASSESSMENT

The first step is to conduct a thorough assessment of caseload needs. Three types of needs are at issue here: client needs, counselor personal-professional needs, and organizational needs. Often these overlap. Client needs, of course, are their requirements for survival, security, love and esteem, and growth. These translate to the basics—food, clothing, shelter, health, employment, and so on.

As important, but often overlooked, are professional counselor and organizational needs. While more than likely survival and security needs are being met, professionals frequently have knowledge and skills deficits, or they may require emotional support to continue in a difficult situation, or they may merely need another professional with whom to discuss new techniques or critical cases. Thus counselors have needs revolving around a desire to be as effective as possible. Similarly organizations have effectiveness needs, which include, naturally, funding, referrals, public relations, community support, and so on[1].

---

[1] While the emphasis in this book is on resources which serve clients' needs, these same resources could easily serve professional and organizational needs. Similarly, the techniques in this chapter are also applicable to professional and organizational needs.

Frequently these needs are already being met through client, professional, or organizational assets, or through existing service agreements with other community agencies. The formal and informal relationships both within and outside the agency or clients' sphere of influence should be examined to determine met needs.

Both unmet and met needs can be determined through a number of sources: (a) interviews with clients, other counselors in the agency, and collateral agencies; (b) caseload reviews; (c) reviews of existing inter-agency service agreements; and (d) self-examination of professional needs and assets. Table 1 is a breakdown of needs assessment approaches and methods, as well as data collection techniques and resources.

POTENTIAL RESOURCE IDENTIFICATION

Once needs have been identified, outside agencies, organizations, and programs should be identified which could potentially serve those needs. The objective at this step should be to identify as many potential vendors as possible for each service need, so that the most efficient, effective decisions can be made. This also lessens the possibility that a particular vendor will be chosen by "default," that is, because it is the only one identified.

Two sources of information about potential resources exist: formal and informal. Formal sources include all printed or published materials about community agencies, such as community assistance directories, information and referral network/databases, telephone books, procedures manuals, and the other public relations materials that individual agencies publish.

Informal sources are those other than published material. Primary among these are the other counselors, supervisors, or professionals–within one's own agency or outside–that form one's professional network. While some professionals may be reluctant to share knowledge that could only be gained after years of experience (Vandergoot & Jacobsen, 1979), a well-cultivated network will provide a wealth of information. As an added incentive, this information will likely include contacts and tactics for working through bureaucracies.

File review from a variety of caseloads constitutes another informal source. Both referral sources and past vendors are potential resources. Personal visits to and from other agencies may be fruitful in both gathering information, and expanding professional networks. Finally, clients and their friends, relatives, and acquaintances may be of assistance.

Table 1. A Guide to Needs Assessment

Assessment Level

International	Geographic community	Specific positions
National	Professional community	Tasks
Regional	Formal organization	Physical resources
State	Informal organization	

Persons to be contacted

Clients	Administrators	Colleagues
Public	Supervisors	Practitioners

Data to be collected

Attitudes	Opinions	Abilities
Values	Knowledge	Demography
Beliefs	Skills	Trends
Feelings		

Method

Key informant/allied professional	Force-field analysis	Knowledge-based
	Stream analysis	Critical incident
Policy analysis	Ecomapping	
Delphi		

Data collection technique

Records audit	Tests	Polling
Nominal/focus groups	Surveys	Sensing
Interviews	Observation	Physical depictions

Diagnostic resource

Data and information

Census studies	Financial records and trends	Complaints and grievances
Audits and exceptions	Personnel-planning data	Absenteeism records
Published trend studies	Situation scans	Job descriptions
Legislative reports	Production records	Task analyses

Organizations

Federal agencies	Community development agencies	Social service agencies
Regional planning agencies	Public health departments	Chambers of Commerce
Community planning agencies	Public welfare agencies	Schools and universities
		Other organizations

Table 2 lists questions that may be considered when examining potential resources, and that will be useful in decision-making and selection of resources. While the intent of this book is to answer some of these questions in the most general sense, specific information gathered by careful examination will be crucial in the selection process.

Table 2. Potential Selection Criteria for Community Resources

General
What is the purpose of the program/agency/organization?
Who is eligible to receive services?
What organizational patterns exist?
What is the nature of funding?
What constraints in service provision does the organization face?
Does the organization have appropriate accreditations?

Services
What services are provided?
Are services available to families?
Are case management services provided?
What emergency services?
What linkages or service agreements does the organization have with others to meet special needs?

Staff Composition
What is the size of the staff?
What is the average caseload size, or staff-to-client ratio?
What are the qualifications of the staff?
Do staff possess required/desired degrees, certifications, licenses, etc.?
What experience has staff had in working with your specific population?

Resources
What facilities are available?
Are locations accessible to clients by a reliable mode of transportation?
If clients must be relocated, are essential/desirable living or support resources available?
Are program facilities accessible to clients?
What equipment (e.g., testing, therapy, training apparatus) is available?

Referral/Utilization
How should referrals be made?
How many people is the agency capable of serving at the same time?
Is there a waiting list? How long is it?
Are regular, meaningful reports issued for clients?

Program Planning
Is there a minimum/maximum length of program?
What post-discharge or follow-up services are provided or available?
Are programs tailored to meet individual consumer needs?
Who is consumer or family input considered in program planning?

Cost
What is the cost per consumer day in the program?
What is the rate/pricing structure (e.g., uniform, cost reimbursement, cost plus fee)?
What discounts are available?

Outcomes
Does organization have an acceptable number of successful outcomes (e.g., consumers placed, trainees graduated, clients detoxified)?
Is there a minimum of unsuccessful outcomes?
What attention is paid to the quality of successful outcomes?
Doe outcomes match organizational goals and objectives?
Do outcomes match a reasonable professional standard?
Does the organization examine unsuccessful outcomes thoroughly?

Consumer/Public Relations
What is the reputation of the program in the community or among other professionals?
Are consumers satisfied with services?
Are consumer families satisfied with services?

Sources: Brolin, 1973; Hagebak, 1982; Hanley-Maxwell & Bordieri, 1989; Lewis & Lewis, 1983; National Head Injury Foundation, n.d.

RESOURCE SELECTION

Having identified needs and potential resources, the most appropriate resources are selected. Selecting the "best" resource requires problem-solving skills and a good decision-making strategy. Two decision strategies have been suggested: optimizing and satisficing.

Optimizing

Optimizing is the examination of as many alternatives as possible to find the most beneficial. McCollum et al. (1979), and Vandergoot and Jacobsen (1979) discuss optimization as desirable in the selection of community resources, while Lewis and Lewis (1983) believe it important to try to optimize in any human service planning endeavor. To optimize, one would first select a number of criteria (perhaps from Table 2) that are most important in a resource for a specific client need, optionally weighting criteria by their relative importance. Next, a wide range of possible alternative resources are identified by "brainstorming." All identified alternatives are then rated or scored on their ability to meet those criteria, with different values assigned to "does not meet," "meets," "partially meets," and "unknown" states. An overall score is arrived at by summing across criterion scores. The resource receiving the highest score is chosen. Presumably, this would be done for each specific client need.

Satisficing

While optimizing is ideal, the process is cumbersome for some decisions and "overkill" for others. A more likely strategy–satisficing–is suggested by Simon (1976), and represents a compromise between consideration of every conceivable alternative and the time and information constraints on such a strategy. In satisficing, a small number of "criteria of value" (p. 98) are established prior to identifying alternatives. Potential alternatives are then examined until one meeting all criteria of value is found, at which time the search stops. For example, in selecting training vendors for clients with brain injury, a counselor might use "experience with the population," "multiple linkages for special needs," as well as a comprehensive list of services offered as criteria of value. Training alternatives are examined until one meeting these criteria is found.

Using Community Resources

DEVELOPING SERVICE DELIVERY SYSTEMS

Once these steps have been accomplished, the counselor/organization can begin to implement specific plans for individual clients. In order to facillitate these plans, an effective and efficient service delivery system needs to be established. Three important parts of the service delivery system are discussed here: utilization of organizational and professional networks, types of fee mechanisms, and preparation of referral letters.

Networks

Human service professionals have long been advised to develop and use "networks" both for their own development and that of their clients. Carroll (1986) defines networking as the development of formal and informal linkages between service providers and agencies to promote resource sharing and information exchange. Three types of networks— often overlapping— can be delineated: personal, professional, and organizational. Personal networks are those friends, relatives, and acquaintances that provide one with support, nurturance, information, and guidance. Professional networks provide information, guidance, and resources, and usually consist of other service providers, professionals, mentors, teachers, and so on.

Organizational networks are usually established through formal linkages among the various service entities that exist in a local community. Hagebak (1982) discusses benefits of organizational networks, including these:

- Local determination–Service integration is often mandated through legislation. By networking, local agencies can determine and control the implementation of that integration.
- Improved cost-effectiveness–By networking, agencies may be able to realize savings from reduced duplication of effort, equipment, staff, and physical facilities.
- Maximized professional relationships–Members working together may develop ideas–synergistically–that no single member could have produced alone.
- Elimination of service gaps–Joint needs assessment and planning ensures comprehensiveness in scope of services and target populations.
- Recruitment activities–Coordination of job listings and manpower planning may ensure that the *community* is able to recruit and retain the most qualified staff.
- Comprehensive data/evaluation systems–Shared data and data-collecting devices may lead to more efficient and effective program evaluation systems.

Even where organizational networks are not established, individual practitioners may realize benefits from professional networking with resource vendors: (a) A network member will better understand typical client needs and counselor expectations; (b) A network member may be more willing to discuss ways of cost containment that would not be harmful to the client's welfare; (c) A member of a network can help cut through "red tape," thus ensuring timeliness of services.

Fee Mechanisms

Thomas and Bordieri (1987) list four of the most common methods of arranging vendor services:
- Service contracts–A service contract is a signed legal document specifying nature of services, method and rate of payment, timelines, and dollar amounts of particular services anticipated to be purchased during the contract period. The contract is legally binding.
- Written purchase of service agreement–Similar to a service contract, a written purchase of service agreement does not obligate purchase of services, but only implies an option to purchase.
- Requests for proposals–RFP's specify services to be provided and special requirements for their provision. They are sent to a number of potential vendors, who bid on them by specifying how services will be provided and projected costs. Chosen vendors are then sent service contracts or service agreements.
- Individual authorization without contract or agreement–As implied in the name, this mechanism authorizes specific services for specified fees. There is no obligation for number of persons served or expected outcomes, although there is usually an understanding of such. In a national survey among state directors of vocational rehabilitation agencies, Thomas and Bordieri (1987)

found that the individual authorization without contract was the most favored mechanism, followed by purchase of service agreement, service contract, and RFP.

Referral Letters

The most effective referral letter is one that follows a phone call to a fellow member of a professional or organizational network. In such a case, the letter reiterates the important points discussed on the phone, clarifies details of service provision, provides supplemental background information on the client, and establishes an often-necessary "paper trail." In discussing the establishment of local community resource systems, Hagebak (1982) lists key reasons for documentation such as referral letters. He included these: (a) A written document can be reviewed and modified; (b) It protects the resource relationship against "memory failure," and staff turnover; and (c) It "locks in" the commitment of parties involved, ethically if not legally. Further, where service contracts or purchases of service agreements are the fee mechanisms, the referral letter is the first document that specifies clients, services to be provided, outcomes expected, timelines, and so on.

Referral letters provide similar information:

1. An introduction of the client–It is important to include   background information that is relevant to the presenting problem, or needed by the vendor in order to effectively serve the client. Clinical impressions and concerns are helpful. In presenting this type of information, care needs to be taken to uphold the policy on release of client information.
2. The specific services needed, or if an evaluation of some type is being purchased, the specific questions in which the referring counselor is interested should be detailed.
3. The monitoring mechanism–Minimally, this includes clearly stated goals and objectives. Terms for renegotiation of service costs, mechanisms for joint case planning, and quality assurance review procedures may be discussed.
4. Timelines, or the date by which the services must be completed or renegotiated, should be specified.
5. Special considerations–A list of the ancillary services needed (e.g., transportation from home, lodging, and case management) should be detailed.

MONITORING

Finally, to remain truly efficient and effective, a service delivery system–whether that system includes a single referral relationship or a comprehensive community network–needs continuous monitoring. While Table 2 can be used as a guide for monitoring, some points require particular attention:

Outcome–Of primary significance in long-term service provision (e.g., training, physical rehabilitation, and psychological counseling), is whether or not the client is making satisfactory progress, and if not, can the vendor provide a satisfactory explanation. If the vendor is providing a short-term service (e.g., vocational evaluation, housing assistance, and financial counseling), the concern is that these were completed satisfactorily. Finally, if the vendor is providing a commodity or equipment (e.g., prosthetic device, food, and modified transportation), the questions are: "Did the client receive the commodity?" and "Does it work as intended?"

Responsiveness to the client's primary and special needs–Clearly important is the vendor's performance in responding to the needs (services, evaluations, special considerations) outlined in the referral letter. Also included here is the vendor's willingness to consider the input of the consumer and the family, as well as overall consumer/family satisfaction.

Responsiveness to referring counselor's needs–Similarly, referring counselors have needs, for regular staffings, having input on planning, receiving useful, timely and accurate reports, and receiving cooperation in cost containment when appropriate.

Responsiveness to organization needs–Finally, a concern relates to whether or not the organization's needs–for timely billing, appropriate data for program evaluation and satisfying legal, funding, or accreditation authorities, and so on–are being satisfied. Additionally, if both organizations are part of a community referral network, the rate at which the vendor is referring clients to the purchasing organization is important.

Summary

This chapter has discussed case management implications of utilizing community resources. A broadened definition of community resource was given, as was a systematic process for identifying, selecting, and using resources. While the benefits for the process herein described are many, it may seem tedious and cumbersome to a few. These persons should bear in mind that a comprehensive needs assessment and resource identification need only be performed once, and that the entire organization can engage in it. Periodic, cursory review of both client needs and available resources can then supplement. Finally, involvement in professional and organizational networks will make the latter activities easier.

References

Abramson, J. (1983). Six steps to effective referrals. In H. Weissman, I. Epstein, & A. Savage (Eds.), *Agency-based social work: Neglected aspects of clinical practice*. Philadelphia: Temple University.

Brolin, D. (1973). The facility you choose . . . . *Journal of Rehabilitation, 39(1)*, 24-26.

Carroll, R.A. (1986). Resource exchange: A catalyst for networking in rehabilitation. *American Rehabilitation, 12(4)*, 3, 18-19.

Hagebak, B.R. (1982). *Getting local agencies to cooperate*. Baltimore: University Park Press.

Hanley-Maxwell, C., & Bordieri, J.E. (1989). Purchasing supported employment: Evaluating the service. *Journal of Applied Rehabilitation Counseling, 20(3)*, 4-11.

Lewis, J.A., & Lewis, M.D. (1983). *Management of human service programs.* Monterey, CA: Brooks/Cole.

McCollum, P.S., Swenson, E., & Hooge, N.C. (1979). Community resources revisited: Sources of support in the rehabilitation process. *Journal of Applied Rehabilitation Counseling, 10,* 72-77.

National Head Injury Foundation, Inc. (n.d.). *What to look for when selecting a rehabilitation facility: A working guide.* Southborough, MA: Author. (Available from NHIF, 333 Turnpike Rd., Southborough, MA 01772).

Rossi, R.J. (1982). *Agencies working together.* Beverly Hills, CA: Sage.

Seider, V.M. (1966). *The rehabilitation agency and community work: A source book for professional training.* Washington, DC: U.S. Department of Health, Education and Welfare, Rehabilitation Services Administration.

Simon, H.A. (1976). *Administrative behavior: A study of decision making processes in administrative organizations.* New York: Free Press.

Vandergoot, D., & Jacobsen, R.J. (1979). Identifying, developing and using community resources in rehabilitation counseling. *Journal of Applied Rehabilitation Counseling, 9,* 159-163.

Weissman, H., Epstein, I., & Savage, A. (Eds.). (1983). *Agency-based social work: Neglected aspects of clinical practice.* Philadelphia: Temple University.

II. Health and Diagnostic Services

Home Health Services

Beverley E. Holland, Rh.D., R.N.

Home health services are on the edge of change in health care provision. Factors that have influenced this rapid growth include increasing numbers of dependent elderly with chronic illnesses, earlier hospital discharges and increased use by doctors. Consumers with increased health awareness and concern are demanding home services as an alternative to institutional care. Another force of growing significance in home health care has been the impact of medical and computer technology. This advanced technology has allowed complex procedures, which before would have been done in the hospital, to be done routinely at home. Cost containment pressures by the government and third-party payers have been a final force providing financial incentive toward growth.

History/Legislation

Home health care had its origins in the United States in New York City. In 1877, the Women's Board of the New York City Mission hired the first nurse to provide skilled nursing care. This nurse also taught cleanliness and provided religious instruction to the sick poor (Bullough & Bullough, 1990). By 1886, other voluntary agencies provided similar home health care services in Buffalo, Boston, and Philadelphia. These agencies would later become Visiting Nurse Associations (Spiegel, 1987).

Metropolitan Life Insurance Company offered home nursing care to its policyholders in the early 1900s. These services became very popular and were soon offered by many other insurance companies. In addition to caring for sick policyholders, prevention was a key focus of care. These programs prospered until the 1940s when they were phased out.

In the late 1940s, a prototype hospital-based home health care program was established at Montefiore Hospital in New York City. This program used a multidisciplinary approach to holistic home care. Home health care was available to anyone discharged from the hospital showing a continued need for care or supervision. Multidisciplinary services included medicine, nursing, physical therapy, occupational therapy, social services, and housekeeping.

By the 1950s and 1960s, home health care providers included government agencies, voluntary health associations, private insurance companies, and hospital-based programs. Since the 1970s, there has been a large-scale entrance into the home health care field by proprietary organizations that operate freestanding agencies.

Growth within the home health care field has been fast. In the past two decades there has been significant legislation passed that influenced the expansion and standardization of the home health care field.

Medicare, passed in 1965, mandated home health care and provided federal definitions and guidelines for care. To meet the guidelines for Medicare reimbursement, the federal government had to appropriate funds to aid home health care agencies in raising their care capabilities.

Other federal programs have mandated or included home health care services as part of their programs. Initially, Medicaid programs did not require provisions for home health care. However, in 1971 new Medicaid regulations stipulated a minimum range of home health services to be a part of their state assistance plans. Home health care services are also available under title XX of the Social Security Act and the Older Americans Act.

Currently, the home health care movement is in an era of growth and increased use. Home health care is becoming an integral part of the health care delivery system.

LICENSURE, CERTIFICATION, AND ACCREDITATION

Due to the fast growth in the field of home health care, there is disagreement about the credentialing needed. The most common credentials discussed in home health care are licensure, certification, and accreditation.

Licensure is legal permission granted, upon meeting certain requirements, to engage in an occupation or activity. It is a regulatory device to protect the public interest. Licensure indicates that the agency meets minimum state standards of care. To obtain specific up-to-date information on licensing requirements in your state, contact your state department of health.

Certification of an agency shows that it has met certain federal standards for patient care and financial management. The agency can receive payment for Medicare home health services and, in some states, for Medicaid/MediCal or other publicly funded home services.

Accreditation is a voluntary process that shows the agency is meeting above-average patient care and operating standards. An accredited agency is evaluated and judged satisfactory against professional standards set by professional organizations that work to promote excellence in home care. Because of the diversity of the home care field, there is no single agency that accredits all participants. There are several nationally recognized accrediting organizations. The Joint Commission on Accreditation of Hospitals (JCAH) accredits home care and hospice services. The National League of Nursing (NLN) accredits home care and community health programs. The National Home Caring Council (NHCC) accredits homemaker-home health aide services, and the Council on Accreditation of Services for Families and Children (COA) focuses on social and mental health agencies. These organizations are voluntary bodies with national reputations. Accreditation can provide a benchmark of quality of care, but accreditation is voluntary and may not be found in many locales.

Purpose/Intent

Home health care can be defined as all the services and products that maintain, restore, or promote physical, mental, and emotional health provided to clients in their homes. The purpose of home health care is to preserve the quality of life for the individual at home by increasing the client's level of independence and reducing the effects of existing disabilities through noninstitutional supportive services (Lundberg, 1984).

People of various ages with a variety of needs use home health care. Home health care can be appropriate for the dependent frail elderly, the urban or rural dweller, children, the handicapped, the chronically ill, the mentally ill, and the terminally ill. Common diagnoses referred for home health care services include the following: cancer, unstable diabetes, heart/circulatory conditions including unstable high blood pressure and pacemaker implant, stroke recovery, respiratory ailments, and postoperative or accident recovery. Home health care is also recommended for clients with arthritis/joint problems, skin problems including bedsores and wounds, bowel and bladder conditions, nerve and muscle disorders, and digestive disorders including those requiring artificial feeding (Nassif, 1985).

TYPES OF HOME HEALTH CARE

Home health care agencies are either nonprofit or proprietary. These labels reveal the extent of an agency's tax obligation not the quality of care provided. Nonprofit agencies may be either voluntary or private. Voluntary agencies are community service-oriented agencies with boards of directors made up of community leaders. Visiting Nurse Association (VNA) is an example of voluntary agency. Private, nonprofit agencies are run by an individual or family or a small board of people. Private agencies can be nonprofit to take advantage of certain tax and state licensing laws. Hospital-based home health agencies could be a private nonprofit agency depending upon the status of the hospital. Proprietary agencies are privately owned profit-making agencies. In many communities, proprietary agencies work cooperatively with nonprofit agencies to provide services.

ADVANTAGES AND DISADVANTAGES OF HOME HEALTH CARE

Home health care is an option that is available for many individuals with health problems. Home health care provides a full range of health care and social services to the client and their family. It promotes dignity, family integrity, and independence and can give a better overall quality of life.

When considering home health care, it is useful to review some advantages and disadvantages for the individual and family.

Advantages

- The individual will receive broad-based care.
- Care is tailored to meet individual needs.
- Home care provides a more comfortable atmosphere.
- Client learning and motivation may be better at home.
- Family is part of the care team.
- Client and family's sense of security are enhanced.
- Clients keep their own identities and sense of usefulness.
- Hospital admissions may be reduced.
- Home care may be less expensive to client and health care system.

Disadvantages

- To be successful, home care must have involvement and commitment of family members.
- Home health care may be started when the family is under stress. The necessary involvement can be viewed as another stressor.
- If the value of a family member's time is included, the indirect costs may be high.

Home Health Care Services

Home health care provides a wide variety of equipment and specific services. Services belong to three major areas: high technology services, client or family care services, and personal care. Use of these service areas is determined according to the needs of the client.

Equipment, high technology, and client or family care services are appropriate to assist for the person, who would otherwise be hospitalized, to remain in their home. These services would involve coordination of a multidisciplinary team of professionals to provide diagnostic, therapeutic, and supportive services.

For the person needing convalescent care, client or family care services and/ or equipment would be appropriate. These services could also be used by individuals recovering from a temporary disability or in need of aid in adapting to permanent changes in health status.

Personal care services can help maintain the individual with long-term care needs in their own home. This service can prevent or postpone the need for institutionalization.

Home health care can provide more than the standard health services. Home health care uses a holistic approach of providing care to the patient with many disciplines working together to resolve identified client needs.

Physician, dental, and pharmaceutical services can be provided to the homebound client. They would be coordinated by the home health care agency.

Skilled nursing care has become the most commonly identified home care service. Skilled nursing is required for the person needing dressings changed or medications administered. It is also used when a person needs to be closely monitored for complications or serious health changes. Skilled nursing may be appropriate to teach patients and their families how to perform procedures for their own home care.

Therapy of many types adds to the spectrum of health services. All therapies aim to restore, maintain, or enhance the abilities of the individual. Physical therapy focuses on the person's physical movement and helps the individual reach their peak ability to function physically. Occupational therapy helps the person overcome problems of daily living that can occur when normal abilities are limited. Speech therapy helps the person with communication disorders caused by speech-production or hearing-related problems and evaluates and treats individuals with swallowing problems. Respiratory therapy provides services to breathing-impaired individuals.

Multidisciplinary services are provided by professionals who have completed a program of study within their field. These professionals hold current licensure or registration and sometimes specialization in their field of practice to provide optimal care for the home health client.

Other disciplines in a multidisciplinary approach would include nutritional services and social services. Nutritional services, provided by Registered Dietitians (RD), assess a client's dietary needs, evaluate current diets, and plan a nutrition program to promote health. Social services, provided by Social Workers (SW), help clients and their families quickly identify and tap into other needed community services. They can aid the client in dealing with the financial side of home care.

Hospice is a concept of care for the terminally ill individual and their family. Hospice services can be provided by a home health care agency and would include social, emotional, and spiritual support for the client and the family.

Often the individual does not need nursing care or therapy. They may only need personal care and housekeeping assistance or companionship to remain in their home. These needs can be met with support service provided by paraprofessionals. Personal care includes help with daily activities which relate to the person's level of functioning. Personal care is provided by home health aides who are trained to provide assistance with bathing, toileting, grooming, dressing, and meals.

Homemaking services involve a full range of household services which keep the home clean and safe and contribute to a person's well-being. The homemaker provides light housekeeping, laundry, food shopping, planning and preparing meals, and paying bills. Chore services, provided by chore workers, help with heavy-duty household tasks that go beyond the scope of homemaking. This includes floor or window washing, yard work, and minor home maintenance and repair.

Companion services provide someone who will read, talk, and listen to the client. These services help to maintain and improve the person's mental alertness and interest.

The paraprofessionals providing support services of personal care, homemaking, chore work, and companionship are trained by their agencies.

ADDITIONAL SERVICES

Diagnostic aids and high-tech treatments which are routine in hospitals are becoming commonplace in home care. Blood or other samples may be taken in the home for later lab analysis, some lab tests can be done in the home. Portable x-rays and cardiographic (EKG) equipment can be brought into the home. Chemotherapy and intravenous (IV) therapy are also available.

Individuals receiving home health care often need medical equipment or supplies. Equipment such as wheelchairs, walkers, and hospital beds may be needed on a long-term basis. These items are considered durable medical equipment (DME) since they will withstand repeated use. Medical supplies such as incontinence pads, syringes, and dressings are nonresuable products. Some agencies can provide DME and/or supplies or provide referral to organizations or companies that can.

PAYMENT FOR HOME HEALTH CARE

Payment for home health care can come from a variety of sources. Often the individual or the family pays for the services. Private and public insurance programs may cover some home care costs. For those whose insurance does not cover home care, some agencies offer a sliding-scale fee schedule. Below are some major payment sources and what they will cover:

Medicare: For those 65 and over, this program pays for home health services, some homemaking services, and some agency-provided medical supplies. The patient must be under a doctor's care and homebound. Services must be provided through a Medicare-certified home health agency.

Medicaid: This medical assistance program for low-income people is administered by the state. Each state has its own set of eligibility requirements. Home care agencies or local social security or welfare offices can provide details.

Veteran's Administration: Veterans with a 50% or more service-connected disability are eligible for home health care coverage. Services must be authorized by a physician to be eligible.

Workers' Compensation: A person injured on the job and in need of home care services is eligible. Workers' compensation representatives have information on eligibility.

Private Health Insurance: Benefits and requirements vary with policy coverage. It is wise to consult both a home health care agency and your insurance carrier to determine the specifics in your case.

BASIC POINTERS FOR DETERMINING NEED AND OBTAINING HOME HEALTH CARE

There are some basic steps that will make the search for the proper home health care easier.

Step 1: Identify your needs
Identify all services you think you will need. Write down a brief description of your situation. The more specific you can be in identifying your needs, the more likely you can get the right source(s) of help faster.

Step 2: Referral sources
The following provides a list of potential referral sources. When you ask for referrals, also ask why they suggested that agency.

Word of mouth: Ask anyone who can help. This includes friends or neighbors and acquaintances, your physician, local clergy, local librarian, or city, county, or state elected officials.

Local hospital, nursing home, or rehabilitation center: Some health care facilities operate home health agencies. If they don't, the discharge planner or social worker can often provide home care information.

Information and Referral (I & R) Services: I & Rs do not specialize in health and home care; but, they are an all-purpose community reference point for a wide variety of local services. Frequently, they can provide a link with the proper service provider.

Religious organizations: Many organizations provide free information and referral, and some provide certain home care services directly.

United Way: This organization funds many community service programs and can refer you to agencies and programs that provide services at a lower cost.

Community (Voluntary) Health Organizations: Voluntary health organizations (e.g., American Cancer Society, Leukemia Society), are devoted to research, public education, and patient services. They have staff that can help you locate services and provide advice about care and self-help.

Step 3: Discussion with the agency
The information obtained, when talking with the health care agency, should provide a basic understanding of the agency and the services they provide. The

following questions can serve as a guide in getting this information. Further information would be necessary based on your individual needs.

Can the agency provide professional references? References should include names of physicians, hospitals, or community social work personnel.

Does the agency limit eligibility for service in any way? Often services are limited geographically, by economic level, or by insurance coverage.

Is the agency accredited, Medicare-certified, or licensed? This does not always imply excellence, but is often important for insurance purposes. Medicare-certified does mean that the agency follows certain requirements in financial management and patient care.

What services are offered? Will the agency help you get other services, if needed, which it does not provide?

When are the agency's services available? How soon before services can begin? Consider the agency's work schedule from the viewpoint of the care you need, not the cost. Additional time may be needed for high-tech care or complex rehabilitation clients.

Does the agency conduct an assessment before developing plan of care and rendering service? An agency has a professional responsibility to conduct its own assessment before developing the plan of care. This assessment should include an in-home visit and thorough assessment of the patient with their family, if possible. A consultation with the doctor or other professionals involved in the situation is necessary too. A detailed plan of care which outlines problems, needed services, and client goals should be presented and discussed before service begins.

What kind of supervision does the agency provide? Good supervision prevents problems and is a key to quality care. This means contact between supervisor, patient, and agency worker to discuss and handle problems as they arise. Frequency of supervisory visits will vary with type of service needed.

Are personnel, professional and paraprofessional, properly trained? Any person employed as a home health aide should have completed a formal aide training program, ideally in home health assisting. The agency should provide inservice training and continuing education to its caregiving personnel.

Can an agency accommodate any special personnel requests? If there are special requests, such as bilingual personnel, someone experienced in kosher cooking, or someone to care for a household pet, this should be discussed with the agency before services begin.

References

Bullough, B., & Bullough, V. (1990). *Nursing in the community.* St. Louis: C. V. Mosby.

Lundberg, C. J. (1984). Home health care: A logical extension of hospital service. *Topics in Health Care Financing, 10*(3), 22-32.

Nassif, J. Z. (1985). *The home health care solution.* New York: Harper & Row.

Spiegel, A. D. (1987). *Home health care* (2nd ed.). Owings Mills, MD: National Health Publishing.

Community Mental Health

Susan Harrington Godley, Rh.D., C.R.C.

History/Legislation

Community mental health services have a relatively brief history. Prior to World War II, mental health treatment primarily took place in mental hospitals. After the war, a convergence of factors led to an emphasis on the community as a desirable locus for mental health treatment. Events related to the war itself influenced attitudes toward mental health treatment. Psychiatrists who worked for the Selective Service system rejected 1,750,000 individuals as not qualified for military service because of neuropsychiatric reasons. This number of rejections was an indication that the incidence of mental problems in this country was greater than was generally believed.

During the war, a number of military personnel experienced mental breakdowns related to their war service. These problems were treated more successfully at the battalion aid station level than at the rear echelon units. These experiences led some to believe that similar successes might occur with civilians who were treated in their community, rather than in a hospital setting (Grob, 1987).

At the same time, a select group of psychiatrists began to believe and work toward addressing mental health needs in the community. With the National Mental Health Act (NMHA) of 1946, the federal government began to play a major role in the development of mental health services. This Act established the National Institute of Mental Health. The three basic goals of the NMHA were to support research related to neuropsychiatric disorders, train psychiatrists, and make grants to states to assist in establishing treatment centers. It also funded research studies on the prevention of neuropsychiatric disorders. The Act provided no financial support for the institutional care of the mentally ill (Grob, 1987).

The Mental Health Study Act of 1955 mandated the development of the Joint Commission on Mental Illness and Health (JCMIH) that would recommend a national policy for mental health. The Joint Commission's final report—*Action for Mental Health*—was published in 1961. John F. Kennedy's tenure as president in the early 1960s coincided with these other developments and his interest in mental health resulted in an expanded federal role in mental health. The Community Mental Health Centers Act became law in 1963 (P. L. 88-184).

The advent of psychotropic medication in the late 1950s also played a role in enhancing the view of the preferability of community mental health treatment. This medication provided a medical treatment that resulted in a rapid change of behavior. Medication provided the opportunity for a quicker transition of an individual from a hospital to the community, or the possibility of treatment in the community (Polcin, 1990).

Massive deinstitutionalization took place during the Kennedy era. The census in mental institutions went from a high of 559,000 in 1955 to 159,000 in 1977 (Grob, 1983). However, deinstitutionalization has not been without its problems. The expectation was that funding for state institutions would decrease. In fact, institutional costs doubled between 1965 and 1980 (Polcin, 1990). The expected transfer of resources from the institution to community mental health centers did not occur. Due to changes in the Medicaid system, many of the elderly individuals who had been hospitalized for mental illness ended up not in the community, but in overcrowded, poorly staffed nursing homes. Many other individuals who have mental illness are part of the country's "revolving door," homeless population who are often repeatedly hospitalized for short periods of time.

The Carter administration attempted to address some of these problems with the Mental Health Systems Act of 1980. This Act emphasized "balanced services" for both prevention and treatment. The Act was quickly repealed as a result of budget cuts during the first year of the Reagan administration (Palmo & Weikel, 1986.)

FUNDING

Subsequent laws to The Community Mental Health Centers Act of 1963 authorized funding of start-up costs for centers. Over 760 catchment areas in the country received federal funding to develop mental health services that could be provided to individuals regardless of their ability to pay. The block grant program combined funding for mental health and substance abuse services into a single grant to states, and transferred the authority for planning and administering the funds from the federal government to the states (Hershenson & Power, 1987). As a consequence, direct federal funding of community mental health centers (CMHC) has decreased.

Sources of funding for community mental health centers include the state mental health agency, other state government agencies, client fees, Medicaid, Medicare, and local government. The percentage of funding from each source varies greatly from center to center within a state, and also between states, since the administrative structure of the mental health centers vary. In some states,

CMHCs are part of the municipal or county government. In other states, they are nonprofit organizations that contract with the state government.

National Institute of Mental Health (NIMH) data suggest that the largest percentage of the centers' funds comes from the state mental health agency (NIMH, 1987). This may be in an arrangement in which the center receives a grant to provide a group of services to a given population, or a fee-for-service arrangement in which the agency is reimbursed by the state on an hourly or daily basis for services delivered.

Community Mental Health Centers attempt to obtain client fee reimbursement through private or government insurance if the individual receiving services has these benefits. Other individuals usually pay their fees according to a sliding scale based on their income.

Since each state constructs its own Medicaid package, Medicaid fundable services vary greatly from state to state. There are presently many opportunities for Medicaid funding, and many states have not taken advantage of the opportunities available to them (Koyanagi, 1990). These opportunities include programs that are optional for the state such as clinic services, the rehabilitation option, and the targeted case management option, all of which can be constructed by a state to allow for the reimbursement of mental health services. In addition, Early, Periodic Screening, Diagnosis, and Treatment (EPSDT) services are mandated. The Omnibus Budget Reconciliation Act of 1989 provides an opportunity through EPSDT to broaden mental health assessment and treatment services for Medicaid-eligible children and adolescents.

Over time, the funding situation for community mental health centers has changed. Community mental health centers are having to develop new methods of marketing and funding to survive. New trends in this area include the development of nontraditional products and services, and participation in managed care contracts.

PERSONNEL

A wide variety of human service professionals and paraprofessionals work in CMHCs. Included among the staff are psychiatrists, other physicians, psychologists, social workers, and registered nurses. A quarter of the professional staff are categorized as other mental health professionals by NIMH (1987) and included are occupational therapists, vocational rehabilitation counselors, and others with at least a bachelor's degree. Paraprofessional staff in CMHCs includes individuals who are licensed practical and vocational nurses, and other mental health workers who have not obtained a bachelor's degree.

Since the development of the CMHCs, a shift has occurred in their staffing patterns. A decrease in the percentage of psychiatrists working at community mental health centers has coincided with an increase in the percentage of psychologists and social workers working in the setting. Increasingly, the type of professional hired by CMHCs is tied to reimbursement mechanisms. A state's Medicaid plan or private insurance require a certain category of professionals to deliver the services for them to be reimbursable under their plans. Psychiatrists, psychologists, and social workers are the professionals most often covered under these plans. Some states license mental health professionals, or have requirements regarding who can be classified as one, and will reimburse other professionals who meet the qualifications.

Mental health counseling is emerging as a distinct profession. Over 100 universities offer a mental health or closely related master degree. The Mental Health Counselors Association (MHCA) offers certification as a mental health counselor through its National Academy of Certified Clinical Mental Health Counselors (CCMHC). The American Association for Counseling and Development (which is the parent of MHCA) also offers certification as a National Certified Counselor (NCC).

Since so many different professions are involved in the mental health field, the academic training of these professionals is highly variable. The Council for Accreditation of Counseling and Related Educational Programs (CACREP) requires the programs it accredits in mental health counseling in community and agency settings to have at least three courses specific to mental health counseling and field work in mental health settings.

Accrediting bodies that would accredit community mental health center service programs include the Joint Commission on Accreditation of Healthcare Organizations and the Commission on Accreditation of Rehabilitation Facilities. Programs which service primarily children's mental health needs might be accredited by the Council on Accreditation of Services for Families and Children. Some states license particular community mental health center programs.

Purpose

RATIONALE

The rationale underlying the development of community mental health centers was that people could, and should, be treated for mental health problems in their home communities, rather than in institutions removed from their community. In addition, local centers could address not only treatment but the prevention of mental health problems. The Community Mental Health Centers Act of 1963 defined CMHCs as places that would be "providing services for the prevention or diagnosis of mental illness, or the care and treatment of mentally ill patients, or rehabilitation of such persons . . . residing in a particular community or communities in or near where the facility is situated" (Title IV, Sec. 401[c], Public Law 88-164).

The original vision for community mental health centers was that they would offer a full range of prevention and mental health treatment services for all segments of the population regardless of their ability to pay. In reality, community mental health centers primarily serve the poor, including those individuals who have the most severe forms of mental illness (Bloom, 1990). Individuals who have more resources often seek treatment through private practitioners, hospitals, or for-profit treatment centers. Many community mental health centers offer multiple services targeted toward the prevention and treatment of mental health problems. Many of their efforts are directed toward preventing unnecessary hospitalization for individuals with chronic mental illness and assisting these individuals in community living.

UTILIZATION

One estimate suggested that the number of persons who were moderately or severely disabled due to chronic mental illness was 2.4 million (estimates were for 1975-1977). Of this total, it was estimated that 6% were in mental health institutions, 31% were in nursing homes, and 63% were in the community. In 1979, there were over 2.6 million persons admitted or readmitted to outpatient or partial care mental health settings. This number represented an increase of about 130% in a 10-year period (NIMH, 1987).

National data on the number of individuals who use community mental health services are not readily available. Part of the reason, is because of the nature of community mental health services. An individual may be seen in one community by one agency for a brief episode for crisis intervention, and then move on and be seen by another agency for another problem episode. In addition, there are inconsistencies in how each state keeps their statistics. NIMH is making an attempt to improve the national data base on mental health services through its Mental Health Statistical Improvement Program (NIMH, 1989).

Client Services

DESCRIPTION OF SERVICES

Community mental health center services are delivered in different ways. Some are like visits to a physician for diagnosis and treatment. Other services are delivered on a per day basis. Still others may be delivered in a residential setting.

The starting point for service should be a comprehensive mental health assessment. While the presenting problem(s) are an essential part of the assessment, examining an individual's history is a critical component of the assessment. Individuals will be asked questions about their personal, family, and mental health, employment, educational, and chemical/alcohol use histories. A psychological evaluation that includes intellectual, personality, or other testing may be part of the assessment. A psychiatric evaluation may also be part of the assessment.

Treatment planning follows the completion of the assessment. It is common practice for treatment planning to include the individual being treated. A treatment plan is formulated with treatment goals specified. Mental health services specified in the plan are tied to the individual's treatment goals.

Actual mental health treatment may consist of various services. These include individual, group, or family therapy or counseling. Treatment may include the prescription and monitoring of psychotropic medication by medical personnel.

Community mental health centers also provide emergency services. Mental health personnel often work with other community agencies like the police or child protective services to help individuals who are in a crisis situation. These may be individuals who are suicidal or a threat to others, and who will require hospitalization. The services described above of assessment, planning, and treatment take place in an abbreviated format during an emergency episode.

Individuals who have had repeated episodes of mental illness and have been hospitalized are most likely to receive psychotropic medication services, rehabilitation services, and support services. The goal for these services is to help these individuals to remain in the community and prevent or avert the necessity of a hospitalization.

Rehabilitation services include skill training, including training in daily living skills or vocational skills. Psychiatric rehabilitation services also include an element of support to aid people in maintaining an independent living situation (Anthony, Cohen, & Cohen, 1983). These services are frequently offered on the basis of a partial or whole day of service.

Some services could be classified as personal care services. These are services that meet the client's needs for food, shelter, and safety. An example of this type of service is a group home for persons who have been repeatedly hospitalized for mental illness. This service would be offered on a 24-hour basis.

Although not a direct service, mental health agencies often are engaged in prevention and consultation activities. Prevention activities include educating the public at large or targeted groups in regards to mental health issues. Consultation activities include consulting with professionals of other human service agencies regarding the mental health needs of their clientele.

SPECIAL CASE MANAGEMENT NEEDS

The need for case management services is directly related to the severity of the mental health problem. The need is most great for a person who has chronic problems with mental illness and who is repeatedly hospitalized. While these individuals may at times function well in the community, the cyclical nature of their mental illnesses will involve periods of severe impairment and they may have great difficulty in caring for themselves and seeking out the resources they need to live independently in the community. Needed services may include medical, social, educational, rehabilitative, or housing services.

Another group that is particularly in need of case management services are children and adolescents who have emotional or behavioral disorders. These children often need services designed especially for them (e.g., educational services), and their families need help in finding those services. Individual needs of children may be neglected as they are caught between the bureaucracies that administer educational, mental health, and social services.

Important components for case management services include assessment, planning, linkage, monitoring, advocacy, and support. Assessment services determine the individual's need for case management services and the medical, social, cultural, and other factors that affect the individual's ability to function. Planning involves the development of a service plan to address the findings from assessment. Through linkage services, the provider facilitates and secures access to the needed services. Monitoring activities include ensuring that the services identified in the service plan are appropriate and delivered in an efficient and dignified manner. Through advocacy, the provider assists the individuals and their families to obtain appropriate services and benefits to which they are entitled. Through support services, the provider maintains an ongoing helping relationship with the individual and may provide problem solving assistance on an ongoing basis and at times of crisis.

Targeted case management is an optional Medicaid service. States who have decided to use this option to serve persons with chronic mental illness, or children with severe emotional disturbances, have constructed their own package of case management services within the Medicaid guidelines. States may also offer Medicaid coverage of case management services through other optional programs like the clinic option.

REFERRAL QUESTIONS

Questions that a mental health worker might ask a referral source will vary with the type of individual referred and the problem. The emphasis of the questions will be to elicit information about the presenting problem and how the individual's behavior has affected his ability to function in different life areas such as employment, school, with family, or socially. A critical piece of information is whether or not the individual is able to live independently and without being harmful to himself or others.

If the individual referred is a child, then referral questions will address those areas which are critical to a child's life. How does the child function at school? How is the relationship with parents, siblings, and peers? Have there been difficulties with the juvenile justice system? Is there a history of drug or alcohol problems? What is the family's commitment to being involved in treatment? Many of the same questions would be appropriate for an adult referral but more emphasis will be placed on those areas of life that are critical for adult functioning.

It is not crucial that a referral source know the answers to all these questions. Referral sources are only expected to describe, as well as they are able, what they have observed in terms of the presenting problem. The mental health worker will obtain much of the information from the individual seeking treatment and, with the individual's permission, seek out the additional sources of information needed to complete a comprehensive mental health assessment.

References

Anthony, W. A., Cohen, M. R., & Cohen, B. F. (1983). Philosophy, treatment process, and principles of the psychiatric rehabilitation approach. In L. Bachrach (Ed.), *New directions for mental health services: Deinstitutionalization*, No 17. San Francisco: Jossey-Bass.

Bloom, B. L. (1990). Managing mental health services: Some comments for the overdue debate in psychology. *Community Mental Health Journal, 24*, 107-124.

Grob, G. N. (1983). *Mental illness and American society 1875-1940*. Princeton, NJ: Princeton University.

Grob, G. N. (1987). The forging of mental health policy in America: World War II to new frontier. *The Journal of the History of Medicine and Allied Sciences, Inc., 42*, 410-446.

Hershenson, D. B., & Power, P. W. (1987). *Mental health counseling: Theory and practice*. New York: Pergamon.

Koyanagi, C. (1990). The missed opportunities of Medicaid. *Hospital and Community Psychiatry, 41*, 135-140.

National Institute of Mental Health. Manderscheid, R. W., & Barrett, S. A., (Eds.) (1987). *Mental Health, United States, 1987*. DHHS Pub. No. (ADM) 87-1518. Washington, DC: Supt. of Docs., U. S. Govt. Printing Office.

National Institute of Mental Health. (1989). *Series FN No. 10, Data standards for mental health decision support systems*. DHHS Pub. No. (ADM) 89-1589. Washington, DC: Supt. of Docs., U. S. Govt. Printing Office.

Palmo, A. J., & Weikel, W. J. (Eds.). (1986). *Foundations of mental health counseling*. Springfield, IL: Charles C. Thomas.

Polcin, D. L. (1990). Administrative update: Administrative planning in community mental health. *Community Mental Health Journal, 26*, 181-192.

Pain Clinics

Bradley W. Kuhlman, Ph.D.
Dennis R. Maki, Ph.D., N.C.C., C.R.C.

Chronic pain is one of the most disabling ailments encountered by health professionals. Many millions of Americans suffer from chronic pain and a substantial portion of these are partially or completely disabled (Turk, Meichenbaum, & Genest, 1983). The statistics are staggering. It has been estimated that, for example, there are 20 to 50 million sufferers of arthritis with 600,000 new victims each year (Arthritis Foundation, 1976). Low back pain alone, one of the most common pain complaints, has disabled an estimated 7 million Americans and accounts for more than 8 million physician office visits per year in the United States alone (Clark, Gosnell, & Shapiro, 1977).

Whereas the majority of this disability group will recover from their pain, 2-5% of this group will continue to seek medical attention (Arnoff, 1985). These individuals will spend an enormous amount of time and energy searching for effective relief for their pain complaints. It is estimated that as many as 80% of all patients who consult physicians do so for pain-related problems (Bresler, 1979).

While the economic costs are great, so are the costs in terms of human suffering. Many people with chronic pain undergo a progressive medical/physical deterioration characterized by numerous physical complaints which may include an exacerbation of symptoms. In addition, many individuals also develop emotional problems such as depression, somatic focusing, and a tendency to deny life problems unrelated to their physical complaints (Bonica, 1985). As the individual moves from professional to professional, he or she experiences hopelessness and despair to the extent that they are usually uncertain as to where else to turn for relief.

Health professionals are also frustrated by the inability to treat and understand chronic pain problems (Keefe & Gill, 1986). Traditionally, health professionals have relied upon conventional methods of treating chronic pain (e.g., medication, bed rest, physical therapy) which often did not result in significant reduction in pain. Patients who do not respond to these treatment modalities are generally either considered poor risks for medical or surgical interventions and are subsequently turned down for treatment, or are referred to other specialists.

Part of the problem in treating chronic pain complaints has been the use of improper knowledge and/or therapies. This is due to both the lack of knowledge of how to treat chronic pain complaints and to the complex nature of chronic pain. It is only in recent years that health professionals have come to realize the critical influence of environmental and psychological factors in the development and maintenance of chronic pain in addition to an original injury (Bonica, 1985). As a result, many health care professionals are just becoming aware of the benefits of utilizing pain clinics in the treatment of chronic pain complaints.

Historical Trends

Chronic pain as described in the literature refers to a pain that persists far beyond the usual course of an acute disease or a reasonable time for an injury to heal, or recurs at intervals of up to several months or years (Bonica, 1985). In the case where injury or exacerbation of a pre-existing condition causes pain, it becomes chronic when the pain is still present after the body is determined to have gone through its normal healing period.

It is axiomatic to emphasize that chronic pain is not a well-defined diagnostic category. Any patient with pain that can not be explained on the basis of organic findings is apt to be diagnosed as "chronic," especially if the pain is prolonged and accompanied by an emotional or behavioral disturbance (Ciccone & Grzesiak, 1984).

One response to this treatment and diagnostic frustration is to judge the patient's behavior solely in terms of how it relates to an underlying organic pathology. Patients who exhibit few organic findings are expected to report few pain problems, and those who exhibit positive findings are expected to report multiple pain problems (Keefe & Gill, 1986). Thus, the more inclusive the findings, the more pain is supposed to be reported. Patients who do not fit within this narrow reductionistic treatment model are subsequently considered poor risks for treatment and are turned down for care or are referred to other specialists. In many cases, patients become stigmatized by the lack of clear findings and are considered malingerers, low back losers, or medical failures.

A large body of data reinforces the view that traditional medical and physical treatment strategies are ineffective in rehabilitating a high proportion of chronic pain patients (Gottlieb et al., 1977; Turk et al., 1983). Sternback and Rusk (1973) have consequently labeled these patients as treatment resistant and generally possessing the following characteristics: complaints of pain for more then six months, inability to work, and a continued search for medical or surgical relief despite previous surgery.

In the past 10 to 15 years, it has become recognized within the treatment community that the initial attempts to identify organic factors within the traditional organic-pathology medical model were failing, and that attention to the behavioral and psychological features of pain reporting was needed to understand the behavior of chronic pain patients. Thus, the emphasis began to emerge to examine psychological factors that may contribute to chronic pain problems.

PAIN CENTERS

In response to the problems associated with effectively treating chronic pain complaints from the traditional medical model, the multidisciplinary pain clinic was developed. Assuming that medical management alone is insufficient or ineffective in alleviating all pain complaints, the pain clinic has developed with an alternative conceptualization of chronic pain. This conceptualization indicates that pain may be understood as one of a constellation of pain behaviors, all of which are related to the pain problem, and all must be addressed to effectively deal with the chronic pain problem. These pain behaviors may include medical, psychological, social, legal, vocational, family, financial, and other related variables.

The multidisciplinary pain clinic offers a structured milieu to its patients which include the use of numerous modalities that are designed to help the chronic pain patient better manage their pain complaints. Services offered within a pain clinic may include medical assessment and management, individual and group counseling, a structured exercise program, physical therapy, work hardening, vocational rehabilitation counseling, family counseling, biofeedback, and relaxation training, as well as educational components. These services are individualized to meet the complex needs of individuals with chronic pain complaints.

PAIN CENTER PERSONNEL

Pain clinic personnel come from a variety of educational and experiential backgrounds due to the complexity of pain complaints and types of modalities offered. Physicians play a key role in the medical diagnosis and treatment planning for chronic pain patients. These physicians usually have experience in the diagnosis and treatment of chronic pain patients.

While physicians play a key role in the diagnosis and planning of chronic pain complaints, they play a lesser role in the actual treatment of chronic pain problems. Other health care professionals are generally involved in direct patient care. These professionals come from a variety of disciplines which include psychologists, biofeedback therapists, recreation therapists, exercise physiologists, physical therapists, rehabilitation counselors, and social workers. These health care professionals all need to be schooled and experienced in the management and care of chronic pain complaints.

TRAINING

Multidisciplinary pain clinic staff members are trained in a variety of different fields. Physicians come from a variety of medical backgrounds including orthopedists, neurologists, surgeons, internists, physiatrists, anesthesiologists, and general practitioners. Similarly, the counseling staff are also quite diverse in training and background which may include clinical, counseling, social, and more recently rehabilitation psychology, as well as rehabilitation counselors and social workers. Other professional staff are trained in such fields as physical therapy, exercise physiology, biofeedback and relaxation training, message therapy, therapeutic recreation, and occupational therapy. The diversity of training adds an important dimension to the treatment of chronic pain complaints as they can offer services from a multitude of approaches.

Purpose/Intent

The basic rationale for the pain clinic is to provide a multidisciplinary approach to complicated medical problems that are not effectively managed by unidimensional health services. The advantages of a multidisciplinary clinic are continuity of care, constant observation and supervision, access to a variety of specialties for consultation and treatment, and an extensive evaluation process.

Treatment goals developed within this setting are determined based upon the needs of individual clients. Common goals may include:
- Learning noninvasive pain coping techniques;
- Increasing physical and social activities;
- Reducing pain medication usage;
- Developing an effective exercise and conditioning program;
- Improving family relationships;
- Reducing the use of the health care system; and
- Vocational rehabilitation counseling and planning.

These goals are then incorporated into the individual's pain management program.

Client Services

Pain clinics provide a variety of services available to help individuals with chronic pain complaints. These services may vary from clinic to clinic. The following will generally appear to be common across settings. Services may include medical assessment and evaluation, individual and group counseling, biofeedback and relaxation training, physical therapy, work hardening and occupational therapy, exercise and conditioning, therapeutic recreation services, and vocational rehabilitation counseling. Other related services may include family counseling, nutrition counseling, and chemical dependency counseling.

MEDICAL ASSESSMENT AND EVALUATION

It is important that an individual be assessed by the program physician prior to entrance into the pain clinic. This assessment is undertaken for several reasons. First, to determine that the candidate is appropriate for services that are provided by the pain clinic, or if there are active disease or injury processes that may be contributing to the chronic pain complaints. If their complaints are due to an active disease process, and if more traditional medical therapies can help ameliorate the pain complaint, individuals may be referred to other specialists that may assist the pain clinic in dealing with the pain problems. Second, it is important to determine medical treatment plans and goals for patients that are accepted into the chronic pain clinic. Services offered by a physician may include consultation for treatment planning with other clinic staff, consultation with other medical specialists on appropriate treatment for complex medical problems, medical assessment and planning for program participants, and prescribing other treatment modalities such as physical therapy and work hardening for clinic patients.

PSYCHOLOGICAL EVALUATION AND TREATMENT

Individuals who are referred to pain clinics may present a variety of emotional problems due to the reaction of encountering long-standing pain complaints. These emotional problems may include reactive depression, anxiety, hypochondriasis, frustration, somatic preoccupation with disease processes, and other personality variables which may act to enhance the development of chronic pain complaints. The goal of the psychologist is to assess and evaluate the presence and effects of these processes, and to explore with the individual methods of ameliorating these complaints, as well as helping them to understand how these processes may be contributing to the pain problems.

The psychologist may also present strategies to individuals regarding more successful coping mechanisms in managing chronic pain complaints. These strategies may be classified under the rubric of coping skills training, and are used to replace ineffective strategies for pain control with more healthy and effective coping mechanisms. In addition, a psychologist provides a setting where the individual can explore the impact of the losses or changes associated with their pain complaints. These services may be provided on a group or individual basis.

PHYSICAL THERAPY

The physical therapist's role and services within the pain clinic are twofold. The first role is to identify physical dysfunctions which may contribute to the pain complaints, and to help restore physical functioning as near to normal status as possible (Yeh, Gonyea, Lemke, & Volpe, 1985). Second, to educate the individual as to what they can do to reactivate themselves physically to increase physical functioning to prevent further physical deterioration (Yeh et al., 1985). The goals of physical therapy are as follows:

- To determine the most effective means of controlling or decreasing the patient's pain problems;
- To help correct, as much as possible, the dysfunctions observed in the evaluation process; and

- To restore the patient's confidence in the ability to move and enjoy physical activity with reduced fear of further injury or pain (Yeh et al., 1985).

This involves techniques to reactivate effective muscle groups, restore muscle length and strength, and to remobilize the body to regain functional movement. This may include the use of heat and cold, soft tissue massage, myofacial pain release, spray and stretch techniques, manipulation of trigger points, and directed exercise and movement therapies.

WORK HARDENING/OCCUPATIONAL THERAPY

To help the individual return to a competitive work environment, a work hardening and occupational therapy program may be warranted. This is especially important if the individual has experienced a prolonged period of inactivity due to pain complaints, or experienced a dramatic injury which may necessitate the retraining of effective muscle groups. A pre-assessment of the individual's present job requirements are critical, along with an assessment of the individual's deficits in motion, strength, and body mechanics.

The goal of work hardening and occupational therapy is to optimize the possibility of returning the individual to their former employment situation or new work activity. Services are usually directed by a physical therapist and may utilize work simulation, exercises to increase motion and trunk strength, endurance training as strength improves, and education and training in the appropriate use of correct body mechanics and energy conservation techniques stressing appropriate lifting and movement functions (Foley & Payne, 1989). Specific goals and strategies are determined by the individual's occupation and physical restrictions.

BIOFEEDBACK AND RELAXATION TRAINING

Another form of treatment for chronic pain complaints commonly seen in pain clinics is biofeedback and relaxation training. These modalities are particularly useful with specific pain disorders that involve the musculoskeletal system (e.g., back pain, myofacial pain, tension headaches), as well as the autonomic nervous system disorders (e.g., hypertension, Raynaud's disease) (Turk et al., 1983).

The therapy sequence usually involves the identification of symptoms and the therapist conducts a careful history with an analysis of the presenting problems. The next phase involves training the patient to develop an increased awareness of the specific physiological responses (e.g., muscular tension, hand temperature, heart rate or blood pressure depending upon the focus of training), teaching the patient voluntary control over his or her physiological responses by means of feedback from various physiological systems, and employing newly acquired techniques and skills in a natural setting (Turk et al., 1983). The ultimate goal is to transfer learning outside the clinic into the home or work setting. As a result, the individual is more aware of the physiological mechanisms influence on pain, and how and when to employ these techniques for pain control.

EXERCISE AND THERAPEUTIC RECREATION

An important goal and component of a pain clinic is to increase the overall activity levels of patients. It is not uncommon for patients to have learned to avoid some or most physical activities associated with previous activity levels as a way of reducing pain and suffering. Patients are often told by health professions to avoid physical activities in the acute stages of an injury or disease process allowing the body time to heal and rejuvenate. However, this is contraindicated with chronic pain complaints as rest and inactivity beyond the healing period can perpetuate or worsen the problem.

The goal of exercise therapy and therapeutic recreation is not to reduce pain by inactivity, but rather to work through the temporary discomfort associated with the effects of disuse; to demonstrate that movement is safe; and to demonstrate the movement can lead to a lessened suffering and a feeling of emotional well-being (Foley & Payne, 1989). This also leads to reactivating persons in their social and leisure activities as the individual finds that the return to activities that were engaged in prior to encountering chronic pain problems is possible.

VOCATIONAL REHABILITATION COUNSELING

Because of the debilitating nature of chronic pain complaints, many individuals have either lost their previous positions or were forced to leave them due to the length and complications of their pain history. These concerns may necessitate vocational rehabilitation counseling. This may be especially important as individuals begin to reactivate their lives beyond the pain clinic. Comprehensive rehabilitation of individuals in pain clinics must include vocational, as well as medical goals.

The role of vocational rehabilitation services may vary depending upon the individual situation. For those returning to a previous position, the role would be one of helping the individual's transition from the clinic setting back to the job. This may involve preparing the individual for the demands of work and working closely with the employer to ensure the success of the individual once they are back on the job.

Another role may be in helping the individual to explore other vocations that may be within the person's physical restrictions, especially if that individual will not be able to return to a previous vocation due to medical restrictions. Many patients are limited to occupations that require light to medium physical demands.

These positions allow for freedom of movement and provide for flexible scheduling in the event of medical complications. Vocational guidance should begin at an early stage of the pain management program and not be reserved for the last days of treatment.

TYPICAL REFERRAL QUESTIONS

Referrals for chronic pain treatment come from a variety of sources which include:
- Physicians who realize that traditional medical interventions may not be effective in treating chronic pain patients;
- Rehabilitation professionals who recognize that their clients are not progressing in a positive direction;
- Individuals who are not satisfied with their progress from more traditional medical therapies; and
- Psychologists who recognize that their patients need more comprehensive services to combat chronic pain complaints.

All of these referral sources have one common element; the need for more comprehensive services for individuals who are not progressing with more traditional therapies.

Because of the complexity of chronic pain complaints, the referral questions will vary with the situational and medical variables. However, it is advisable that the referring professional provide sufficient information about the individual so that the pain clinic personnel are able to effectively evaluate and determine appropriate programming. Some typical referral questions may include:
- What is the nature of the chronic pain problem and how long has it existed?
- What types of therapeutic modalities have the individual been involved with and what was the result of the treatment?
- What medical complications exist that may impact on the individual's pain management program?
- What is the individual's level of motivation to participate in a pain clinic?
- Does the individual have an active disease process or medical problem that may need immediate attention?
- Has the referring professional sent all relevant background medical, psychological, and vocational information?
- Is the person currently addicted to pain medications or other controlled substances?
- Are there any cognitive or emotional impairments that may affect the individual's participation in a pain clinic?
- What is the individual's current activity and tolerance levels?
- Is the individual's family supportive of the rehabilitation efforts?
- Is the individual returning to a previous position, or will a new vocational direction be sought?

Summary

Because of the complex nature of chronic pain complaints the multidisciplinary pain clinic was developed. These clinics are centered on an alternative conceptualization of chronic pain which indicates that pain can be understood as one of a constellation of pain behaviors all related to the pain problem, and all must be addressed to effectively deal with the chronic pain problem.

The pain clinic offers a structured milieu to its patients which includes the use of several modalities that are designed to help remobilize the patient to a more active lifestyle. These modalities are provided by a staff of rehabilitation professionals trained in a variety of specialty areas with an emphasis on chronic pain management. The rationale for a pain clinic is to provide goal-directed, multidisciplinary services for complicated medical problems that cannot be effectively managed by one-dimensional services, and to help individuals take control over and better manage their pain complaints.

Individuals with chronic pain complaints can be treated through a variety of services and procedures that can be individualized to meet the demands of presenting problems. Thus, active communication between referring professionals and pain clinic staff is essential to provide the best possible combination of services for the individual. Hence, it is important for the referring professional to provide appropriate background information and referral questions to assist the pain clinic staff in developing treatment programming. Finally, it is essential that the referring professional have a working knowledge of how a pain clinic can assist them in delivering the best possible services for persons with chronic pain and to help prepare their clients for their experience with the pain clinic.

References

Arnoff, G. M. (Ed.) (1985). *Evaluation and treatment of chronic pain.* Baltimore: Urban & Schwarzenberg.

Arthritis Foundation. (1976). Arthritis, the basic facts. In D. C. Turk, D. Meichenbaum, & M. Genest (Eds.), (1983), *Pain and behavioral medicine: A cognitive-behavioral perspective.* New York: Guilford.

Bonica, J. J. (1985). Importance of the problem: Introduction. In G. M. Arnoff (Ed.), *Evaluation and treatment of chronic pain* (pp. 1-12). Baltimore: Urban & Schwarzenberg.

Bresler, D. E. (1979). *Free yourself from pain.* New York: Simon and Schuster.

Clark, M., Gosnell, M., & Shapiro, D. (1977). The new war on pain. *Newsweek, 89,* pp. 48-58.

Ciccone, D. S., & Grzesiak, R. C. (1984). Cognitive dimensions of chronic pain. *Social Science in Medicine,* 1339-1345.

Foley, K. M., & Payne, R. M. (1989). *Current therapy of pain.* Toronto: B.C. Becker.

Gottlieb, H., Strite, L. C., Koller, R., Madorsky, A., Hockersmith, V., Kleeman, M., & Wagner, J. (1977). Comprehensive rehabilitation of patients with chronic low back pain. *Archives of Physical Medicine and Rehabilitation, 58,* 101-108.

Keefe, F. J., & Gill, K. M. (1986). Behavioral concepts in the analysis of chronic pain syndromes. *Journal of Consulting and Clinical Psychology,* 776-783.

Sternback, R. A., & Rusk, T. N. (1973). Alternatives to the pain carrier. *Psychotherapy: Theory, research and practice, 10,* 321-324.

Turk, D. C., Meichenbaum, D., & Genest, M. (1983). *Pain and behavioral medicine: A cognitive-behavioral perspective.* New York: Guilford.

Yeh, C., Gonyea, M., Lemke, J., & Volpe, M. (1985). Physical therapy: Evaluation and treatment of chronic pain. In G. M. Arnoff (Ed.), *Evaluation and treatment of chronic pain* (pp. 251-263). Baltimore: Urban & Schwarzenberg.

Alcohol-Drug Programs

Mark D. Godley, Ph.D.
Brian C. Cronk, M.A.
Eugene Landrum, M.D.

Treatment services specifically for the client with alcohol or other drug related problems are provided by the growing substance abuse field. It is estimated that one in 11 adult Americans suffers a severe addictive problem, and one in six teenagers has an addictive problem. The cost of these addictions in terms of lost productivity, health care, and so on, is over $53 billion dollars a year (Cummings, 1979). Statistics such as these are plentiful, and are frequently over-used. The important fact to be gleaned from this data, however, is that addictive problems are of epidemic proportion in America today, and that many different people suffer the effects, whether directly (family and friends) or indirectly (social costs).

Persons with substance abuse problems *will* be encountered by helping professionals, regardless of a counselor's area of specialty. Most counselors will have occasion to refer a client to some sort of alcohol or drug treatment program. The purpose of this chapter then is to provide a practical, working knowledge of how the alcohol and drug abuse treatment system works, what to expect from it, and how to help a client use it when the need arises.

History/Legislation

HISTORY

The substance abuse treatment field is a complex area of the larger human services field. There are numerous distinct etiological theories, treatment approaches, and types of addiction. Each approach has some merit, yet the connection between theories and approaches is often hard to establish. Approaches to addiction treatment can best be understood as the history of four different model types: legal, medical, traditional, and other approaches (Guydish, 1982).

The Legal Model

In the late 1800s, addictive behavior was viewed mostly as a moral problem. Addicted individuals were seen as evil, morally weak, or as being possessed by evil spirits. Thus, the early 1900s saw widespread anti-alcohol movements, both in Europe and America. In America, Carrie Nation and the Women's Christian Temperance Union were seeking a "legal cure" to alcoholism by initiating prohibition.

For drugs other than alcohol, the Harrison Act of 1914 was implemented to regulate widespread opium use. It has been suggested that the Harrison Act and subsequent similar legislation has resulted in the development of a substance abuse subculture and black market. It is from this subculture and black market that many of the larger social consequences of drug addiction arise.

The Medical Model

Alcoholism was first labeled as a disease by Dr. Benjamin Rush in 1785. It was not until 1957, after the failure of prohibition and the "legal cure," that the medical profession turned its attention to alcoholism. In 1957, the American Medical Association (AMA) endorsed the concept of alcoholism as a disease. Soon afterward, an influential book, *The Disease Concept of Alcoholism* was published by Jellinek. Jellinek (1960) noted that alcoholism follows a similar course in many individuals. He suggested that it was useful to *conceptualize* alcoholism as a disease.

The medical model has led to several different pharmacotherapy interventions for alcohol and drug abuse. Some professionals believe that alcoholics drink to relieve stress. To counteract this, many doctors prescribed tranquilizers or antidepressants as alternatives to alcohol. Another medical intervention is to prescribe Antabuse® (disulfiram) which acts as a deterrent to drinking by making the patient violently ill when he or she drinks alcohol.

Perhaps the most widely used application of medical services in the medical model is in medical detoxification. This is the process in which an alcoholic or other drug addict withdraws from foreign substances under medical supervision, occasionally with the brief use of tranquilizers.

While the medical model and disease approach have reduced the social stigma and punishment arising from alcoholism, it has also caused problems. The sole reliance on this model has allowed abusers to escape responsibility for their behavior and rehabilitation. Unfortunately, the passive nature of this approach does not serve the rehabilitative process well. Rehabilitation from drug or alcohol dependence requires a great deal of personal effort.

The Traditional Model

During the period from the end of prohibition (1932) and the formal recognition of alcoholism as a disease by the AMA in 1957, alcoholics themselves were working on a treatment model for their disease. It was through these efforts that the traditional model arose. Alcoholics Anonymous (AA) began in 1935 when two alcoholics began to help one another. AA's treatment goal is abstinence from alcohol, and is adhered to using the "twelve steps of AA." AA functions with small groups of alcoholics helping each other. Narcotics Anonymous (NA) and Cocaine Anonymous (CA) are other applications of the traditional model in the treatment of addiction to drugs other than alcohol. It should be noted that most 12-step groups are comprised of individuals who have used more than one substance, and that the different groups exist more to provide a group experience that will be sure to *include* a particular individual rather than to *exclude* those who use more than one drug. So, a client who uses cocaine and alcohol would be welcome in AA and CA.

Marty Mann established the National Council on Alcoholism in 1944 after undergoing her own recovery from alcoholism. She went on to publish *Primer on Alcoholism* (Mann, 1950) and, later, *New Primer on Alcoholism* (Mann, 1958) which became the centerpiece of the traditional model. In this book, terms such as loss of control drinking, compulsive drinking, denial, and rationalization are used to describe the alcoholic. These notions then became easily accessible to counselors because of the popularity of the books. Psychotherapeutic intervention consequently often uses the concepts of the traditional model, and characterizes much of the treatment for addiction which exists today.

The traditional model is the most frequently used model. This model has been developed by people who have successfully completed treatment, so it includes the techniques that have worked the best, as well as embracing the concept of relapse prevention. The traditional model is evolving as new techniques are shown to be effective. Both the medical and traditional models rely on the disease concept of substance abuse, and both can use drugs such as Antabuse® to control drinking.

Other Models

Behavioral models view addictive problems as a series of behaviors that are learned through classical and operant conditioning. The key to treatment lies in counter conditioning (e.g., modifying the reinforcing properties of drugs [through aversion therapy]) (Rimmele, Miller, & Dougher, 1989). Operant conditioning approaches seek to enhance personal competence (e.g., social skills training), improve relationships (e.g., marriage counseling), and assist the client to alter his social and interpersonal environment such that substance abuse results in "time out" from these enhancements (Azrin, Sisson, Meyers, & Godley, 1982). This model has brought to the substance abuse field the methodological advantages of a behavioral approach, but has not been widely used by substance abuse treatment providers.

Another approach through which to view the etiology and treatment of alcohol and drug abuse is suggested by White (1990). In this approach, entry into alcohol or drug abuse is based on multiple pathways, including cultural, biological, and psychosocial reasons. The premise of this approach is that before recovery can take place, certain elements of a person's behavior and thinking have to change. These aspects are referred to as the culture of the individual, and consist of the person's dress, language, music, social support system (family and friends), and job. The cultural approach addresses each of these issues, as well as the traditional issues in treating the substance abuser.

LEGISLATION/AUTHORITY

Some of the early legislation related to the treatment of alcohol and drug abuse was the 1970 Hughes Act. This act created the National Institute on Alcoholism and Alcohol Abuse (NIAAA) which is a prominent resource for workers in the substance abuse field. In more recent years, the federal government has taken a renewed interest in the substance abuse field by passing the anti-drug acts of 1986 and 1988.

The confidentiality of the substance abuser who seeks treatment was protected by federal legislation in the early 1970s (42 U.S.C. §§ 290dd-3 and §§ 290ee-3), and the Department of Health and Human Services issued regulations in 1975 (42 C.F.R. Part 2 modified in 1987) which governed the release of identifying information in a substance abuser's records. Essentially, these regulations protect the substance abuse client's privacy by prohibiting treatment providers from disclosing patient identifying information except under extraordinary circumstances.

FUNDING

Funding for chemical dependency programs is somewhat complicated because it can vary dramatically from state to state. Because payment for treatment can be a very expensive proposition, it is necessary to provide in some detail an understanding of funding mechanisms that will affect every substance abuse referral a counselor makes. In recent years, some states have mandated that insurance companies pay for substance abuse treatment. Even in states where this is not mandatory, many private insurance companies now provide coverage for alcohol and drug abuse treatment.

Each state typically commits a portion of its general revenue to services for alcohol and other drug abusers. States will use either grant-in-aid or a purchase of care mechanism for treatment financing. The organizations that receive state tax dollars to provide substance abuse treatment services are usually private, not-for-profit agencies, local, or state government agencies. The states commit their tax dollars to treatment services to make such services available to chemically dependent individuals who do not have the ability to pay for services.

Many, if not most, private insurance carriers will pay for inpatient rehabilitation for chemical dependency. Policies vary regarding the type and extent of coverage, and the counselor is advised to know the benefit limits of the client's policy when seeking admission to a substance abuse facility. It is less common for private insurance to cover intensive outpatient services (day treatment). Outpatient services, if covered at all, will frequently carry a 50% copayment (amount the client is responsible for). Hospital-based and freestanding proprietary chemical dependency treatment facilities are typically not subsidized by state or federal government. Therefore, they are not likely to facilitate admission for clients *unless* they are covered by private insurance or otherwise have the ability to pay for their treatment.

PERSONNEL

Substance abuse professionals come from a variety of disciplines and backgrounds. In general, the staff can be classified as counseling staff or medical staff. Within each of these classifications, staff can have backgrounds in social work, rehabilitation, psychology, nursing, or can have life experience with substance abuse.

Physicians, while playing a critical role in the management of medical and psychiatric problems which arise out of substance abuse, play a small role in substance abuse treatment itself. Physicians are likely, however, to play a role in the initial medical detoxification of the client and, in certain cases, may provide medical consultation to treatment staff. Beyond this, however, the nonmedical staff of the substance abuse treatment center generally have responsibility for client care. Such staff include a primary counselor, who will be responsible for treatment planning and counseling, and auxiliary staff (e.g., recreation therapist, technicians, educational staff, tutors).

Training

Substance abuse professionals may be either degreed or nondegreed. Degreed staff have been trained in a human service field (e.g., social work, rehabilitation, psychology, nursing), and have chosen substance abuse treatment as their area of expertise. There are few post-secondary training programs which specialize in substance abuse, however, so most degreed individuals obtained general education in the human services, and gained expertise in the substance abuse field later. The second type of substance abuse professional is the nondegreed staff member. Most of these individuals are recovering from substance abuse themselves, and acquired their skills through life experience and their own recovery, and training after being hired by a treatment center. Each of these different types of staff has a different perspective to offer, thus enhancing the flexibility of the system to respond to a wide variety of clients.

Certification, Licensing, Accreditation

Although the National Association of Alcoholism and Drug Abuse Counselors (NAADAC) is working toward forming a national certifying body for substance abuse staff, none currently exists. Many states have voluntary counselor certification boards operated by private, not-for-profit corporations to provide the public assurance of professional competence.

The quality of substance abuse programs is monitored by outside agencies in two separate ways: licensure and accreditation. The *licensure* standards of each state provide the consumer the assurance that the treatment center meets the minimum acceptable standards for life safety, confidentiality, and treatment. Each individual treatment component of the substance abuse center is usually licensed separately (e.g., inpatient, outpatient, intensive outpatient, detox). *Accreditation* of substance abuse centers is voluntary, and recognizes compliance with state-of-the-art standards for treatment, facilities, and staff. Accreditation comes from two primary sources: the Joint Commission on Accreditation of Health Organizations (JCAHO) and the Commission on Accreditation of Rehabilitation Facilities (CARF), both of which are private organizations.

Purpose/Intent

GOALS OF TREATMENT

Centers which provide services for drug and alcohol abusers strive to return the client to a normal level of functioning. To obtain this end, abstinence from the use of drugs and alcohol is required. Additionally, centers which apply the traditional model attempt to return the client to a state of *serenity*. The first proponents of the 12-step model discussed this concept of serenity in terms of a feeling of connection with a *higher power*. The higher power is a spiritual concept that may or may not involve traditional religious ideas of spirituality. Nevertheless, proponents of the 12-step model are typically convinced of the importance of the higher power in personal recovery programs.

SPECIAL CASE MANAGEMENT NEEDS

Very few clients presenting at a substance abuse treatment facility are lucky enough to suffer from substance abuse alone. For this reason, the task of the substance abuse counselor is far more rich than simply monitoring the abstinence program of a client. The special nature of substance abuse treatment requires human service staff to address a wide variety of problems, including family counseling, relationship and marriage counseling, women's issues, and special problems of treatment with adolescent clients. In addition, substance abuse treatment utilizes all of a trained counselor's skills in assessment and possible referral to other practitioners.

Substance abuse treatment is currently on the leading edge of research and implementation of services for such diverse and socially important challenges as the dually diagnosed (i.e., clients who have substance abuse problems in addition to mental illness), cocaine addicted women and their infants, and individuals infected with HIV.

Client Services

DESCRIPTION OF SERVICES

Drug and alcohol abuse treatment centers provide a variety of services. Most centers provide assessment services and one or more of the following: inpatient, outpatient, and aftercare. Additional services which many centers offer include detoxification, intensive outpatient, and educational programs. The major treatment modalities are described below.

Detoxification

Frequently, the first referral a substance abuse client needs is to a detoxification center. All general medical hospitals are capable of providing this service, however, their willingness to do so will depend on the availability of physician expertise. Hospitals with substance abuse specialties or other freestanding substance abuse treatment units should be consulted as to the availability of detoxification services and cost information.

Detoxification programs usually last from three to five days unless medical complications require an extended hospital stay. During this time the client will receive supportive nursing care and pharmacotherapy for withdrawal, if necessary. During the detoxification process, many therapists and concerned others have found that substance abusing individuals are remorseful and more likely to accept additional assistance (e.g., outpatient or inpatient substance abuse therapy). In any event, it is important to stress with addicted individuals that detoxification is *not* substance abuse treatment. It only gets the individual ready to enter substance abuse treatment. Ideally, the client will be entering a substance abuse treatment program immediately after discharge from the detoxification unit.

Outpatient

Substance abuse outpatient clinics are commonly found in state-subsidized treatment facilities. Less frequently, such clinics may be found in hospital or freestanding substance abuse clinics. Outpatient treatment is a less costly alternative to residential substance abuse treatment. In addition, it allows the client to continue working and maintaining other daily activities. Accordingly, it is the least restrictive and intrusive treatment alternative the substance abuser has available. Like all substance abuse treatment modalities, outpatient treatment seeks to focus the client's initial efforts on maintaining abstinence. Both traditional and behavioral methods to promote abstinence may include: (a) 12-step work; (b) attendance at AA; (c) disulfiram therapy; and (d) relapse prevention training. Most clients require ongoing support from some combination of therapist, other recovering persons, family, or friends for staying drug free. However, once the client has demonstrated some ability to do this, outpatient therapy may begin to assist the client and significant others in healing damaged relationships and facilitating adjustment to a lifestyle free of alcohol and other drugs.

Outpatient treatment is not recommended for clients whose substance abuse has progressed to the point where there is almost no stability in life functioning or social support. Outpatient treatment is most useful for those individuals whose drinking or other drug use is beginning to or periodically interferes with one or more aspects of their life (e.g., relationships, employment, health, legal). Outpatient therapy is often the first treatment experience because of low cost and unintrusiveness on the client's life. Should the client's alcohol or other drug use not show significant improvement while in outpatient treatment *and* deterioration in one or more life/health areas continues, then referral to a detoxification or inpatient treatment unit is indicated.

Inpatient

Inpatient substance abuse treatment programs may be found in many hospitals. In addition, many large cities have freestanding proprietary and not-for-profit residential treatment centers. To a lesser degree, state-subsidized, inpatient treatment units are available and provide services to clients without adequate insurance coverage. The model length of stay for clients of inpatient units tends to be 28 days. Inpatient treatment provides a controlled, safe environment. Such an environment removes the client from the substance-using environment and permits the initial stages of recovery to begin. During inpatient treatment, clients will receive medical monitoring and intervention when indicated, psychological assessment, and nutritional assessment and diet.

The substance abuse intervention component to inpatient treatment tends to follow the traditional model. Most inpatient programs are highly structured and provide intensive substance abuse education, individual and group therapy, and self-help group meetings. Clients are typically oriented to the 12-step approach to recovery and their individual therapist monitors, advises, and supports their progress in "working the steps" toward recovery. Family or significant other involvement in the client's treatment is usually required during the course of the residential stay. Nearly all inpatient programs offer some form of post-discharge follow-up counseling or aftercare. Because addictive disorders are similar to other chronic illnesses (i.e., compliance to lifestyle modifications), aftercare monitoring and counseling is essential.

TYPICAL REFERRAL QUESTIONS

The referral questions asked by treatment centers will vary. Some centers may want to know in-depth information about a client while others will ask relatively few questions. In any case, the referring human service worker should be prepared to provide information addressing the following questions:

What is the nature and severity of the client's substance abuse problem?

The substance abuse counselor or intake manager will need to know what drugs the client uses, including alcohol and prescription medications; how long each substance has been used; the maximum amount the client has habitually used; what social consequences the client has experienced as a result of substance abuse; especially legal difficulties associated with substance abuse, and whether there is a diagnosis of mental illness concurrent with substance abuse.

What is the extent of family involvement?

Substance abuse itself and substance abuse treatment are family oriented. Families suffer along with the substance abuser, and families should be involved with the treatment process in order to enhance the client's chances for success. Treatment agencies will want to know what family members are available to assist the assessment and treatment process with the client. Referring agencies should prepare families for their role in collaborating in the recovery process with the client.

Are there any medical complications associated with substance abuse?

Treatment agencies will ask if the client has any active medical complications associated with or affected by substance abuse. Most, but not all, nonhospital-based substance abuse treatment facilities have limited resources available to manage acute medical problems. Typical questions may include references to pancreatitis, diabetes, hepatitis, HIV infection, concurrent mental illness, prescribed medications, and pregnancy.

References

Azrin, N. H., Sisson, R. W., Meyers, R., & Godley, M. D. (1982). Alcoholism treatment by disulfiram and community reinforcement therapy. *Journal of Behavior Therapy and Experimental Psychiatry*, *13*, 105-112.

Cummings, N. A. (1979). Turning bread into stones, our modern antimiracle. *American Psychologist*, *34*, 1119-1129.

Guydish, J. (1982). Substance abuse and alphabet soup. *Personnel and Guidance Journal*, *61*, 397-400.

Jellinek, E. M. (1960). *The disease concept of alcoholism.* New Haven: Hill House.

Mann, M. (1950). *Primer on alcoholism.* New York: Holt, Rinehart and Winston.

Mann, M. (1958). *New primer on alcoholism.* New York: Holt, Rinehart and Winston.

Rimmele, C. T., Miller, W. R., & Dougher, M. J. (1989). Aversion therapies. In R. Hester & W. Miller (Eds.), *Handbook of alcoholism treatment approaches: Effective alternatives* (pp. 128-140). New York: Pergamon.

White, W. (1990). *The culture of addiction: The culture of recovery.* Bloomington, IL: Lighthouse Training Institute Publications.

Peer Self-Help Groups

John J. Benshoff, Ph.D.

Peer self-help groups have grown to occupy a prominent place in the retinue of available community services. Generally modelled on the success of Alcoholics Anonymous, these groups offer guidance, support, and solace to individuals suffering from a variety of societal, behavioral, or medical conditions. They are typified by their absence of formal, professional leadership, acceptance of all comers who indicate an interest in change, and their emphasis on change occurring through participation within the structure of the program.

Alcoholics Anonymous

The best known and oldest peer self-help group is Alcoholics Anonymous (AA). The founding of Alcoholics Anonymous can be traced to the chance encounter in 1935 of two recovering alcoholics, Dr. Bob Smith and Bill Wilson. Smith and Wilson had tried many avenues seeking their own recovery, and were determined in that fateful meeting in the kitchen of the Smith home in Akron, Ohio to divine a successful method for recovery from alcoholism. From that humble beginning, AA has grown to include 1.5 million members in 115 countries around the world.

The sole criteria for AA membership, as articulated in AA Tradition 3, " . . . is a desire to quit drinking." There are no dues except for the dollar bills dropped in the basket when it is passed to help pay for the ubiquitous coffee and snacks, and literature for new members. The local meeting or group is the keystone of AA. Members may choose to affiliate with a *home* group, or may choose to attend a variety of groups. In general, most individuals select a group in which they feel comfortable.

In urban areas, there are special meetings for alcoholics of all persuasions: professional groups, old-timer groups, gay groups, Hispanic groups, physician groups, women's groups, and so on. Most AA meetings, and there are thousands occurring daily, are *Open Meetings*, as the name implies, open to all comers, both alcoholic and nonalcoholic. In more populated areas, *Newcomer's Meetings* cater to AA beginners; Big Book Meetings center on discussion from *Alcoholics Anonymous* (Alcoholics Anonymous World Services, 1976), the aptly named AA bible; Step and Tradition Meetings focus on the Twelve Steps and Twelve Traditions of AA; *Closed* meetings are limited to members of local groups or visiting members from other groups to provide a forum for those unique and common problems faced by all recovering alcoholics. Meeting times and places are often advertised in the daily paper and, generally, a local phone number will be listed to provide information about meetings. Meetings are generally held in church basements, community centers, group halls, or other public locations. Meetings are also held in hospitals and chemical dependency treatment centers, for the convenience of individuals in treatment. These meetings, while hosted by the institution, are conducted according to the tenets of Alcoholics Anonymous and are viewed as a service for the host institution.

A member's participation in AA is grounded in the Twelve Steps:

1. We admitted we were powerless over alcohol—that our lives had become unmanageable.
2. Came to believe that a Power greater than ourselves could restore us to sanity.
3. Made a decision to turn our will and our lives over to the care of God *as we understood him.*
4. Made a searching and fearless moral inventory of ourselves.
5. Admitted to God, to ourselves, and to another human being the exact nature of our wrongs.
6. Were entirely ready to have God remove all these defects of character.
7. Humbly asked Him to remove our shortcomings.
8. Made a list of all persons we had harmed and became willing to make amends to them all.
9. Made direct amends to such people wherever possible, except when to do so would injure them or others.
10. Continued to take personal inventory and when we were wrong promptly admitted it.
11. Sought through prayer and meditation to improve our conscious contact with God *as we understood Him*, praying only for the knowledge of his will for us, and the power to carry that out.
12. Having had a spiritual awakening as the result of these steps, we tried to carry this message to alcoholics, and to practice these principles in all our affairs.

From a clinical perspective, the Twelve Steps of AA neatly encapsulate the treatment issues of problem recognition, insight, help seeking, restitution, stress reduction, and assumption of a healthy, nonegocentric lifestyle. Perhaps, however, the Twelve Steps are best understood in the words of Nan Robertson (1988), Pulitzer Prize-winning journalist, and longtime AA member:

> We admit we are licked and cannot get well on our own. We get
> honest with ourselves. We talk it out with somebody else. We try

to make amends to people we have harmed. We pray to whatever greater power we think there is. We try to give of ourselves for our own sake and without stint to other alcoholics, with no thought of reward (p. 26).

Fundamental to the belief system espoused by AA is the concept that alcoholism is a lifelong illness, for which there is treatment resulting in remission of the disease through abstinence, but not cure. Consequently, AA members refer to themselves as recover*ing* alcoholics, not recover*ed* alcoholics.

Just as individual participation centers on the Twelve Steps, the Twelve Traditions of AA guide the functioning of the organization:

1. Our common welfare should come first; personal recovery depends upon AA unity.
2. From our group purpose there is but one ultimate authority—a loving God as He may express himself in our group conscience. Our leaders are but trusted servants; they do not govern.
3. The only requirement for AA membership is a desire to stop drinking.
4. Each group should be autonomous except in matters affecting other groups or AA as a whole.
5. Each group has but one primary purpose—to carry its message to the alcoholic who still suffers.
6. An AA group ought never endorse, finance, or lend the AA name to any related facility or outside enterprise, lest problems of money, property, and prestige divert us from our primary purpose.
7. Every AA group ought to fully self-supporting, declining outside contributions.
8. Alcoholics Anonymous should remain forever nonprofessional, but our service centers may employ special workers.
9. AA, as such, ought never be organized; but we may create service boards or committees directly responsible to those they serve.
10. Alcoholics Anonymous has no opinion on outside issues; hence the AA name ought never be drawn into public controversy.
11. Our public relations policy is based on attraction rather than promotion; we need always maintain personal anonymity at the level of press, radio, and films.
12. Anonymity is the spiritual foundation of all our traditions, ever reminding us to place principles before personalities.

As the Traditions suggest, the local group is the basic functional unit of AA. It is independent and autonomous from other groups, often fiercely so. There are no membership applications, requirements for a quorum, conformity to rules and regulation of meeting decorum, subservience to an overseeing body, or obeisance to professional groups. Indeed, the long form of the Traditions suggest that where two or three members are gathered for sobriety, a meeting may occur. Obviously, a group as wide-ranging as AA cannot exist in a totally unstructured state. At the group level, officers may be elected for short terms as chairperson, secretary, or treasurer, or to various committees with responsibility for carrying on the logistics of the meetings.

In larger communities, Regional Service Boards exist to coordinate group meeting times and places and to deal with issues which concern the welfare of groups within the region. Often, for example, Regional Service Boards will sponsor quarterly or annual breakfast or dinner meetings bringing together all of the members of all of the groups in a region.

Overall responsibility for the service standards of Alcoholics Anonymous rests with the General Service Board, based in New York City. This 21-member board is composed of both AA members and nonalcoholic members, with the unique feature that only nonalcoholic members can assume positions of financial responsibility within the board. This longstanding tenet is based upon Bill Wilson's recognition that even the most firmly committed AA member can experience a slip, a temporary relapse from sobriety. Wilson's fear was that a slipped alcoholic with fiscal responsibilities could do great financial and moral damage to the Fellowship. The Board oversees the operation of the General Service Board, the publishing and supporting arm of AA, and serves as a central clearinghouse for information. In recent years, the General Service Board has assumed responsibility for devising strategies to underserved minority groups, both within the US and around the world. AA's only paid staffers work for the General Service Office.

ANONYMITY—THE ESSENCE OF AA

The late Bill Wilson wrote in *AA Comes of Age* (Alcoholics Anonymous World Services, Inc., 1957), "Moved by the spirit of anonymity, we try to give up our natural desires for personal distinctions as AA members both among our fellow alcoholics and before the general public. As we lay aside these very human aspirations . . . each of us takes part in the weaving of a protective mantle that covers our whole society and under which we may grow and work in unity." The anonymity principle serves to keep the new AA member focussed on the newly recovering self, and for controlling urges for power and prestige, urges that are seen as contrary to the notion of a sober life.

Secondly, anonymity allows the newly recovering person safe haven from the stigma of alcoholism. Despite the recent gains which have been made in society's understanding and perception of alcoholism problems, negative social, economic, and familial consequences from the former alcoholic lifestyle exert pressures which can be damaging to sobriety. Anonymity does not, however, provide an excuse or alibi for past irresponsible or harmful behaviors. Indeed, AA members are called throughout the Twelve Steps to assume individual, personal responsibility for their behavior, past and present.

Finally, the anonymity principle promotes participation by individuals from all walks of life, with anonymity the great leveler. Members are asked to give only their first names in meetings and all are viewed as fellow travelers on the road to sobriety. No member, by virtue of experience, rank, or expertise, is placed above any other member, and the Fellowship has been quick to separate itself from those who flaunt their recovery for personal aggrandizement or gain. Indeed, anonymity is seen as a method for members to develop a new, humble sense of self, devoid of the ego demands which are felt to lead to a return to drinking behavior.

The only role that members can assume which distinguishes individuals from one another is the role of sponsor. New members are commonly encouraged to find a sponsor, in effect a mentor, who can provide guidance, support, and understanding, both in normal and trying times. Typically, sponsors should have several years of quality sobriety and an interest in providing empathic guidance and assistance. The organization establishes no formal guidelines for sponsorship, nor does it provide any training except that which occurs serendipitously through attending meetings and observing other individuals in action.

Consistent with the anonymity principle, Alcoholics Anonymous has steadfastly refused to have its name associated with *any* other organization, nor does it accept donations, believing to do either could divert the organization from its primary purpose. Many alcoholism treatment programs will advertise themselves as AA model programs, an appellation which is self-ascribed, and which should not be construed as AA endorsement. Similarly, AA has refused to allow bumper stickers, jewelry, trinkets, and the like to be imprinted with the AA logo or other identifying marks. Recently a series of bumper stickers, T-shirts, and other paraphernalia have appeared with AA slogans on them (e.g., Easy Does It, I'm a Friend of Bill's, One Day at a Time), however, the feeling of the membership and the General Service Board was that these sayings were sufficiently unknown to the general public and, hence, not a danger to any member's anonymity. Alcoholics Anonymous supports itself primarily through the sale of books and pamphlets about AA, all of which are inscribed "AA General Conference-approved literature."

WHO JOINS AA?

The sole criteria for AA membership is a desire to quit drinking. In its early days, Alcoholics Anonymous meetings were apt to be filled with middle-aged, white, male alcoholics. As drug use has grown more prevalent, the composition of the membership has expanded to include younger individuals, and individuals from a variety of ethnic backgrounds. Similarly, more women are now seen in AA meetings. In the past the lead speaker might have started his address with the statement "Hello, my name is Joe, and I'm an alcoholic." Today, it is equally probable that the lead speaker will say "Hello, my name is Joanne, and I'm an addict and an alcoholic."

This changing composition has not always been greeted enthusiastically by individual members. Many "old deacons," long-time recovering alcoholics, regard this new breed of member with a history of multiple addictions to multiple substances with some disdain. Fortunately, these individuals nearly always are in the minority, and there is growing, explicit recognition that, just as society has changed, so too have addictive diseases, and consequently the membership of AA.

Ogborne and Glaser (1981), in a review of the literature on affiliation with AA suggested that members tended to be white males, middle-aged, and from upper- or middle-class backgrounds. In addition, they tended to be binge drinkers, with a physical dependence on alcohol and a history of loss-of-control drinking. Membership has also been associated with external locus of control, strong affiliation needs, and the loss or threatened loss of a lifestyle because of drinking.

More recently, Emrick (1987) has suggested that successful participation (i.e., development and maintenance of sobriety) among AA members is related to leading meetings, having a sponsor and acting as a sponsor, and working Steps 6 through 12 following residential treatment. Frequency of attendance was also correlated with sobriety status and duration. Hoffman, Harrison, and Belille (1983) reported the efficacy of AA as an aftercare strategy, correlating weekly AA attendance with preservation of sobriety. As one might expect, "AA members who are more active in the organization, both with frequency of attendance and participation in the organization's therapeutic mechanisms, have an outcome status that is as good as and probably better than those members who attend or participate less actively." (Emrick, 1987, p. 420)

From an empirical perspective, aside from the studies previously mentioned and a handful of others, relatively little is known about the treatment efficacy of AA. The anonymity principle, while fostering membership growth and participation, also effectively hinders an in-depth research understanding of who attends meetings, for how long, and how often. Little is known, for example, about the recovery success of individuals who attend a few meetings for a short time and then drop out, or about individuals who attend meetings sporadically over a number of years. Moreover, meager knowledge exists about persons who attend one AA meeting, and never go back. AA freely admits that the program is not for all people. It concedes that AA is not for the individual who is unwilling to frankly admit to being an alcoholic, or who cleaves to the notion of a return to social drinking.

Peer Self-help Programs for Codependents

Alcoholism has been generally conceptualized as a family disease, affecting not only the identified alcoholic, but also the family, with recurrent problems evident. Individuals affected by, and enmeshed in the problems of an alcoholic are broadly considered to be *codependents*. They include spouses, children, teen-agers, and most recently adult children of alcoholics. The best known peer self-help group for codependents is Al-Anon.

Begun in the early 1950s in response to the need to provide support and guidance for spouses in alcoholic marriages, the program has grown to include 25,000 groups worldwide. Just as a basic premise of AA is that the alcoholic is powerless over alcohol, Al-Anon members learn that they are powerless over alcohol and the alcoholic. The Al-Anon recovery program emphasizes independence, abandonment of previously held control notions, and detachment, a willingness to allow the world to run itself (Young, 1987). Just as in AA, the membership of Al-Anon has grown increasingly diverse. No longer are meetings attended only by white females in their middle age. Males, minorities, and younger people make up a significant proportion of the membership today.

Although not formally affiliated with Alcoholics Anonymous, Al-Anon uses a 12-step model, and meetings are frequently scheduled concurrently with AA meetings. There are no dues, no membership lists, and no requirements for participation. Some Al-Anon members join because a loved one has joined AA. For others, Al-Anon provides support and guidance about living with a family member who is continuing to drink. Teenagers from alcoholic homes can receive support and guidance from Alateen. Again, there are no dues, and no rules and regulations governing membership, however, adult leadership is provided, often from a recovering individual or spouse.

In the late 1970s, clinicians identified a complex set of characteristics which were found in adults who had been raised in alcoholic homes, and the Adult Children of Alcoholics (ACOA) movement was born. Children who grow up in alcoholic homes have to learn a complex set of survival skills to cope with the exigencies of living with an alcoholic parent. They learn to live and adjust to shifting, and generally dysfunctional, patterns of communication, intimacy, behavior, and relationships. Unfortunately, these survival skills, which served them well as children, may result in problems in adult life. Frequently, adult children of alcoholics experience difficulties with interpersonal relationships, intimacy, trust, and an inability to develop a healthy sense of self-esteem and personal identity. Because they have been raised in homes full of turmoil, their lives may be characterized by disorder, thrill-seeking, and risk-taking. Finally, there is a high incidence of alcoholism among this group. Adult Children of Alcoholics groups are found in most areas of the country, and a considerable popular press has emerged concerning the problems of ACOAs.

Narcotics Anonymous, Cocaine Anonymous, and Other Peer Self-help Groups

The history of Narcotics Anonymous (NA) can be traced to the late 1940s and early 1950s when concerned recovering drug addicts, recognizing the success of AA, realized that a similar program could be beneficial to drug addicts. Just as in AA, NA is a fellowship of sufferers, hence, leadership and authority within NA flows from the bottom up, not the top down. NA maintains its own World Service Board and has evolved its own Twelve Steps and Twelve Traditions. In part, NA originated in response to the implicit, and occasionally explicit, rejection of addicts and the problems they faced by AA. Today, however, NA members often attend AA meetings and vice versa, and just as in the AA community, relatively few *pure* addicts are seen.

The core belief of NA is that members suffer from the disease of drug addition, without specific recognition of any particular drug. This addiction is thought to be a life-long addiction for which the only treatment is abstinence from *all* potentially addicting substances including alcohol. As the group name implies, the focus tends to be on the universality of potential problems caused by addicting drugs—narcotics—rather than on the unique problems of individual members. From an ideological viewpoint, NA is intolerant of any drug consumption, other than that which is medically necessary, although slips (relapses) are recognized as intrinsic elements of the addictive process. Addicts who slip are allowed to remain in the fellowship, provided, of course, that they cease using drugs.

NA meetings include testimonial meetings in which lead speakers deliver speeches about their addiction and subsequent recovery, step-study and tradition-study meetings, and discussion meetings often focussing on questions and answers about NA and addiction (Peyrot, 1985). Both open and closed meetings are held, and are advertised in local newspapers and directories of human services.

The expanding cocaine epidemic of the 1980s has resulted in the establishment of a number of treatment alternatives for cocaine and crack addiction, including the formation of Cocaine Anonymous. Modelled on traditional 12-step, peer self-help principles, this fellowship provides assistance, guidance, and support specifically for those addicted to cocaine and its derivatives. Cocaine Anonymous groups tend to be found in large urban areas, but as cocaine addiction continues to expand, groups are forming in less populated areas.

The peer self-help model has proven popular for treating a variety of other social ills. Gamblers Anonymous serves individuals with compulsive gambling disorders; Overeaters Anonymous provides support for individuals with eating disorders. These, and other groups, are widely available throughout the country.

Peer Self-help Groups and the Professional Counselor

For the counselor seeking help for a client with an alcoholism or addiction problem, peer self-help groups present a number of advantages. They are easy to refer to, and there is never a waiting list. Indeed, often regional service boards or individual groups will arrange for newcomers to be accompanied to meetings by veteran fellowship members. Peer self-help groups present the additional advantage of being free, also, an important consideration in these times of escalating health care costs.

This cost-free benefit may have a multiple impact. Not only is the identified client spared the direct cost of services, but the dollars which are saved can be used to purchase other services or to provide services to other clients. Finally, the popular literature, and the nonempirical-based professional literature strongly suggest the efficacy of peer self-help groups. Part of their success may rest with a preconceived notion that clients and counselors may have that the treatment will work.

Despite these advantages, counselors need to guard against the assumption that peer self-help groups will work for every patient every time. For some individuals that will be the case, but peer self-help groups are not a panacea for all ailments. Indeed, in most cases they should serve as an adjunct to the already established therapeutic relationship.

Peer self-help groups are not for all clients. Addicts or alcoholics who are unwilling or uninterested in stopping all alcohol or drug consuming behavior—those individuals who wish to drink or use drugs socially—are not good candidates for peer self-help groups. Individuals whose recovery will require close monitoring, generally will not make good peer self-help group members initially. The leaderless, anonymous characteristics of these groups make close scrutiny and accountability difficult in many instances. Groups will provide feedback about individual attendance if asked, usually through the mechanism of a signed note from the group secretary. Counselors requiring feedback information should establish a procedure for getting this information from the local group or meeting, and should not place this logistical burden on the client. At best, it may raise the anxiety level of the first time group participant and serve as a deterrent to group participation. At worst, clients in denial of their addictive disease may take advantage of the situation and not attend meetings, but return notes signed by friends or family.

Peer self-help assistance is based on a unitary premise: abstinence from chemicals. Clients presenting multidimensional problem (e.g., dual addictive disease, psychiatric diagnoses) will require more intervention than a peer self-help group may be capable of giving. While group participation may be a useful adjunct for therapy, peer self-therapy cannot substitute for the intensive therapy often needed in these situations, or for required psychotropic medications.

Counselors need to carefully monitor clients who are taking psychotropic or other therapeutic medications and who are attending AA or NA meetings. While these groups recognize and support the consumption of medication for valid medical or psychiatric purposes, individual group members may espouse a totally different philosophy to the detriment of clients who require medication to function in society.

Finally, counselors who choose to refer clients to peer self-help groups should become aware of the value structures, mores, and cultural traditions of local groups. Almost by definition, peer self-help groups represent a microcosm of society, reflecting both that which is positive and that which is negative. Groups, while espousing an openness to all, may have taboos about race, gender, gender preference, or other issues which may alienate certain individuals.

Despite these cautions and disadvantages, peer self-help groups represent a vital, growing, and effective way for many individuals to cope with the problems of life. They serve as a useful adjunct to therapy and, for some clients, may be the critical element in achieving recovery from addiction or alcoholism.

Useful Addresses

Alcoholics Anonymous World Services
Box 459 Grand Central Station
New York, NY 10163
(212) 686-1100

Al-Anon Family Group Headquarters, Inc.
Box 182 Madison Square Station
New York, NY 10159-0182
(212) 683-1771

National Association for Children of Alcoholics
Box 421961
San Francisco, CA 94142
(415) 431-1366

Narcotics Anonymous World Services Office
Box 622
Sun Valley, CA 91352

References

Alcoholics Anonymous World Services, Inc. (1957). *AlcoholicsAnonymous comes of age: A brief history of AA*. New York: Author.
Alcoholics Anonymous World Services, Inc. (1976). *Alcoholics Anonymous* (3rd ed.). New York: Author.
Emrick, C. D. (1987). Alcoholics Anonymous: Affiliation processes and effectiveness as treatment. *Alcoholism Clinical and Experimental Research, 11*, 416-423.
Hoffman, N. G., Harrison, P. A., & Belille, C. A. (1983). Alcoholics Anonymous after treatment: Attendance and abstinence. *The International Journal of Addictions, 18*(3), 311-318.
Ogborne, A. C., & Glaser, F. B. (1981). Characteristics of affiliates of Alcoholics Anonymous: A review of the literature. *Journal of Studies on Alcohol, 42*(7), 661-675.
Peyrot, M. (1985). Narcotics Anonymous: Its history, structure, and approach. *The International Journal of Addictions, 20*(10), 1509-1522.
Robertson, N. (1988, Feb. 21). The changing world of Alcoholics Anonymous. *New York Times Magazine*, pp. 24-26, 47, 57, 92.
Young, E. (1987). Co-alcoholism as a disease: Implications for psychotherapy. *Journal of Psychoactive Drugs, 19*, 257-268.

III. Social Services

Social Security Disability Insurance/ Supplemental Security Income

Wanda D. Bracy, M.S.W.

History/Legislation

Both the Social Security Disability Insurance (SSDI) program and the Supplemental Security Income (SSI) program were enacted under amendments of the Social Security Act. The Social Security Disability Insurance program was enacted into law on August 1, 1956, and the Supplemental Security Income program was established by the 1972 amendments to the Social Security Act, and enacted into law on October 30, 1972.

The Social Security Act of 1935 is considered landmark legislation, and has undergone decades of evolution since its enactment in 1935. The major objectives of the Social Security Act is to provide for the material needs of individuals and families, to protect the aged and disabled, to keep families together, and to provide children with the opportunity to grow up in health and security; its programs account for most of the cash support received by Americans.

There are two major categories of programs included in the Social Security Act. They are the social insurance programs of which the Social Security Disability Insurance (SSDI) program is one, and the public assistance programs which include the Supplemental Security Income (SSI) program. Social insurance programs are distinguished from public assistance in that social insurance is considered a right of the individual, and designed to protect individuals and families from a loss of income due to no fault of their own. It is seen as a right because workers contribute a portion of their wages in the form of payroll taxes for the purpose of this protection. Public assistance programs usually carry a stigma, and are seen less as a right than as a gift by the government. Eligibility for these type of programs are based on need and recipients must undergo a means test demonstrating that they lack necessary resources and income to support and maintain themselves. Eligibility for social insurance programs is based on meeting the cirteria of insured worker status and, in the case of the SSDI program, meeting the requirement for disability. There is no means test to determine need. The concept of social insurance carries with it the idea of protection against presumed risk.

ADMINISTRATION

Both the SSDI and the SSI programs are administered by the Social Security Administration which was established in 1946 when its predecessor, the Social Security Board, was abolished. The Social Security Administration is located in the Department of Health and Human Services (DHHS) and the Commissioner of Social Security is directly responsible to the Secretary of Health and Human Services. The Social Security Administration, whose mandate is to provide benefits to those entitled to the provisions of the Social Security Act and to protect the Social Security Trust Funds, is one of the largest components of the Department of Health and Human Services. The central office is located in Baltimore, Maryland where the Office of Central Records Operations is also housed. This office is responsible for maintaining the records of individuals' earnings and preparing benefit computations.

The operations of the Social Security Administration are decentralized to provide appropriate services at the local level. There are 10 regional offices headed by a regional commissioner, who is responsible for providing services directly to the public and coordinating regional operations so that they are consistent with national requirements. The regional offices are located in Atlanta, Boston, Chicago, Dallas, Denver, Kansas City (Missouri), New York City, Philadelphia, San Francisco, and Seattle.

Each of the regions contain a network of district and branch offices and teleservice centers that serve as contact centers between the Social Security Administration and the public. These offices are responsible for providing information on the purposes and provisions of social security programs, informing claimants and beneficiaries of their rights and responsibilities, assisting claimants and beneficiaries, developing and adjudicating claims, and making rehabilitation service referrals.

Within each region there are local district offices where a person can apply for social security benefits. There are also a number of teleservice centers that handle telephone inquiries and make appropriate referrals. In addition to these offices, there are also program service centers that house and service the records of individuals who are receiving social security benefits. These program service centers are processing centers and is where determinations as to entitlement on many claims for social security benefits are made.

To further ensure public access, the Social Security Administration operates contact stations in outlying areas to serve people who live a distance from a city or town in which an office is located. A schedule of staff visits to these locations can be obtained at the nearest local social security office. The Social Security Administration will also send a representative to make a home visit in the case of illness or infirmity.

The Office of Hearings and Appeals is responsible for the supervision of hearings held, and decisions made, on appealed cases. This function is actually performed by a national association of administrative law judges who conduct independent hearings, and decide on appealed determinations of benefits. The Office of Hearings and Appeals is responsible for providing administrative direction to this national organization. There is also an Appeals Council responsible for reviewing appealed determinations and rendering the final decision.

SOCIAL SECURITY DISABILITY INSURANCE (SSDI)

The Social Security Disability Insurance (SSDI) program is part of the Old Age, Survivors, and Disability Insurance (OASDI) program and has been in effect since 1954. The purpose of this program is to replace loss of income when the wage-earner is no longer able to work. The Disability Insurance program insures against the loss of income due to the worker's physical or mental disability.

Funding

The SSDI program is funded by earmarked payroll taxes that are deposited in a Disability Insurance Trust Fund. Any revenues not immediately needed to finance current benefit levels are invested in interest-bearing United States Treasury securities, and the interest on these securities are accrued to the trust funds.

Until recently, this form of taxing was considered regressive because the burden fell disproportionately on the lower income households. This was due to the flat-rate tax which did not exempt low-paid workers and those with large families and required higher income earners to pay taxes on only a portion of their income. This method of taxation, however, did benefit the low income because they disproportionately received a much higher percentage of their Average Indexed Monthly Income (AIME). In the 1980s, the burden of the payroll tax for the upper income was increased when Congress, through social security amendments, raised the ceiling on the amount of earnings subject to payroll taxes to the point that the cap now covers the total earnings of most workers.

Benefits

Disability insurance benefits for disabled workers are in the form of cash payments and "protections." Benefits in the form of cash payments are paid monthly by check or direct deposit to insured individuals, or to their representative payee if the beneficiary is incapable of managing his or her own funds.

The Old Age, Survivors, and Disability Insurance program is the largest of all the social welfare programs, and has grown enormously over the years due to the decision by Congress to tie increases in social security benefits to the nation's rate of inflation. Under this law, if the inflation rate exceeds 3% from the first quarter of one year to the first quarter of the next, social security benefits automatically increase at the rate of inflation shown by the Consumer Price Index (CPI).

In July 1990, monthly cash benefits were awarded to 305,358 persons under the Old Age, Survivors, and Disability Insurance Program, and 13% of these awards were to disabled workers. The average monthly payment in July 1990 for disabled workers was $570.93.

In 1990, some benefits became subject to federal income tax if the adjusted gross income plus nontaxable interest and 50% of benefits exceeded the base amount. The base amount in 1990 for an individual was $25,000, and for a married couple it was $32,000 if they filed jointly, and zero if they filed separately.

Benefits in the form of protections establish a period of disability which protects the disabled worker against a loss or reduction in the amount of disability benefits, and provides for hospital and supplementary medical insurance protection, as well as vocational rehabilitation services. There is, however, an initial five-month waiting period required before disability insurance benefits will be paid. Benefits are payable for the sixth month, however, if a worker becomes disabled within 60 months after termination of disability benefits, this individual may be paid for the first full month of the disability after reentitlement.

After benefits have been received for 24 months, the beneficiary is eligible for Medicare protections to help pay for hospital, doctor, and other medical bills. This 24-month waiting period is in addition to the five-month waiting period after the onset of disability. The 24 months in the qualifying period need not be consecutive. Months from a previous period of disability may be counted in determining when Medicare benefits begin. Individuals who were previously entitled to Medicare may be immediately eligible for Medicare upon reentitlement to disability benefits. Also, if there was no previous entitlement to Medicare, previous months of disability benefit entitlement may still be counted in determining when the individual has been entitled for 24 months.

Eligibility for Benefits

To be eligible for disability benefits, an individual must have disability insured status, have not attained the age of 65, have a disability that falls within that which is defined by the Social Security Act, have filed an application for the period in which the disability is effective, and have completed a five-month waiting period. Medical proof is also required to determine that a disability rules out gainful employment.

Eligibility is based on the number of years an individual has contributed to social security. To be fully insured, a person must have contributed through payroll taxes for 40 quarters (10 years). To be eligible for Disability insurance,

20 quarters is the minimum period of time for contributions. In some cases, people 18 and over can qualify for disability insurance even though they may not have contributed through payroll taxes. These persons are eligible if they were totally and permanently disabled before age 22, and she or he had been a dependent of an insured worker who is currently disabled, retired, or deceased.

The persons who are eligible for disability benefits are as follows:

- An insured worker with a disability who is under age 65.
- A spouse of a disabled worker who is entitled to benefits, who is age 62 or over, or has in their care a child under the age of 16, or if over 16, are disabled. This person is entitled to benefits under the worker's social security.
- A divorced spouse of a disabled worker who is entitled to benefits, if age 62 or older, and married to a worker for at least 10 years.
- A divorced spouse of a fully insured worker who has not yet filed a claim for benefits, if both are age 62 or older, were married for at least 10 years, and have been finally divorced for at least 2 continuous years.
- A dependent, unmarried child of a retired or disabled worker entitled to benefits, or of a deceased insured worker if the child is: a) under age 18; b) under age 19 and a full-time elementary or secondary school student; or c) age 18 or over, but under a disability which began before age 22.
- A disabled, surviving spouse (including a surviving divorced spouse in some cases) of a deceased insured worker, if the widow(er) is age 50-59, and becomes disabled within the specified period.

Vocational Rehabilitation Benefits

When a claimant applies for disability benefits, information about the claimant, and his or her impairment, is sent to the State Vocational Rehabilitation agency as required by law. The claimant may be contacted about services that may help regain the ability to work. If the claimant receives rehabilitation services, disability benefits will continue until the impairment improves and the beneficiary returns to work.

Definition of Disability

Disability, for the purpose of entitlement to disabled workers' benefits, is the inability to engage in any "substantial gainful activity (SGA) by reason of any medically determinable physical or mental impairment which can be expected to result in death, or which has lasted, or can be expected to last, for a continuous period of not less than 12 months." Impairment must be the primary reason for the inability to engage in substantial gainful employment, although age, education, and work experience are taken into consideration. The claimant/beneficiary must not be able to engage in any work which exists in the national economy, regardless of whether such work exists in the immediate area, whether a specific vacancy exists, or whether the person would be hired.

For the purpose of Social Security, blindness is defined as either central visual acuity of 20/200 or less in the better eye with use of a correcting lens, or a limitation in the fields of vision so that the widest diameter of the visual field subtends an angle of 20 degrees or less.

Period of Disability

The period of benefits will continue for as long as impairment has not medically improved and the beneficiary is not able to work. Cases will be reviewed periodically to make sure all requirements for disability are being met.

If a person has disability insured status, the period of disability begins on the date the disability began, however, the impairment must have lasted or be expected to last for a continuous period of not less than 12 months. Disability ceases when there has been medical improvement and the individual is deemed able to engage in substantial gainful activity, or when the individual demonstrates, by working, the ability to engage in substantial gainful employment. Disability can also be ceased when the person does not cooperate with the Social Security Administration, or fails to follow prescribed treatment. The Social Security Administration also has the right to cease disability when they cannot locate the individual. Also, if the beneficiary is disabled at 65, benefits as a disabled worker will automatically be changed to retirement benefits, generally in the same amount.

Determination of Disability

The determination of disability is done by the Social Security Administration and must be based on all the facts in an individual's case. Medical evidence is necessary for this determination and may be sufficient to establish that a person is, or is not, disabled for purposes of receiving any type of disability benefit, or for establishing a period of disability.

The medical evidence for an individual's mental or physical impairment should include a report signed by a duly licensed physician, osteopath, or licensed or certified psychologist. This medical evidence should also include a copy of, or abstract from, the medical records, if any, of a hospital, clinic, institution, sanatorium, or public or private agency. Also included as part of medical evidence are the clinical findings, laboratory findings, diagnosis, and prescribed treatment, as well as the prognosis.

A severe impairment may not automatically qualify a person to be determined disabled. If treatment could be expected to restore the person's ability to work, the person would be considered disabled if, despite the treatment, the impairment meets the severity requirement and is expected to last for 12 months. The person, however, would not be considered disabled if they refuse treatment.

In some cases, the Social Security Administration may require a consultative examination to clarify the clinical findings and diagnosis, or to obtain technical or specialized medical data not otherwise available. This consultation will also be requested to resolve a conflict or inconsistency in the medical evidence, or to resolve any issue regarding the ability of the person to engage in substantial gainful activity. When these consultations are required, it is at the government's expense.

Disability Reviews

Social security law requires that all disability cases must be reviewed to make sure that people receiving benefits are still disabled and meet all other requirements. The frequency of these reviews depends on the nature and severity of the impairment, and the likelihood of improvement. The frequency can range from six months to seven years. There are several situations that may warrant these reviews. For one, if medical improvement can be predicted when the benefits begin, the first review should take place between six and 18 months later. If medical improvement is possible, but cannot be predicted, the review will be about every three years, and if improvement is not expected, then the case will only be reviewed about once every five to seven years. Reviews also occur when there are substantial earnings posted to a beneficiary's employment record, or when a beneficiary or a rehabilitation agency reports medical improvement.

A beneficiary will receive a review notice and will be interviewed either in person or via the phone. The social security representative will explain the review process and appeal rights, and beneficiaries will be asked to provide information about medical treatment and any work activity. The beneficiary will also be asked to describe the condition that constitutes impairment preventing him or her from engaging in substantial gainful activity. This information will be submitted to the state agency that makes disability decisions on behalf of social security, and an evaluation team which includes a disability examiner and a doctor will review the file and medical reports. In most cases a decision is made based on reports, however, if reports are deemed to be incomplete or dated, the beneficiary will be asked to undergo special tests and/or an examination. The beneficiary will receive written notice of the decision of this review.

If the decision is that the beneficiary is no longer disabled, he or she has the right to file a written appeal within 60 days after receiving a notice. The case will be reconsidered and independently reviewed by people not involved with the decision to stop benefits. If the beneficiary does not file an appeal, he or she will receive a benefit for the last month of disability and two additional months.

Trial Work Period

Social security offers encouragement and help to those who want to return to work and offers provisions to ease the transition. If a person attempts to return to work, they can continue to receive benefits for up to nine months while testing their ability to work. Beginning in 1990, only months in which over $200 in gross wages were earned counted towards trial work months. The nine trial months need not be consecutive. At the end of this period a decision is made as to whether a person is able to engage in substantial gainful activity.

SUPPLEMENTAL SECURITY INCOME PROGRAM

History and Legislation

The Supplemental Security Income (SSI) program was authorized by title XVI of the Social Security Act, and is a public assistance program administered by the Social Security Administration. This program was established to provide cash assistance to individuals who have limited income and resources, and who are age 65 or older, blind, or disabled.

The SSI program was created in 1972 (to be effective in January 1974) to meet the needs of the blind, disabled, and aged persons who were not covered by the Social Security Disability Insurance (SSDI) program, or those who receive SSDI benefit payments below the level determined as the safety net. The basic purpose of SSI is to assure a minimum level of income to people who are aged, blind, or disabled.

Beginning in 1974, the SSI program replaced the prior federal/state matching grant program of assistance to the blind, aged, and disabled. Prior to SSI, states operated these programs in a similar manner to the Aid to Families with Dependent Children (AFDC) programs. The federal government contributed a share of the cost, however, state and local governments assumed responsibility for the majority of the costs, administered the programs, and determined eligibility benefit levels. These benefit levels varied widely from state to state.

When the SSI program went into effect in January 1974, those who were eligible for benefits under the prior federal/state matching grant program in December 1973 were "grandfathered." Congress established special "grandfather" provisions because they did not want anyone to be disadvantaged by any conversion to SSI.

Administration and Funding

The Supplemental Security Income program is administered by the Social Security Administration and operates in the fifty states, the District of Columbia, and the Northern Mariana Islands. The SSI benefits are financed from the general funds of the United States Treasury and are *not* paid out of the social security or Medicare trust funds.

States may supplement the basic SSI benefits, and any state may enter into an agreement to have the Social Security Administration administer its supplementation program and pay the state supplementary amount along with the basic SSI benefits.

There are two types of state supplementary payments—mandatory and optional. Mandatory payments are for individuals converted to SSI from state assistance programs. The law requires that the benefit level for a person under SSI should not be less than that received under the prior federal/ state assistance program. In these cases, states are required to supplement the benefit so that it is at the same level as under the prior program. These payments may be issued directly by the state, or the state may elect to have the Social Security Administration combine this payment in one check issued by the federal government. All but seven states provide state supplementation.

Optional supplementary payments are provided by most states, however, they vary from state to state, and reflect the cost-of-living differences in the various regions. The law gives the states the option to have the federal government administer the state supplementation, and in those states a single application covers both federal and state payments. There are 26 states that administer their own supplement.

Eligibility

The Supplemental Security Income program is based on a public assistance model in that eligibility is dependent upon demonstration of need and fulfillment of requirements for disability. The eligibility requirements and the federal income floor defining the minimum amount of payment are the same regardless of the geographical area in which the recipient resides. However, recipients must demonstrate that their resources and income are limited because payments are made only to persons whose income and resources are below specified amounts.

The Supplemental Security Income program has three categories of persons eligible for assistance. These categories are: the aged, defined as 65 or older; the blind, as defined by the program; and the disabled, as defined by the Social Security Disability Insurance program.

Since the Supplemental Security Income program is based on need, the amount of a person's income and resources is used to determine both eligibility for SSI benefits and the amount of this benefit. To be eligible, an individual cannot have monthly countable income in excess of the current federal benefit rate (FBR). The federal benefit rate is set by statute and is subject to annual increases as dictated by cost-of-living adjustments. As of January 1989, the FBR for an individual is $368, and $553 for a couple. These amounts, however, may be supplemented by states.

For SSI purposes, income is anything an individual receives during a calendar month and can use to meet his or her needs for food, clothing, or shelter. Income is divided into two categories: earned and unearned. Earned income includes wages, net earnings from self-employment, income tax credit payment, or income from a sheltered workshop. Unearned income includes social security benefits, workers' or veterans' compensation, pensions, in kind support or maintenance, annuities, rent, or interest. In kind support or maintenance includes such items as food, clothing, or shelter, or something a person can use to get food, clothing, or shelter.

Countable income is the amount remaining after eliminating all items that are not income from consideration and after applying all appropriate exclusions to the items that are income. Countable income is determined on a calendar month basis. Although some of the person's earned income is counted against the SSI income limit, benefit amounts are not reduced dollar-for-dollar as the result of income from work. This provision encourages those who can work, to do so, and the blind and disabled are referred to vocational rehabilitation agencies for services to help them enter the labor market.

In 1990, unearned income of less than $406 per month qualified a person for federal SSI benefit payments, and for a couple this amount was $599. In this same year, earned income of up to $657 per month for an individual, and $1,243 for a couple qualified persons for the federal SSI benefit payment.

Eligibility for SSI is also dependent on a person's resources (cash or other liquid assets) which can not be in excess of a specified amount. Resources, for the purpose of SSI, is cash or other liquid assets and any other real or personal property that an individual owns and could convert to cash for the purpose of support or maintenance. The limit on the resources a person is allowed to own is set by statute and has been increased over the period of the existence of SSI. In 1990, a single person could own $2,000 in resources, and a couple $3,000 and still receive an SSI check.

Further requirements for eligibility require that an individual be a resident of one of the 50 states, the District of Columbia, or the Northern Mariana Islands; be a citizen of the United States or an authorized alien; and not be a resident of a public institution throughout a month with some exceptions. A person must also not be absent from the United States for more than a calendar month, and must accept appropriate available treatment, and not refuse vocational rehabilitation services. The claimant or recipient must also file for any other benefits for which she or he is potentially eligible since SSI is a program of last resort.

Benefits

In order to receive SSI benefits, a person must file an application with the local social security office. A parent or guardian can apply for a blind or disabled child under 18 years of age. When applying, the following information will be requested:

- Social security card or record of the social security number.
- Birth certificate or other proof of age.
- Information about the home where claimant resides, such as mortgage or lease, and landlord's name.
- Payroll slips, bank books, insurance policies, car registration, burial fund records, and other information about income and resources.

- Names and addresses of doctors, hospitals, and clinics that have treated claimant, and the names and addresses of social workers or institution superintendents.

The Social Security Administration is responsible for providing individuals with a written notice of potential eligibility for other benefits, and the individual has 30 days from the date shown on the letter to file for other potential benefits.

A person's right to SSI benefits, how much he or she can get, and under what conditions, are defined in title XVI of the Social Security Act. If, however, an individual disagrees with the decision on the case, he or she can obtain an administrative review of the decision. Several independent reviews of a case are provided for a person who is dissatisfied with the determination or decision made by the Social Security Administration. Each review is a step in the administrative appeals process, and each must be requested within the prescribed limits of time. If the individual is still not satisfied with the results of the review, he or she may initiate court action.

The SSI benefit is in the form of a cash payment, in check or direct deposit, paid directly to the eligible person or to a representative payee if the person is incapable of managing benefits. Having a permanent residence is not a requirement for eligibility and, therefore, the homeless are eligible for SSI benefits. Special arrangements can be made for delivering checks to the homeless, and an organization can serve as a mail drop. The social security law also requires that payments to disabled drug addicts and alcoholics be made through a representative payee, and an organization can volunteer to be a representative payee.

In July 1990, 4,717,100 persons received federally administered SSI payments and the average payment was $289. By category of eligibility the average payment for the aged was $210, for the blind was $335, and for the disabled it was $324.

The SSI benefits are paid under conditions that are as protective as possible of people's dignity, and there are no restrictions, implied or otherwise, placed on how people spend their SSI benefits.

While the federal SSI benefit rate is the same for all categories, some individuals may fit more than one category and the difference in income/resource exclusions for the blind or disabled may result in higher benefit than that for the aged. For example, a person may be blind and disabled, or aged and blind. In the case of the individual who is 65 or older and blind or disabled, the blindness or disability must have been established at least one month prior to attaining age 65 to qualify for the higher exclusions.

A number of work incentive provisions have been incorporated in the SSI program that enable blind or disabled persons to either return to work, or increase their levels of work activity without the loss of SSI disability status. These persons also have their SSI benefits protected from reduction based on the increased earnings and, in most states, they also permit continued Medicaid coverage.

A plan for achieving self-support can help an individual establish or maintain SSI eligibility, and can also increase the individual's SSI payment amount. Establishing this plan allows a disabled or blind SSI recipient to set aside income and/or resources for a specified period of time for a work goal such as education, vocational training, or starting a business. Individuals can set aside funds to purchase work-related equipment and the income and resources that are set aside are excluded from the SSI income and resource test. Also, the plan does not affect a substantial gainful activity determination.

The plan must contain a feasible work goal, a specific savings/spending plan, and a clearly identifiable accounting for the funds which are set aside. This plan must be in writing and have a specific time frame that must be followed by the individual. Revisions can be negotiated as needed.

Individuals may receive assistance in the development of this plan from such persons as vocational counselors, social workers, or employers. The Social Security Administration is responsible for evaluating the plan, determining its acceptability, and, when necessary, helping the individual put the plan in writing.

The SSI program also offers special benefits to disabled persons who work at substantial gainful activity levels. SSI disabled and blind individuals with earned income may continue to be eligible for cash SSI benefits. This incentive allows special SSI cash payments to disabled persons in place of their regular SSI payments, when their earned income is at the amount designated at the substantial gainful activity level. To qualify for this incentive, the person must continue to have the original disabling impairment under which eligibility for SSI was initially determined, and currently meet all other eligibility rules, including the income and resource tests.

Disabled and blind recipients can also maintain eligibility for Medicaid. Maintaining Medicaid status is important because it protects Medicaid benefits when earnings are too high for cash payments, but not high enough to offset the loss of Medicaid. States have three options as to how they treat SSI recipients in relation to Medicaid eligibility. The law allows the Social Security Administration to enter into agreements with states to automatically cover all SSI recipients with Medicaid eligibility. Under this arrangement, the SSI recipient is not required to make a separate application for Medicaid. There are 30 states that have chosen this option, and the SSI recipients in these states account for approximately 75% of all SSI recipients nationwide.

Under the second option, states elect to automatically provide Medicaid eligibility for all SSI recipients, but only if the recipient completes a separate application with the state agency which administers the Medicaid program. Six states have chosen this option, they are Alaska, Idaho, Kansas, Mississippi, Nevada, and Oregon, and this arrangement affects about 2.5% of SSI recipients nationwide.

The third, and more restrictive, option permits states to impose Medicaid eligibility criteria which are more restrictive than SSI criteria, so long as the criteria chosen were part of the state's approved Medicaid State plan in January, 1972.

Except in Wisconsin and California, SSI beneficiaries may qualify for food stamps if they meet the food stamp income and assets requirements. In the two states (California and Wisconsin), the food stamp program is "cashed out," meaning that these states have chosen to increase state SSI supplemental payments in lieu of food stamps.

Summary

The Social Security Disability Insurance program and the Supplemental Security Income program were enacted by the Social Security Act and administered by the Social Security Administration. The primary difference between the two programs is that the SSDI program is a social insurance program funded through payroll taxes and placed in a Disability Trust Fund for the purpose of paying benefits. As an insurance program, eligibility is determined on the basis of insured status and meeting requirements of disability, not on financial need.

The Supplemental Security Income program is a public assistance program, and eligibility is based on established need. This program is funded through the General Tax Fund, and recipients must meet certain income and resource requirements to become eligible for this program.

Both programs offer cash benefits, as well as in kind benefits or protections. For SSDI, the cash benefit is based on the contributions made through payroll taxes, and the cash benefit for SSI is determined by the amount of income and resources of a claimant or beneficiary.

The Social Security Administration is required by law to provide information on how to apply for programs and to inform claimants and beneficiaries about their rights and responsibilities. This information is provided to individuals, as well as organizations and institutions acting on behalf of individuals. For specific information regarding the services, the Social Security Administration can be contacted at 1-800-234-5772.

Sources

Social Security Administration. (1988). *A summary guide to Social Security and Supplemental Security Income work incentives for the disabled and blind.* Washington, DC: Government Printing Office.

U. S. Department of Health and Human Services. (1988). *Social Security handbook–1988* (10th ed.). Washington, DC: Government Printing Office.

U. S. Department of Health and Human Services. (1990). *A guide to SSI for groups and organizations.* Washington, DC: Government Printing Office.

U. S. Department of Health and Human Services. (1990). *Your Social Security rights and responsibilities: Disability benefits.* Washington, DC: Government Printing Office.

U. S. House of Representatives, Committee on Ways and Means. (1989). *Background material and data on programs within the jurisdiction of the Committee on Ways and Means.* Washington, DC: Government Printing Office.

Medicaid

Garry A. Toerber, Ph.D.

History/Legislation

Government involvement in health care in the United States has had a long and involved history. It, nonetheless, has largely been piecemeal. Generally, the role of government has been to step in where the private purchase of health care has failed. For example, one of the first government sponsored programs involving major providers of health care services (e.g., hospitals, physicians) was the state sponsored workman's compensation program.

The federal government first became directly involved in the provision of health services for the general civilian population in 1921, when the Sheppard-Towner Act was passed providing federal grants-in-aid to states for maternal and child health services. Although the Sheppard-Towner Act was discontinued in 1929, due to lack of appropriations, it was reactivated by title V of the Social Security Act, passed in 1935, providing the same set of benefits that the Sheppard-Towner legislation had provided during the 1921-1929 period.

Additional piecemeal federal programs were soon passed providing services to selected, presumably needy, groups. The Federal Emergency Relief Administration provided assistance through grants-in-aid for medical care to those receiving unemployment relief. The Farm Security Administration developed a medical program for low-income farmers. Although these programs proved to be generally abortive efforts, they did lay the ground work for government involvement in the provision of health care services to medically needy populations.

However, it was not until the 1960s that the federal government passed legislation, sufficiently broad in scope, that general population categories received support for their health care needs. First in 1960, President Dwight Eisenhower signed the Kerr-Mills Bill (Medical Assistance Act). With its passage, the federal government first recognized the concept of medical indigency, and did so quite logically, through expansion of the public assistance section of the Social Security Act. The Medical Assistance Act permitted federal grants to states to stimulate state expansion of their medical care programs for those low-income aged who did not qualify for the categorical old-age assistance program.

In 1965, the Medical Assistance Act was replaced by the Social Security Amendments which introduced the Medicare and Medicaid Act. While the Medicare program generally provides medical assistance for individuals who qualify for Social Security benefits, the Medicaid program replaced the Kerr-Mills program and provides benefits to welfare beneficiaries and certain other low-income individuals.

The Medicaid program is a federal-state, means-tested entitlement program. It is jointly funded by federal and state contributions. Within federal statute and regulation, states have certain latitude to implement state specific elements into somewhat unique individual state programs. Thus, state Medicaid programs are quite different in design, individuals eligible, and services provided. In fact, each state operates a unique program. No two states provide the same set of benefits, or offer services to the same type of eligibles. However, all states, the District of Columbia, as well as the territories of American Samoa, Guam, North Mariana Islands, Puerto Rico, and the Virgin Islands have developed a Medicaid program.

Funding for the state Medicaid programs comes from general revenue of the federal government and from revenue of the participating states, the District of Columbia, and the territories. The level of federal contributions to individual state programs varies according to a formula from 50% federal dollars to 83% at the federal maximum level, although, currently, no individual state receives the maximum 83% level. The formula is determined by the per capita income in each individual state compared to the per capita income of the United States as a whole. The lower the state's per capita income, the higher the federal matching rate. The higher the state's per capita income, the lower the federal matching rate. A state whose per capita income matches the federal per capita income would receive a 55% federal matching rate.

Expenditures under the Medicaid program have grown rapidly from $1.5 billion in 1966, to approximately $51.5 billion in federal fiscal year 1991. From a different perspective, individual expenditures have grown from about 3.3% of total national health expenditures, to about 10% today. Of the $51.5 billion in total expenditures, the federal share equals approximately 55%, with the state share the remaining 45%.

The number of Medicaid beneficiaries totals approximately 25 million, with a beneficiary defined to be an individual who received any Medicaid-covered service during the fiscal year. Eligibility for Medicaid is dependent upon categorical inclusion and limited income and resources, with each state having the authority to determine its income and resource limits, subject to federal rule and regulation.

Purpose/Structure

When the Medicare and Medicaid programs began in 1966, Medicare was generally considered to be the more significant of the two programs. While expenditures under the Medicare program remain the larger of the two programs, Medicaid has grown rapidly as well, and today could arguably be considered as having equal or greater impact upon the health of medically needy persons.

The intent of the Medicaid program is to provide medically necessary services to low-income persons. Nonetheless, by federal statute and regulation, Medicaid is categorically based. Since the enactment of the Medicaid program in 1965, eligibility has been largely linked to cash assistance under the federal welfare program. Eligibles have had to meet the welfare definitions of age, blind, disability, or membership in a family where one parent is absent, incapacitated, or in some cases unemployed. Since the Medicaid program is categorically based, many persons cannot qualify for Medicaid regardless of their financial condition. Single persons and childless couples who are not blind, disabled, or aged typically are not eligible for Medicaid. In addition, intact families (two-parent families) typically do not qualify unless the principal breadwinner is unemployed.

The definition of low income varies by state. Income and resource limits can vary dramatically across the states. For example, income eligibility for families with dependent children (AFDC) can vary by hundreds of dollars a month for a typical family with three members. Income eligibility for Medicaid services for aged, blind, or disabled persons can also vary across state lines, but such variability has typically been far less than for AFDC families.

In addition to income limits on eligibility, persons eligible for Medicaid must have limited resources. Resource limits vary across states and across eligibility categories, but in general AFDC families are limited to $1,000 in equity. Aged, blind, or disabled persons are limited to $2,000 per individual, and $3,000 per family. However, a person's home and a car for transportation are typically excluded, as are personal clothing and furniture.

In addition to the population described above, all states have made many persons in nursing homes eligible. Federal law and regulation allow persons in nursing homes to be eligible if their income is no more than 300% of the federal Supplemental Security Income (SSI) level. The reason for making the so-called 300 percenters eligible relates to the emphasis in Medicaid upon long-term care services and the cost of such services. As such, the intent of this optional coverage was to allow persons in nursing homes where income was below the cost, or more directly the price, of nursing home care to be eligible for nursing home services through Medicaid. Conversely, persons in nursing homes whose income was in excess of 300% of the SSI benefit level were supposed to be able to purchase nursing home services out of their own income. However, nursing home costs have been rising at a faster rate than the SSI benefit level so that, currently, persons can have income above the 300% standard, but below the cost of nursing home services.

These persons fall into the so called "Utah gap." They can neither qualify for nursing home services as a Medicaid recipient, nor afford the cost of nursing home care.

States also have the option to provide Medicaid coverage to persons in foster care, persons who receive an additional state supplemental cash payment, and who meet federal definitions of categorical eligibility, as well as some other minor eligibility groups.

Another major eligibility category that represents an optional group for Medicaid coverage is the medically needy. These are persons who, except for income and resources, fall into one of the categories described above. These persons, by federal law and regulation, cannot have income above 133-1/3% of the state's AFDC program standard, except if they have medical expenses that force them to spend down to the medically needy standard (spend all excess resources above the 133-1/3% standard for medical services). These persons are seen as medically needy, and thus the basis for the income category.

Nonetheless, to date, due to conditions of categorical eligibility along with income and resource limits, less than half of persons across the country who live at or below the federal poverty level can qualify for Medicaid. Obviously Medicaid was not designed, nor has it yet evolved to a position of providing necessary medical services for the indigent of the country.

While historically the Medicaid program has been tied closely to the receipt of welfare cash assistance, recent federal mandates have begun to delink Medicaid and welfare programs. Beginning with the Omnibus Budget Reconciliation Act (OBRA) of 1986, certain new target groups have been identified for the Medicaid program to cover. Foremost among these groups have been pregnant women and young children in AFDC-like or intact families. New federal law and regulations have mandated that pregnant women and infants to age one must be covered in families up to 133% of the federal poverty level. Additionally, states have the option to cover pregnant women and infants, to age one, up to 185% of the poverty level.

With more recent OBRA legislation, states are now being required to cover all children born after September 30, 1983, who are in families at or below the federal poverty level, to be covered up to their eighteenth birthday on a phased-in basis. That is, as these children age, federal law and regulation mandate that these children remain eligible until they reach age 18.

A second major target group are aged, blind, and disabled persons who qualify for the Medicare program. By 1995, states will be required to purchase the Medicare premiums for aged, blind, or disabled persons whose income falls below 120% of the federal poverty level. In addition, the coinsurance and deductibles will be paid for by the Medicaid program.

While these new federal mandates provide significantly broader coverage for the Medicaid program, the mandates also signify a growing interest in the country in using the Medicaid program to selectively provide medical coverage for particularly deserving groups. These recent mandates may well be followed by new federal mandates expanding Medicaid coverage to additional deserving groups.

The addition of these eligible groups to the Medicaid roles has not occurred without significant controversy, as state coffers have been severely strained to accommodate the additional medical expenses of these persons. Significant debate has recently raged between Congress and state legislatures over the expanded mandates that states have had to accommodate within their budgets. Nonetheless, at this time, Congress appears set on a course of continuing to mandate coverage to new deserving groups to provide medical care for additional populations, much to the consternation of states which struggle to provide essential state services.

ADMINISTRATION

Administration of the Medicaid program occurs at the state level. Each state must select a single state agency to administer the Medicaid program. In most states, the social services agency or a combined health and social services agency is selected to be the single agency to administer the Medicaid program.

At the federal level, the Health Care Financing Administration (HCFA) of the Department of Health and Human Services administers the Medicaid program. The federal HCFA office writes rules and regulations allowed or required by federal statute, to which state operation of the Medicaid program must adhere. The federal HCFA office consists of a central office in Baltimore, Maryland and 10 regional HCFA offices situated throughout the country.

The agreement between each state and the HCFA office is spelled out in the Medicaid State Plan. This state plan describes the state's basic list of eligibles, the services provided, the reimbursement protocols, and administrative policies of the state. Whenever a change in state policy occurs, or new federal regulations are promulgated, a new state plan must be submitted by the state. Failure to submit a timely state plan change can result in the loss of federal matching funds by the state.

In the state administration of the Medicaid program, each state must establish a Medicaid Advisory Committee (MAC), made up of providers and recipient representatives, to review and make recommendations on policy and state plan amendments. The MAC is intended to assure that the interests of the Medicaid recipients and Medicaid providers are considered in the state administration of the program.

Notwithstanding the single state agency requirement, the Medicaid agency, if not a social services (welfare) agency, must have an agreement with the state welfare agency for eligibility determination. Likewise, if the Medicaid agency is not the State Health Department, it must have been an agreement with the health department to advise on provider certification and quality of care standards.

Client Services

The Medicaid program provides a wide variety of medical and health care services. The service package is divided into federally mandated services and state optional services. Federally mandated services must be provided by the state and territories if federal matching funds are to be available to the state. State optional services may be chosen by a state, and if so chosen, federal matching funds will be available.

FEDERALLY MANDATED SERVICES

The list of federally mandated services includes both institutional services and ambulatory services. The institutional services required are inpatient hospital services, outpatient hospital services, and nursing facility services for persons 21 years of age and older. While hospital services are traditionally provided through insurance arrangements or through government programs like the Medicare program, nursing facility service coverage is quite unique and makes the Medicaid program a major funder of the long-term care institutional services. In most states, 50% or more of total dollars earned by nursing homes come from the state Medicaid program.

The ambulatory care services available include physician services, rural health clinic services, nurse practitioners' services including nurse midwife services, family planning services, and early and periodic screening, diagnosis, and treatment services for persons under 21 years of age (EPSDT).

Physician services represent the key to the provision of services in the Medicaid program. All services authorized for payment must be provided by a physician, or ordered and authorized by a physician. Rural clinic services are mandated due to the frequent access problems encountered by recipients in medically underserved areas of the individual states where rural health clinics are located.

Recently, the services of nurse practitioners, including nurse midwives, have been added to the list of mandated service providers. Again, the rationale has been to increase access of Medicaid recipients to necessary care.

Family planning is the only Medicaid service that is viewed by the federal government so positively that the federal matching rate equals 90% of total family planning service expenditures.

EPSDT represents a unique benefit for persons under 21 years of age. The EPSDT program requires that states set up a periodic screening program for children. Medical problems uncovered through the screening process must be diagnosed and treated regardless of whether the medical or dental procedure required is otherwise a benefit of the Medicaid program. The periodicity schedule set up for screening is age sensitive so that young infants would be expected to be screened more frequently than adolescents. States are free to choose the periodicity schedule considered appropriate, so long as it meets federal requirements and is clinically based.

STATE OPTIONAL SERVICES

In addition to the list of mandated services, states can choose from a menu of 31 optional services that they may wish to provide with federal matching funds assured. The list of optimal services is headed by prescribed drugs. All states and territories, with the exception of Puerto Rico and the Virgin Islands, have chosen to include prescribed drugs within their basic benefit package.

Other services that almost all states elect are the services of optometrists, services for speech, language, and hearing disorders, prosthetic devices, eyeglasses, intermediate care facility services for the mentally retarded (ICF-MR), nursing facility services for persons under 21, and transportion services. Other optional services which states can choose range from the services of dentists, podiatrists, and chiropractors, to physical therapy, occupational therapy, and hospice services.

The range of optional services selected varies, from some states which cover almost all optional services, to other states and territories which cover very few optional services. Interestingly, no two states or territories have the exact same list of optional services. Furthermore, states are free to place restrictions on the optional services so that an optional service such as prosthetic devices may be limited to those devices that are surgically implanted.

CASE MANAGEMENT REQUIREMENTS

With a broad range of Medicaid-funded services available, states have typically found abuse and misuse of services common. As such, numerous states have turned to managing the provision of services. Management strategies generally include pre-admission and/or concurrent review for hospital and nursing home services. Prior authorization of services (prior to the services being provided) for such ambulatory services as drugs, physician services, dental procedures, home health, and nonemergency transportation services are common utilization control strategies.

To control consumer demand, client co-pays have been adopted by some states. However, client co-pays have been of minimal impact since the providers of Medicaid services cannot elect to deny services because a recipient does not pay the co-pay. Federal law and regulation require that the services be provided regardless of the actual payment of the co-pay (requirement intended to assure the provision of services regardless of whether the client has the ability to pay). The result has been that the imposition of co-pays has more often than not merely been a reduction in reimbursement to Medicaid providers.

The difficulties in the control of misuse and abuse of services have led numerous states to develop more direct case management protocols. Arizona has developed a unique Medicaid program that requires all services be provided under prepaid capitation arrangements. Organizations have been set up in all geographic parts of Arizona to enroll Medicaid recipients and provide services under risk contracts with the state of Arizona (risk contracts refer to a contractual arrangement whereby the contracted agency receives a pre-determined level of reimbursement and must, by contract, provide all the medical services required by the Medicaid recipients).

A number of other states have also signed pre-paid capitation contracts with Health Maintenance Organizations (HMOs) in their respective states. The popularity of these HMO contracts can be traced largely to the predictability of state expenditures under a contract with an HMO, and to the greater control which the HMO can assert on utilization of services for recipients. HMOs typically utilize case management techniques for these clients in order to reduce the risk that HMOs assume under the contract with the state.

Due to the limited number of HMOs around the country, penetration ratios (percentage of Medicaid recipients enrolled in HMOs) have typically been less than 10%. In response, several states have sought special federal approval to develop alternative physician case management arrangements. Primary care physician case management arrangements have been set up in a number of states. These primary care case management arrangements have been approved by the federal government under the terms of the Omnibus Budget Reconciliation Act of 1981 which allows a waiver of recipient federal freedom of choice of provider requirements. Under this federal waiver program, states can require that a primary care physician provide, or refer to other providers including other physicians, a specific set of services, if payment under the Medicaid program is to be received. As such, the primary care physician controls the services that the recipients receive, and thus controls abuse or misuse of services. The types of services that a primary care physician case management program has found to be effective in controlling are misuse of hospital emergency room, doctor shopping, as well as drug misuse. Case management has been effective in controlling the cost of care, as well as improving the quality of care.

Another area of case management has been in the long-term care arena. Again, the Omnibus Budget Reconciliation Act of 1981 allowed home- and community-based waivers to be granted. Under these waivers, states have been able to provide a coordinated set of noninstitutional services to be provided to a specific group of individuals. Typically, states have elected to provide case management and personal care to recipients in their own homes, who would otherwise require nursing home admissions. Significantly, the cost of the set of noninstitutional services cannot be more expensive than would have been the cost of institutionalizing the client. As such, the client is provided community- and home-based services (frequently strongly preferred by the client), at less cost than would have been incurred if admission to the nursing home would have occurred.

REIMBURSEMENT FOR SERVICES

Perhaps the most significant and controversial part of the Medicaid program is the flexibility allowed to states in provider reimbursement strategies.

Reimbursement strategies are critical to states, in that states frequently attempt to limit their financial obligations through restrictive reimbursement strategies.

However, levels of reimbursement can, and do, have a significant impact upon the availability of participating medical service providers within the program. Physician participation, owing at least in part to the level of physician reimbursement, has been a significant issue, if not a very critical problem. With states frequently limiting the level of reimbursement to physicians, the federal government has recently instituted requirements for higher reimbursement for primary care physicians, particularly for pediatric care and obstetrical care. While such requirements will strain state budgets, the impact upon the participation of physicians and, thus, the availability of physician services, could be significant.

Nonetheless, the approach to reimbursement will remain a significant part of state Medicaid program strategies. Reimbursement strategies will remain a state-selected technique for controlling state Medicaid program expenditures. As such, state Medicaid program reimbursement strategies will join the eligible population and the benefits available in defining a state's Medicaid program.

TYPICAL REFERRAL QUESTIONS

Typical referral questions depend upon the agency or individual asking the questions. However, from a potential client perspective, the following questions frequently occur:

What is the difference between the Medicare program and the Medicaid program?

The Medicare program serves clients who generally qualify for social security. Persons who have contributed to social security are generally eligible for Medicare benefits. The set of benefits under the Medicare program are generally inpatient and outpatient hospital services and physician services. The Medicare program is administered by the Federal Health Care Financing Administration. In contrast, the Medicaid program is a means tested entitlement program. Welfare recipients, other low-income, pregnant women and young children, as well as other selected low-income persons can qualify for a wide set of acute care and long-term care services. The Medicaid program is administered by an agency of state government.

How do I become eligible to receive Medicaid services?

Eligibility for the Medicaid program is available through two techniques, depending upon the application procedures selected by the individual states. In some states, application for Supplemental Security Income benefits (SSI) carries with it eligibility for Medicaid. In other states, a separate application must be filed with the appropriate state or county social service agency.

Application for Aid to Families with Dependent Children will generally be filed with state or county social service agencies. Finally, many states are now allowing applications to be taken by some medical care providers (e.g., hospitals) that serve a high number of low-income recipients.

From the medical care provider perspective, the most frequently asked question is generally:

How can I participate in the Medicaid program, and how do I get paid?

Participation in the Medicaid program is almost always based upon filing an application with the single state Medicaid program, or in some states with the organization that processes Medicaid claims. Appropriate licensure and/or Medicaid certification is necessary for a provider to participate in the Medicaid program. Once an application is filed and approved, bills must be submitted on claim forms approved by the state Medicaid agency. Claims are generally submitted to the state fiscal agent, which is either the single state Medicaid agency or an agency that contracts with the state agency to process Medicaid claims.

Sources

Holahan, J. F., & Cohen, J. W. (1986). *Medicaid: The trade-off between cost containment and access to care*. Washington, DC: The Urban Institute Press.

Spiegel, A. D., & Podair, S. (Eds.). (1975). *Medicaid: Lessons for national health insurance*. Rockville, MD: Aspen Systems.

Toerber, G. A. (1972). *An evaluative analysis of medical care financing systems with particular emphasis on a national health insurance*. Health Care Research Services No. 20. Iowa City, IA: University of Iowa Graduate Program in Hospital and Health Administration.

U. S. Congress, Subcommittee on Health and the Environment, Committee on Energy and Commerce. (1988). *Medicaid source book: Background data and analysis*. Washington, DC: U. S. Government Printing Office.

Children and Family Services

Karen M. Sowers-Hoag, Ph.D.

Bruce Thyer, Ph.D.

History/Legislation

Prior to the 1900s, children were considered little more than chattel of their families and were often referred to as "it" rather than by name or gender. Although reported criminal cases in the United States involving child abuse have been recorded as early as 1655, it was not until about 1825 that a general recognition of the right and duty of the public authorities to take action in cases of parental cruelty and gross neglect arose (Watkins, 1990). Removal of a child from the home often meant placement in almshouses and indentured servitude. In the early 1900s, children accounted for about one-third of the annual mortality rate and about one-fifth of the children who died were babies less than one year old. Children from poor families and children who had no families were cared for in almshouses and were required to work to repay the community for their expense. In fact, all children were to expected to work, whether they lived at home or in an almshouse. Children in almshouses suffered from inadequate diet, and lack of sanitation, education, and normal family life. It was not until the late 1700s to mid-1800s that public charitable orphanages became established throughout the country. Despite the creation of orphanages as a result of the public outcry against the conditions of the almshouses, abuse and neglect of children in many institutionalized settings continued to occur (Rothman, 1971). It was, perhaps, because orphan asylums used indentures as one of the principal forms of placing children, that adoption did not become prominent until the early 1900s.

In 1853, Charles Loring Brace established the Children's Aid Society of New York for the purpose of effecting foster home placements for children. Advocates for foster care rather than institutionalization, argued that for most children maintenance in a normal home was better than institutionalization, and the apparent success of the Children's Aid Society led to the organization of other child-saving agencies employing similar foster home placement methods (Axinn & Levin, 1982). Today, institutions are seen as appropriate for groups of children whose needs are best met in a group setting, or who cannot be served by other means, such as children who are emotionally disturbed, mentally deficient, or severely physically disabled.

The past 75 years have seen a change in the nature of children receiving foster care. Initially, the parents of children receiving foster care were either poor or deceased. Today, the composition of children in foster family care has changed from destitute children to those whose parents are unable to care for them due to social and emotional problems, rather than simply economic disruption of the family. As more women who once offered foster homes enter the primary labor market, and as the needs of children placed in foster homes have shifted from economic to psychological, the problem of finding adequate foster homes has increased. To adapt to these changes, social workers have developed group foster homes, and small family settings staffed by house parents, and have trained women receiving Aid to Families with Dependent Children for their own children to be foster parents for other children. The current federal mandate emphasizing permanency planning for the child has placed responsibility on child and family service agencies to work with the biological family, whenever possible, to ensure return of the child as soon as possible, or when it is not possible to return the child to the home, to provide for an adoptive family for the child. Thus, permanency planning seeks to shorten the amount of time children remain in substitute care and increase the probability that children will secure a permanent home and family.

In the past, adoption services in this country primarily focused on serving white, middle-class couples wishing to adopt infants. With the current availability of legalized abortion and the reduced stigma of out-of-wedlock pregnancy and single parenthood, fewer infants are available for adoption. Today, adoption agencies are finding a growing need to recruit adoptive homes for older children, sibling groups, racial and ethnic minority children, and children with special needs such as children with emotional, mental, and physical disabilities.

LEGISLATION/AUTHORITY

At the urging of the first White House Conference on Children, convened in 1909, the federal government established the Children's Bureau. Legislation creating the Children's Bureau charged it with investigating and reporting upon all matters pertaining to the welfare of children and child life among all classes of people and to investigate the questions of infant mortality, the birth rate, orphanages, juvenile courts, desertion, dangerous occupations, accidents and diseases of children, employment, and legislation affecting children in all the states. The delegates at this conference went on record as supporting the principle of maintaining children in their own families whenever possible and not depriving them of home life, except for urgent and compelling reasons. The Children's

Bureau took as its highest priorities the registration of all births in the United States in an attempt to begin investigating infant-maternal mortality, distribution of child and maternal health care publications, and the promotion of subsidized maternal and infant health care. The 1909 White House Conference on Children also focused on placement of children and declared carefully selected foster homes for normal children the preferred placement to institutionalization (Kadushin, 1974). Gradually, foster family care placements became the responsibility of social welfare agencies, public and private, rather than being left to private charity, and subsidized foster care became the norm. In 1961, title IV-A of the Social Security Act authorized the Aid to Families with Dependent Children (AFDC) program to provide federal funds for the care of children in out-of-home placement. In June 1980, legislation was passed which replaced title IV-A with title IV-E and title IV-B providing for maintenance of children in foster care placement, foster care for AFDC-eligible children and for adoption subsidies for special needs children.

Despite the fact that laws providing for the protection of children appeared to exist since 1655, it was not until 1825 that state statutes were adopted that established a public duty to intervene in cases of cruelty or neglect of children. With the passage of the Social Security Act in 1935, child protection became a mandate of public social service agencies. However, it was not until the late 1960s that legislation had been enacted in every state mandating the reporting of suspected maltreatment. In 1974, the Child Abuse Prevention and Treatment Act was signed into law, establishing the National Center on Child Abuse and Neglect to coordinate the federal response to child maltreatment. The reporting statutes of the Child Abuse Prevention and Treatment Act require mandatory reporting of suspected child maltreatment, and places responsibility for protecting children to a wide range of professionals including medical, psychiatric, social work, education, counseling, and law enforcement professionals.

Legal adoption in the United States did not exist until the mid-nineteenth century. The first adoption law in the United States was passed in 1850 in Texas and provided for adoption by deed, signifying a transfer of property. In 1852, Massachusetts passed an adoption statute which became a model for the other states. The law provided for court procedures and guidelines and clearly established, for the first time, that the child's welfare should be a primary consideration in adoption. In addition, the law stressed the obligation of the court in protecting the biological parents from coerced relinquishment, and the prospective adoptive parents from making a hasty or uninformed decision (Cole, 1987). By 1929, all states had passed adoption laws. In 1980, the Adoption Assistance and Child Welfare Act Law was enacted which created a conditional ceiling on federal funding for foster care maintenance payments, authorized funding for adoption subsidies for children with special needs, and provided fiscal incentives and penalties related to the development of preventive and reunification services. This act requires states to establish case review mechanisms to insure that reasonable efforts are made to prevent placement, to arrange placement in the most appropriate setting, and to discharge children to permanent homes in a timely manner. Although twentieth century adoption practices evolved to serve white infants born to unmarried parents (Benet, 1976), the civil rights movement and the marked decline in availability of infants, due to the use of birth control and abortion, served to place a growing emphasis on older, minority, and handicapped children who needed to be placed for adoption.

FUNDING

Federal payments to states for adoption assistance and foster care are made available through title IV-E funds for foster care for AFDC-eligible children and for adoption subsidies for AFDC- and SSI-eligible children who have special needs. Children who receive federally reimbursed subsidies are also eligible for Medicaid. States are required to make reasonable efforts to prevent placement and to provide reunification services as a condition for title IV-E funding. Federal funding is also available to states through title IV-B which has been used mainly to pay for the cost of maintaining children in foster care.

Funding for, and the provision of, services to children and families differs from state to state. Only three services (intra-familial/quasi-familial child protective services, foster family care services, and adoption) are provided universally on a state-wide basis by public child welfare agencies. Most states commit a portion of its general revenue to services for children and families. Some cities and counties may also provide services from the local tax base. States tend to use either grant-in-aid as a purchase of care mechanism or general revenue funds for provision of services. Organizations which receive state tax dollars to provide services to children and families are generally private or voluntary not-for-profit agencies, and city, county, or state government agencies.

PERSONNEL

Child and family welfare professionals come from a variety of disciplines and backgrounds. In general, the staff can be classified as counseling staff from backgrounds in social work, psychology, rehabilitation, education, or sociology. Direct service workers in child and family services, at the baccalaureate level, usually provide investigative, assessment, community referral, and support functions. At the master's level, child and family service workers tend to provide staff supervision and training, and provide direct services in the form of individual, group, or family treatment to children and their families. A national study of some 900 child welfare workers conducted in 1981 found that 41% of the workers covered an integrated child welfare caseload and 47% covered a specialized caseload. Among those whose primary caseload assignment is specialized, the most frequently indicated fields were protective services (22%), foster care (10%), shelter care (6%), and adoption (5%) (Vinokur, 1983).

There has been a decrease over the past 10 years in employment opportunities for child welfare workers in general, and an increase in the percentage of workers without previous training in child welfare. Civil service positions have, in many cases, been reclassified to delete the requirements of educational credentials for access to entry-level positions (Kadushin, 1987). A 1989 national survey of state-level human service agencies found that almost 90% of the states report difficulty in recruiting staff for child welfare positions, and that shortages are most acute among direct service workers in child protective services. More than half of the states were found to be dissatisfied with the administrative structures for screening and hiring child welfare staff. Approximately 25% of the states reported that educational requirements for some positions in direct service required less than a college degree and only 9.3% of the states reported educational requirements for supervisors at the master's level. States reporting authorized, but unfilled, child welfare positions cited a lack of qualified candidates, hiring freezes, budgetary constraints, staff turnover, unappropriated funds, and recruitment and retention difficulties due to low salaries and high caseloads as primary factors (American Public Welfare Association, 1990).

Purpose/Intent

GOALS OF SERVICE PROVISION

Child and Family Services is accorded sanctioned responsibility by the community to focus on children and families needing services in response to a particular set of social problems and situations. In general, the child and family social service system provides preventive and rehabilitative services in the event that parents are unable to provide appropriate care for their children due to unemployment, death, imprisonment, or problems due to emotional/psychological instability, substance abuse, and physical disability.

Recently, the child and family services field has reallocated its priorities with the provision of supportive and supplementary services designed to promote maintenance of the family as its highest priority. Keeping the child in the home whenever possible and supporting the permanence and continuity of a caring relationship has become the primary focus of services. Likewise, providing permanence through adoption when families cannot be reconstituted has also become a high priority. Foster family care has diminished in priority and, with continued emphasis on deinstitutionalization and normalization, institutions now have the lowest priority among substitute care services (Kadushin, 1987).

SPECIAL CASE MANAGEMENT NEEDS

Case management services are important in all child welfare cases because most families receiving child welfare services have diverse problems whose resolution requires assistance from multiple providers. Responsibility for assisting families with problems may be shared by attorneys, psychiatrists, mental health practitioners, school guidance counselors, social workers, and child welfare workers. Some services providers may move in and out of a client's life as need dictates. To ensure that clients receive needed services in an efficient and timely manner, one person (generally a case manager in a child welfare service agency) may assume responsibility for the evaluation of the family and the coordination and monitoring of all services. This coordination ensures that all providers are working toward mutually accepted goals, and that services are provided in a timely manner. The case manager must be an expert in the wide array of community services available, service eligibility requirements, and must be able to link clients with needed services. In addition, the case manager must often act as an advocate for the client systems in seeing that sufficient and effective services are provided (Stein, 1987).

Client Services

CHILD PROTECTIVE SERVICES

Reports of child abuse and neglect are usually reported to child protection divisions of public social service agencies for investigations. Child abuse and neglect generally include physical abuse, sexual abuse, emotional abuse, or inadequate provisions for housing, clothing, food, adult supervision, medical attention, or school attendance. Reports are made by a wide variety of concerned individuals including extended family members and neighbors and by working professionals such as physicians, law enforcement officers, teachers, and school social workers. Reports of suspected child abuse, neglect, or both, are investigated and if substantiated, plans to effectively intervene are developed and implemented. Intervention plans may include removal of the child from the home in cases in which the worker finds that the well-being of the child is at risk (e.g., severe physical abuse, sexual abuse, neglect). Under these circumstances, the worker develops plans with the parent(s) or guardian to aid them in successfully alleviating the original problems leading to removal of their child with the primary goal of returning the child to the home. Whether the child remains in the home or is removed, intervention plans for families may include therapeutic services (e.g., family therapy, psychotherapy, parenting training) and concrete services (e.g., housing, job placement, financial assistance). The protective service worker is responsible for the development of the treatment plan and the coordination of services. The provision of direct services by the protective services unit differs throughout the country. However, most typically, the protective service worker provides some direct services—such as intake, investigation, or counseling—and coordinates additional services through the use of referrals to community service agencies such as mental health centers and public assistance housing programs.

FOSTER CARE

Foster care refers to full-time, substitute care of children outside their own homes. All states operate foster care programs. Substitute care may be provided directly by the state's public welfare agency, purchased by the state from a voluntary agency, or both. Foster caretakers may be related or unrelated adults other than a child's biological parents. Foster care of children occurs in family homes, groups homes, and institutions. In recent years, significant changes have been made in the foster care system. Federal policy now reflects the importance of maintaining children in their own homes, whenever possible, and supporting efforts toward permanency planning for children in substitute care.

Children may be placed in foster care voluntarily, through a contract between a parent and child care agency, or involuntarily, by court order. Most children are in foster care under court order. Precipitating factors usually associated with involuntary placement include child abuse or neglect, while factors associated with voluntary placement include family conflicts, substance abuse of a parent, parental absence, parental illness or disability, or financial hardship.

The overarching goal of foster care programs is the reunification of the family and, as such, the bulk of services are directed toward the child and biological family to help them resolve the difficulties that necessitated placement. Services provided generally include parent education, respite services to provide time-out from ongoing child care responsibilities to reduce stress, supportive self-help groups, counseling, and case management services to coordinate the use of referral agency providers such as legal services, medical services, housing, job placement services, and mental health services.

ADOPTION

Adoption is one of the oldest of child welfare services and will probably always be necessary. Adoption involves becoming a parent through a legal and social process, rather than through a biological process. For the child, adoption involves a permanent change in family affiliation. Adoption social services are the necessary array of professional assistance services offered and coordinated by an agency to place a child in an adoptive family, and to preserve and strengthen the adoptive family (Cole, 1987). The key assumptions undergirding the provision of adoptive social services include:
- All children, regardless of age, sex, race, and physical, intellectual, or emotional status, are entitled to a continuous, caring environment;
- For most children, the biological family, in its broadest definition, provides the best environment;
- When a child's family of birth is not able or willing to nurture him or her, the child is entitled to a timely placement with a stable, caring family;
- For most children, adoption provides a new family, better than any other form of substitute parenting; and
- Adoption is a means of finding families for children and not of finding children for families.

The emphasis is on the child's needs (Child Welfare League of America, 1978).

Social agencies providing adoption services are directly concerned with finding an appropriate adoptive home, evaluating the home and prospective parents, and supervising and monitoring the adoptive placement for a period of time after the child is placed. Adoption workers typically interview persons and families interested in adopting a child and assess the prospective parent(s) with respect to their motivation for adoption, their understanding of children, experiences with children, the history of interpersonal interactions, employment and education history, patterns of social participation, attitudes of extended family members toward adoption, and attitudes toward working with the adoption agency. Interviews may be followed by a series of home visits to assess the home, neighborhood, and physical resources. After applicants have been approved for adoption, adoption workers attempt to match the child and prospective parent(s) in terms of ethnic background, physical appearance, temperament, and intelligence potential. When a potential match is developed, the prospective parent(s) is called in and given background information on the child and, if agreeable, the worker schedules time for the child and prospective parent(s) to meet.

Adoption workers also prepare extensive histories of the child, including medical and personal information when available. With older children, workers help in preparing them for the adoption and may arrange a gradual placement, including overnight and weekend visits.

After the placement is made, there is usually a trial period of six months to a year when the child remains under the legal guardianship of the agency. At the end of the trial period, if it is agreeable to the adoptive parents, the agency, and the child (if the child is old enough), the final adoption takes place through appropriate court action.

Summary

Despite the past initiatives designed to promote family stability and permanency planning and reduce the need for out-of-home placements for children, no systematic efforts were made until the past two decades. In the past, and even to some extent today, families with children at risk for out-of-home placement are viewed more as part of the problem, rather than as part of the solution. A recent trend in the field of child and family services has been a growing emphasis on the provision of intensive family preservation services, characterized by highly intensive services, delivered generally in the client's home, for a relatively brief period of time. These services focus on the enhancement of strengths within the family and the immediate access and utilization of community resources to provide supportive services to the family. The primary goals of this approach include the protection of children, the maintenance and strengthening of family bonds, and immediate intervention. Although only a few states have, to date, adopted a statewide family preservation focus for child and family services, the initial data from these projects indicate some promising results, with a reduction in the need for out-of-home placements for children and a reduction in recidivism of child maltreatment. In addition, there is some indication that the use of a family preservation model reduces turnover of direct line workers because workers have fewer cases and are allowed to work intensively with fewer families. This approach fosters the development of in-depth casework with families, allowing the worker and families to realize improved conditions more rapidly, thus reducing burnout and frustration and providing more immediate positive reinforcement. Currently, several additional states are considering the adoption of a family preservation focus for the delivery of child and family services.

Note: Preparation of this chapter was facilitated by a NIMH Faculty Scholar Award (MH-19079) and a University of Georgia University Affiliated Program Faculty Fellow grant received by Dr. Thyer.

References

American Public Welfare Association. (1990). *Factbook on public child welfare services and staff*. New York: Author.

Axinn, J., & Levin, H. (1982). *Social welfare: A history of the American response to need* (2nd ed.). New York: Harper & Row.

Benet, M. (1976). *The politics of adoption*. NY: Free Press.

Child Welfare League of America. (1978). *Standards for adoption service* (rev. ed.). NY: Author.

Cole, E. S. (1987). Adoption. In A. Minahan et al. (Eds.), *Encyclopedia of social work*, Vol. 1. (18th ed.). Silver Spring, MD: National Association of Social Workers.

Kadushin, A. (1974). *Child welfare services* (2nd ed.). New York: MacMillan.

Kadushin, A. (1987). Child welfare services. In A. Minahan et al. (Eds.), *Encyclopedia of social work*, Vol. 1. (18th ed.). Silver Spring, MD: National Association of Social Workers.

Rothman, D. J. (1971). *The discovery of the asylum: Social order and disorder in the new republic*. Boston: Little, Brown.

Stein, T. J. (1987). Foster care for children. In A. Minahan et al. (Eds.), *Encyclopedia of social work*, Vol. 1. (18th ed.). Silver Spring, MD: National Association of Social Workers.

Vinokur, D. K. (1983). *The view from the agency: Supervisors and workers look at in-service training for child welfare*. Ann Arbor, MI: National Child Welfare Training Center, University of Michigan School of Social Work.

Watkins, S. A. (1990). The Mary Ellen myth: Correcting child welfare history. *Social Work, 35*(6), 500-503.

Women's Centers

Lenore Patton, M.A.

History/Legislation

Before the mid-1970s, women who were battered or raped had no place to turn for help. There were no community services available to them, nor, in fact, was there any recognition by most of society that there was any need to provide such services.

Wife beating, or what we now call domestic violence, was not looked upon as a crime, but was one of those situations referred to as a "family matter" and beyond the purview of government or social service agencies. Some women who found themselves victims of battering turned to friends and family for help. Most suffered in silence, afraid to admit to their victimization and unsure of the reaction even of those closest to them.

Few instances of battering were ever reported to police. Police officers and others in the law enforcement community were reluctant to involve themselves in what many still see as a private domestic dispute, moreover one in which the intervenor is often in personal danger. On those occasions when police were called to the scene of what many still refer to as a "domestic disturbance," their standard response was to send the batterer off for a walk "to cool down" and to lecture the victim about behaving in a manner that provoked the abuse.

Social service agencies did not provide much more help to battering victims. Spouse abuse or domestic violence victims were not recognized as a category of people needing social services, and no services were available to them. Social service agencies, the courts, churches, and most of the community often blamed the abuse on the behavior of the victim and suggested that by changing her behavior, she could make the battering stop.

Throughout history, society's traditional responses to the plight of rape victims ranged from indifference to blaming the victim for her own victimization. In no other situation in our society is the victim considered to bear the responsibility for a crime against herself. The guilt and shame society forced on sexual assault victims, combined with the trauma of the original violation, usually kept rape victims silent.

The insensitivity of a legal system which often focused on the lifestyle, dress, or previous behavior of the victim, and made it seem that the victim was on trial rather than the perpetrator, reinforced the conviction of rape victims that there was no justice for them in the courts and discouraged them from even reporting, let alone prosecuting, incidents of rape.

Many early domestic violence and rape victim services were provided by former victims and volunteers and a handful of feminist lawyers and social service workers. Victims often felt themselves disbelieved by the establishment, and felt the need to help themselves and others in the same situation. Feminists saw attitudes toward abuse victims as reflecting women's lower status and position in society and as part of the strategy by those in power to keep women from achieving equality (Schecter, 1982).

They realized, too, that it was not enough to provide help to those already victimized, but that it was necessary to make fundamental changes in society which would empower women, to change public attitudes about the victimization of women, and to lobby state and federal legislative bodies to enact new laws which would provide protection to future victims of abuse.

Support groups became more structured, providing training in legal advocacy, seeking out financial support and writing grant proposals for operating funds, forming state and regional coalitions, and working with sympathetic legislators to draft legislation which would establish programs to provide services to victims.

As the feminist message of the victimization of women began to be heard and understood by professionals in the field of social service, law enforcement, medicine, and government, many of the early activists expressed deep concern about the loss of feminist ideology that would likely occur if the movement were taken over by professionals. This concern was not without foundation. With success in achieving new legislation and increasing availability of both government and private funding, came the new need to be accountable to outside agencies. Debate still exists among members of the movement as to just how much autonomy must be lost in order to comply with governmental regulations and community restrictions and, thus, ensure the best possible service to victims. It may be a problem without a solution that is satisfactory to everyone.

SHELTER MOVEMENT

The first stirrings of the shelter movement arose in England with the opening of Chiswick Women's Aid in 1971. Less than one year later, Women's Advocates in St. Paul, Minnesota, and Haven House in Pasadena, California, opened the first shelters for battered women in the United States.

With the beginning of a strong feminist movement in the mid-1970s, came the increased awareness of, and support for, victims of domestic violence. Very slowly, women began to reach out to their sisters who had been victims of battering, to encourage them to speak out about the violence, and to make a public issue of a subject society had long kept hidden. The feminist contention that women had the right to control over their own bodies provided the impetus for the organization and growth of self-help groups for abuse victims. As women began to provide for one another the support and protection they could not get from established agencies and organizations, the grass roots safe-home networks which were the seeds of the shelter movement began to appear (Dunwoody, 1982).

Pennsylvania established the first state coalition against domestic violence in 1976. In that same year, the Pennsylvania legislature became the first state legislative body to adopt a statute providing for orders of protection for victims of domestic violence.

From the handful of programs and shelters that began to provide services, often operating on shoestring budgets and staffed by volunteers, have come the more than 1,400 shelters, counseling programs, and hotlines that are in operation in the United States today.

Today, while some women's centers and shelters are still housed in inadequate, shabby facilities, many programs have moved into comfortable quarters where victims can feel supported and reassured that they do not have to face their victimization alone. Most programs are staffed by highly trained professionals. While many still rely heavily on volunteers to supplement services, those volunteers are well trained in listening and communication skills and crisis counseling. Funding, too, remains a problem. Center staffs find themselves spending large amounts of time searching for money to continue operating—time that could be more usefully spent in providing direct service to victims.

RAPE CRISIS MOVEMENT

The rape crisis movement also developed out of the feminist movement of the late 1960s and early 1970s. Rape victim support groups and rape crisis hotlines began to appear in various locations around the country as women began to work together to change old stereotypes and outmoded responses to the needs of sexual assault victims. Survivors of sexual assault worked closely with other feminists to provide counseling, advocacy, and support to victims, and to help them to empower themselves to become survivors.

Although the beginnings of the rape crisis movement are not well documented, it is believed that the first community-based rape crisis center to open was the Bay Area Rape Crisis Center in Berkeley, California, in 1969. During the next year or two, a handful of other centers were founded in other parts of the country. By 1974, there were 61 rape crisis centers operating in 27 states. The latest national directory of victim/survivor programs, published in 1989, lists 2,700 programs in 50 states providing direct service to victims of sexual assault (Webster, 1989).

LEGISLATION

The earliest federal funding dealing with family violence prevention came through the Law Enforcement Assistance Administration (LEAA) of the Department of Justice who, during the early 1970s, provided some discretionary funding to anti-rape programs (West & Christ, 1982). However, the criticism of LEAA by the domestic violence and rape crisis movements was that the main emphasis of their concern and the bulk of their funding were always provided to the law enforcement community rather than being directed to programs that could assist victims with counseling and advocacy.

In April 1979, President Jimmy Carter created the Interdepartmental Committee on Domestic Violence. One of the mandates of the committee was to report to the President ways to increase the responsiveness of government agencies to the needs of battered women. At that same time, President Carter also established the Office on Domestic Violence (ODV) as a part of the Department of Health Education and Welfare. However, neither the ODV nor the committee on domestic violence had any legislative mandate to provide funding directly to programs providing service to violence victims.

The first federal financial support for battered women came from title XX funds which could be used by states to provide emergency shelter. Other federal agencies such as the Department of Housing and Urban Development (HUD) and the Community Services Administration also provided some, very limited, funding for services to victims of domestic violence and rape (Moore, 1985; Mettger, 1982).

In 1984, citing Bureau of Justice statistics which determined that more than 2 million women were abused and 1,300 women killed by their husbands or boyfriends each year, Congress passed the Family Violence Prevention and Services Act. Under this legislation, the federal government provided assistance to states to develop and maintain programs aimed at prevention of family violence. Included in the legislation were provisions for shelters, programs to provide technical assistance, and training of personnel to provide assistance to family violence victims.

In subsequent years, the Act has been extended and improved (Copeland, 1987). When it was reauthorized in 1987, the Act provided funding for research into individual characteristics related to family violence. It also authorized the collection of data on victims of family violence and their children, even in cases where charges are not brought against the abuser, and provided funds to train law enforcement, medical, and social service personnel to encourage them to be more sensitive to the needs of domestic violence victims. Due in large part to the work of a loose coalition of domestic violence and rape crisis workers, legal services attorneys, feminists, community activists, and some law enforcement officials, the last 15 years have seen a rapid growth in legislation to both provide protection and options to battered women and rape victims and to fund services for those victims.

Currently, 49 states and the District of Columbia have laws allowing battered women to obtain civil protection orders against their abuser independent of any domestic relations proceedings, in most cases providing for the eviction of the abuser from jointly occupied premises. Many states have adopted model protocols for law enforcement response to domestic violence. The status of legal protection for battered women, however, varies from state to state, and continues to change; therefore, a comprehensive description by state is not available at this time (Lerman, 1982; Lerman & Livingston, 1983).

Laws dealing with the handling of sexual assault incidents and protection for the rights of victims, too, vary greatly among the states. Although most states have rape shield laws, protecting victims from hostile questioning about past behaviors, and many states protect the confidentiality of rape crisis workers and center files, rape victim advocates continue to lobby legislatures to modify often outdated criminal justice responses to rape victims.

SHELTER AND CRISIS CENTER PROGRAMS

Who Works in Programs

Although domestic violence and rape crisis centers began as a grass roots response to the victimization of women and grew out of the feminist movement and although most still employ the feminist empowerment counseling model; thanks to increased funding and support by communities and legislative bodies as well as the legal, medical, and educational communities, most shelters across the country are staffed by professional counselors and support personnel, augmented by highly trained paraprofessional crisis intervention volunteers.

Philosophy and Mandate

While most programs in the United States are largely autonomous and self-governing, the philosophy and mandate do not differ very much from program to program or state to state. In the main, they view their mandate as the temporary protection of women and children who are victims of family violence and sexual assault, the empowerment of women to enable them to take back the control of their lives that has been taken from them by their abusers, and the education of the community to raise the level of understanding about the societal causes of violence against women.

Few programs for battered women or rape victims employ the therapeutic counseling model. Most use supportive empowerment counseling to attempt to facilitate the return of control over their lives to women who have been controlled by their abusers. Staff members and volunteers work with victims to recognize and build individual abilities and strengths, to safeguard and obtain their rights through the legal system, and to secure a future free from abuse and control by others.

Services Available

Like everything else about domestic violence and rape crisis programs, the extent and type of services available to victims vary from center to center and from state to state. At the very least, most programs offer free counseling 24 hours a day over crisis hotlines. Ongoing individual and group supportive counseling services are usually available to victims of battering and sexual assault and to their significant others. In addition, many programs provide advocacy and accompaniment services to victims who must deal with other community systems such as the medical, legal, or criminal justice systems. The overwhelming majority of domestic violence programs also offer emergency shelter to violence victims and their children, either in a staffed shelter or through an informal network of "safe homes." The costs of many services to domestic violence and sexual assault victims are based on a sliding scale, and regulated by the victim's ability to pay. In fact, in a number of states, all services of domestic violence and rape crisis centers are free to any state resident, regardless of ability to pay.

REFERRAL INFORMATION

Because so much variation exists both in availability of services for victims and in types of services provided to them, a social service worker would do well to investigate the resources available in his or her immediate area before making referrals of either battered women or rape victims. In fact, many women's centers acquire most of their clients through self-referral and may prefer to communicate directly with a victim before accepting a referral.

Leaving an abusive situation is often a long, complex process. Most battered women leave and return to a violent relationship many times before making the final break (Okun, 1986). Leaving the first time may be only a test to see if the action shocks the abuser into getting help, or a way of finding out just what services are available in the community. Social service workers who refer victims before they are themselves ready to make a change, can expect to see the client reject the referral or not to follow through for very long.

Sexual assault victims, too, must be ready themselves to deal with the issues of their victimization before a referral to a rape crisis center is useful. Many victims use denial as a way of surviving their victimization and trying to put their lives back in order. A victim may insist that she is handling the situation and doing just fine not only immediately after an assault, but for a long time thereafter. Since the focus of supportive empowerment counseling is the attempt to put the victim back in control of her life, giving her the option of when, or even whether, to call the domestic violence or rape crisis center is seen as an empowering act, and the first step on her path to healing.

Both the National Coalition Against Domestic Violence, which operates a 24-hour referral and crisis hotline, and the National Coalition Against Sexual Assault can serve as initial contacts for the referring social service worker. Either of the two organizations can provide the referring agency with information about services available in a particular state or community.

National Coalition Against Domestic Violence
P. O. Box 34103
Washington, DC 20043-4103
(202) 638-6388 (office)
(800) 333-SAFE (national hotline)

National Coalition Against Sexual Assault
P. O. Box 21378
Washington, DC 20009

References

Copeland, L. (1987). Congressional reauthorization of federal domestic violence programs. *Response*, *10*(4), 20.

Dunwoody, E. (1982). The National Coalition Against Domestic Violence: A grass roots movement. *Response, Special Winter Issue, 5*, 15.

Lerman, L. (1982). Court decision on wife abuse laws. *Response, 5*(3), 3.

Lerman, L., & Livingston, F. (1983). State legislation on domestic violence. *Response, 6*(5), 1.

Mettger, Z. (1982). More than a shoestring budget: Survival and growth for family violence programs. *Response, 5*(3), 1.

Moore, J. M. (1985). Federal funding for family violence programs. *Response, 8*(3), 24.

Okun, L. (1986). *Women abuse: Facts replacing myths*. Albany, NY: State University of New York.

Schecter, S. (1982). *Women and male violence*. Boston: South End.

Webster, L. (1989). *Sexual assault and child sexual abuse: A national directory of victim/survivor services and prevention programs*. Phoenix: Oryx.

West, L., & Christ, K. (1982). Federal initiatives on family violence blocked. *Response, Special Winter Issue, 5*, 4.

Family Planning

Vicente N. Noble, Ph.D.

The health care system in America is largely based on private medical care and access to private physicians varies significantly in the United States. Nonmetropolitan areas of the country are less well served than are metropolitan areas. A person's ability to have consultation with a private physician also varies by his or her ability to pay for care and, in the absence of a national health insurance program, medical care is funded through a patchwork of systems. In 1984, seven out of 10 women of reproductive age were covered by private health insurance and nine in 10 men and women had private insurance through their employment. However, some people do not have health insurance covered through their employment or cannot afford private insurance. They encompass several million low-income families and teenagers who do not have access to private health care.

History/Legislation

Organized efforts to address population growth, birth control, and family planning issues were initiated at the turn of the century in America. The first birth control clinic opened in New York City in 1916, but was shut down 10 days later as a violation of obscenity laws. Nonetheless, court decisions by 1918 made it possible for health care personnel to provide information and methods on birth control. Margaret Sanger, the noted proponent of women's emancipation, was credited with coining the phrase *birth control* and she was the president (1917) of what is now the Planned Parenthood Federation of America (PPFA), a private, nonprofit organization. PPFA provided women with contraceptive information at a time when physicians were unable or reluctant to do so. Eventually, private physicians began offering contraceptive advice and services, and private clinics provided contraceptive services for poor women who were unable to receive assistance from public health services.

Religious and political controversy, as late as the 1950s, excluded local, state, and federal tax support for family planning services. However, the climate of change during the 1960s helped to promote the passage, in 1970, of the national Family Planning Services and Population Research Act, commonly known as title X—The National Family Planning Program, which authorized funding to establish a network of clinics. The 1960s was also an era where there was an increased demand by women for effective contraceptives, smaller size families, and a recognition of the need of family planning services for low-income women, teenagers, and the reduction of high-risk and unintended pregnancies. Family planning services reached its height during the mid-1980s. At that time, there were approximately 2,500 agencies operating clinics at more than 5,000 sites in the country for almost 5 million patients.

The majority of family planning clinic patients are poor women (83% have incomes below 150% of the poverty line), and metropolitan areas are better served than nonmetropolitan areas. The majority of family planning clinics are operated by public health departments. Planned Parenthood, a private, nonprofit organization composed of approximately 180 agencies, serves an average of 1,400 patients per site and approximately 600 community organizations (i.e., neighborhood health centers, women's health centers) serve about 21% of all family planning clinic patients.

FUNDING

Congress used a health approach to justify public support for family planning and did not formulate a domestic population policy. This approach warranted family planning services as a means to reduce undesired births, decrease high-risk pregnancies, and potentially reduce congenital birth defects, mental retardation, and infant mortality. As such, title X—The Family Planning Services and Research Act of 1970—was passed by Congress by an overwhelming majority. Title X provided funding to public agencies or private, nonprofit community groups for comprehensive family planning clinic services with a requirement that low-income persons and teenagers be given priority. Inasmuch, a survey of funding sources for family planing services in 1987, indicated that Medicaid has exceeded title X as the largest source of family planning funds. Approximately one-half of Medicaid family planning funds are used to reimburse private medical service personnel who provide contraceptive services to Medicaid recipients. Other sources of funding include the Maternal and Child Health Program, foundations, and private corporations. Family planning services also receive funds from state budgets in addition to federal funds. However, the number of title X grants declined from 300 in 1972 to 83 in 1988, which has been noted as a change in policy from renewed religious and political controversy on the issue of abortion.

PERSONNEL

Family planning clinics are supervised by full- or part-time physicians. However, because of expenses, many clinics have heavily relied on nurse-practitioners to provide family planning services under a doctor's standing orders. Clinics vary in size and composition depending on patient load. Bean, Anderson, and Tatum (1971) described the typical clinic as composed of a physician, nurse-practitioner, health educator, social worker, and clinic and community aides. However, many clinic salaries are not competitive with other medical facilities and there has been some difficulty recruiting and retaining physicians and nurse-practitioners. Family planning clinics located near colleges and universities have, in some instances, utilized college student-interns or trainees from the fields of counseling, psychology, and social work to provide family planning counseling and advisement services.

Clinical aides and community aides, as paramedical personnel, have served to strengthen a number of family planning agencies by freeing the physician and nurse for other responsibilities. The outreach worker in the community provides education and follow-up services to ensure continuity of use and maintenance of medical care. In many situations, these workers are instructed through short-term, specialized courses and in-service courses.

Medical personnel, physicians and nurses, require formal education from accredited institutions. Other nonmedical personnel (i.e., health educators, public health workers, social workers) are typically college graduates who have chosen to work in family planning or population growth services.

At present, there is not a national organization for certifying workers in family planning services. However, for a number of the degreed roles (i.e., physician, nurse, social worker, counselor) many, if not most, states have certification boards which provide licensure for these occupations.

The quality of many family planning programs if often monitored by outside funding agencies (e.g., Medicaid, title X) which have a number of built-in requirements and assurances.

Purpose/Intent

Family planning programs generally strive to provide education and medical and family planning assistance. Nonprofit family planning organizations and public health agencies focus on the needs of low-income women and unmarried teenagers, as well as special populations of non-English speaking immigrants, native American Indians, and rural poverty patients, to enhance family planning strategies and reduce the risks of unintended pregnancies for those who cannot afford private medical care. In most publicly funded situations, family planning services are not intended to provide comprehensive medical and reproductive health care, although a wide range of services are available for preventive and reproductive health care, testing, counseling, advisement, educational materials, and referral to appropriate providers.

Organized efforts that have addressed many of these services have been carried out by private medical services, private family planning agencies, and state-federal publicly funded agencies.

PRIVATE MEDICAL SERVICES

Seventy-four percent of women of reproductive age are covered by private health insurance, and nine out of 10 men and women have health coverage through their employment. The majority of persons in this situation are most likely to receive family planning consultation from their insurance-covered physician. This would include preventive reproductive services ranging from birth control methods, contraceptives, and referral for sterilization or abortion services. However, one in four physicians are not likely to provide contraceptives to minors without parental consent and this lessens a minor's chance to obtain confidential services. Thirty-one percent of abortion services are provided by nonhospital clinics, although they account for 83% of all induced abortions (Henshaw, Forrest, & Van Vort, 1987).

PRIVATE FAMILY PLANNING NONPROFIT ORGANIZATIONS

The leadership for developing a national family planning program in America came largely from the efforts of the Planned Parenthood Federation of America (PPFA). Government agencies and private medical services did not have significant involvement until the middle portion of the twentieth century. PPFA affiliates, community health centers, community-based poverty programs, women's clinics, free clinics, adolescent health centers, and emerging community-based organizations constitute approximately 2,400 provider agencies who operate about 5,000 sites in the country. These organizations account for 28% of services to family planning patients. The principal effort of their activities is to make family planning services available to low-income persons where charges are either free or based on their income. However, 92% of these agencies charged some or most of the family planning patients with some fee.

STATE-FEDERAL PUBLICLY FUNDED AGENCIES

The primary thrust of publicly funded agencies is to provide family planning services to women who cannot afford private physicians. Title X—the Family Planning Services and Population Research Act (1970)—authorized funding to establish a network of clinics which would ensure the provision of comprehensive family planning services in a location within the reach of a target population of low-income persons and teenagers who are given priority. The majority of family planning clinic patients are women who are below the poverty level and teenagers. The latter account for approximately one-third of the caseload. The majority of publicly funded family planning clinics are run by public health departments and they constitute 1,400 health departments with an average of two sites each.

Planned Parenthood agencies, as well as a sizeable number of the organizations mentioned in the private family planning nonprofit organizations, are also funded by title X funds, in addition to obtaining funds from the corporate and foundation sectors. Planned Parenthood agencies are often located in metropolitan areas, while health departments typically provide family planning services in nonmetropolitan areas.

UTILIZATION CRITERIA

Private medical family planning care may provide a full range of reproductive and preventative health care services with variations accounted for by health care insurance and affordability. However, most nonprofit organizations and publicly funded agencies typically do not offer a full range of health care services, and many clinics refer patients to other providers who offer particular services.

Clinics receiving title X funding must provide services at no charge to any patient with a family income under 100% of the poverty level. Nonetheless, one out of four clinics often require income substantiation, beyond the patient's own statement of income, to quality for services. Clinicians in most family planning clinics generally prescribe and provide oral contraceptives and diaphragms, as well as information on nonprescription contraceptives and other family planning educational materials. However, about half of the clinics generally set an upper age limit of 35 for women requesting the pill.

SPECIAL CASE MANAGEMENT NEEDS

The typical patient at a nonprofit organization or public health department is generally poor, a teenager, or both. This may require the coordination and referral of financial and social support services, as well as addressing personal, family, and relationship counseling, educational and vocational problems, examining women's issues, and attention to legal and developmental concerns of adolescent patients. In addition, some of the religious and political controversies that attended the inception of family planning programs have resurfaced, which create social challenges for both prenatal patients and staff in family planning settings.

Client Services

Family planning services, whether private, nonprofit, or governmental, offer a variety of services These services have included education, medical screening and counseling, and medical assistance and referral to appropriate resources.

EDUCATION

Almost all agencies disseminate printed educational literature which range from birth control methods and considerations, how to recognize and deal with relationships, family problems, personal and social concerns, pre-and postnatal care, and wellness and disease issues. In addition, most agencies also provide individual and group family planning education meetings. Group meetings have been supplanted by individual attention which expedites patient screening and education. This assures that a patient has given informed consent in receiving only the educational service regarding the risks and benefits of a chosen method, including alternative methods. Approximately two-thirds of all family planning patients decide on the pill as their choice of birth control. Subsequently, a patient may choose to proceed to a physical examination and medical tests where it is appropriate to their situation.

A number of family planning services also have programs and disseminate literature regarding prenatal care, programs for pregnant teenagers, nutrition, teenage parenting, AIDS education and prevention, sex education, and materials describing the role of self-concept in relationships and sexuality. Some programs have utilized direct mailings to teenage males about the impact of knowledge, attitudes, and sexual behavior in regard to condom usage.

Teenagers currently constitute a sizeable percentage of the patients at family planning services. It has been estimated that teenage mothers will more than likely have a higher risk of single parenthood, incomplete educational status, and experience poverty, unemployment, and welfare dependency. They are also at higher risk of being separated and divorced if married, and teenage rates of pregnancy are higher in America than in other industrialized countries.

In many clinics, friends and parents of the patient are the primary source of referral for first family planning visits. Approximately one-fourth of a sample of teenage patients reported that their first visit was due to a suspicion of their pregnancy which is the leading reason for visiting clinics. In most instances, these patients also report that they chose to visit family planning services rather than a private doctor because of expense, fear that the doctor would inform their parents, and unfamiliarity of a doctor to provide services.

MEDICAL SCREENING AND COUNSELING

Family planning services funded by title X allocations are required to offer pregnancy diagnosis and counseling, as well as refer pregnant women who request information to other sources of prenatal care, delivery, infant care, foster care, adoption, and abortion.[1] Many family planning clinics also require for inclusion in their services that patients have a physical examination which includes screening for sexually transmitted diseases, infections, cancer, high blood pressure, and infertility.

A number of family planning clinics are not open on a daily basis, and the average site is open for approximately 30 hours a week. Some are open during evenings and fewer are open on Saturday. Most clinics require an appointment for services.

---

[1] Note: Recent Supreme Court rulings may affect counseling options in federally funded programs.

Family planning services require a physician's supervision but a good number of clinics rely on nurse-practitioners to provide services under a physician's orders.

Family planning clinics generally train a number of their personnel to provide counseling about the risks, benefits, use, effectiveness, and alternatives of their choice of available methods. Unmarried women, teenagers, and college students currently represent the majority of patients, and surveys indicate they know more about reproduction and birth control than an earlier generation of patients. Today, many patients know which method of birth control they prefer, and individual counseling can be addressed to specific needs. The focus of counseling is to assist a patient make an informed choice, help them determine and strengthen their future, as well as promote more secure and rational decision making in their sexual conduct. A little over half of the family planning clinics offer infertility counseling, and less than half of the clinics offer genetic counseling and programs for adolescent mothers.

Title XX—the Adolescent Family Life Act of 1981—was enacted to fund innovative demonstration programs regarding teenage pregnancy and childbearing. It addressed two areas: adolescent pregnancy prevention programs and care for pregnant or teenage parents. Approximately 45 projects were funded and the Act mandated that they provide 10 specific services directly or through referral. Stahler, DeCette, and McBride (1989) noted that

> ...the services included pregnancy testing and maternity counseling, adoption counseling and referral services, primary and preventive health care services including prenatal and postnatal care, nutrition information and counseling, referral for screening and treatment of venereal disease, referral to appropriate pediatric care services, education in sexuality and family life, referral to appropriate educational and vocational services, family planning counseling and referral, and referral to mental health services or other appropriate health services. Additionally, some supplemental services are eligible for funding for child care, consumer education and homemaking, counseling for extended family members, transportation, and outreach programs. (p. 123)

The goals and services provided are laudably comprehensive.

Namerow, Weatherby, and Williams-Kay (1989) have described the effectiveness of a counseling approach which is termed *contingency planning*. Contingency-planning counseling submits that family planning counseling should go beyond the traditional approach of information dissemination and help in decision making. Contingency-planning counseling is described as:

> ...including a focus during counseling on the patient's behavior and the circumstances she will face after she leaves the clinic with a method of contraception and aims to help a patient consider and plan for contingencies—such as side effects, pressure from someone to stop using her method and financial difficulties in getting methods are care—that could potentially interfere with effective contraceptive use. Contingency planning supplements by

adding a focus on factors that will affect a women's ability to maintain her decision to practice contraception over an extended time and the counselor and patient develop an individual plan for pregnancy prevention. The goal is to increase contraceptive and clinic continuation and avoid unwanted pregnancies by focusing not only on the individual's current perception of birth control but also on her past experiences and projected experiences with the method selected. (p. 115)

MEDICAL ASSISTANCE AND REFERRAL

More than two-thirds of all clinic patients have chosen the pill as their method of contraception. As a requisite for family planning medical services, many women are required to have a physical examination which includes screening for high blood pressure, cancer, venereal disease, and infections. Public health agencies or nonprofit agencies provide medical examinations that are offered at a free or low cost to the patient depending on their income. The clinicians generally prescribe oral contraceptives and diaphragms and the clinics often furnish the supplies, as well as information on nonprescription contraceptives. Approximately one-half of the clinics set an upper age limit for pill use at 35 for women.

A little more than the majority of clinics offer infertility counseling but only 20% provide infertility treatment. Prenatal care services are also offered on a limited basis and only one-fourth to one-half of the clinics provide this service.

Generally, specialized treatments such as adoption, abortion, and sterilization are referred to other appropriate sources in the community. A significant number of private physicians and hospitals in the regular American health care system do not provide abortion services.

Sterilization services are also not widespread, and only one general practitioner in four are able to perform vasectomies and one in five perform tubal sterilizations. Vasectomies are less difficult than tubal sterilizations and the majority of vasectomies are performed in a doctor's office.

The majority of private medical practitioners will provide contraceptives to minors without parental consent. However, a sizable number of doctors, depending on the state and area, will not provide this service to minors. Subsequently, a large number of minors seek such services from public health agencies or nonprofit family planning clinics where there is generally a madate for confidentiality.

TYPICAL REFERRAL QUESTIONS

Family planning services may be located in private medical facilities, local public health departments, nonprofit family planning clinics, or community women's or health centers. Subsequently, the referring human service worker is advised to become familiar with information regarding some of the following questions:

Where can I obtain family planing services?

Information about family planning services and programs can usually be obtained from local public health departments. They should have a listing of nearby, available centers or clinics such as the Planned Parenthood Federation of America. An appointment is usually required with the centers or clinics as they are generally not open every day or evening.

What are the financial charges for services?

The referring service worker will need to know if the patient will use a private medical facility or nonprofit agency. Private medical facilities are typically for-profit services and the charges are usually determined by community standards. In some instances, some private medical facilities receive funding from title X and can provide free or low-cost services for low-income women and teenagers. As mentioned earlier, confidentiality for teenagers may be an issue that will require determination prior to the patient's first visit, if this is of concern to that person. Nonprofit organizations and public health facilities generally operate on a low-fee schedule and, if funded by title X funds, will give priority to low-income women and teenagers at a free or low-cost fee.

If I am a teenager, will my family be notified of the services provided to me?

The majority of states have enacted laws that ensure confidentiality of minors over the age of 12 with regard to health services. However, some states still assign this responsibility to the attending physician and the service worker should predetermine the state laws governing confidentiality of minors. The vast majority of publicly funded, nonprofit agencies do adhere to the right of a minor to have confidential treatment.

REFERENCES

Bean, L. L., Anderson, R.K., & Tatum, H. J. (1971). *Population and family planning manpower and training.* North Haven, CT: Van Dyke.

Henshaw, S. K., Forrest, J. D., & Van Vort, J. (1987). Abortion services in the United States, 1984 and 1985. *Family Planning Perspectives, 19*(3), 63-70.

Namerow, P. B., Weatherby, N., & Williams-Kaye, J. (1989). Effectiveness of contingency-planning counseling. *Family Planning Perspectives, 21*(3), 115-119.

Stahler, G. J., DuCette, J., & McBride, D. (1989). Evaluation component in adolescent pregnancy care projects: Is it adequate? *Family Planning Perspectives, 21*(3), 123-126.

IV. Rehabilitation Services

Vocational Rehabilitation

Richard R. Wolfe, Ph.D.

History/Legislation

The relative success of the Smith-Sears Act—also known as the Soldier's Rehabilitation Act—set the stage for the first civilian vocational rehabilitation act, the Smith Fess Act, signed into law June 2, 1920. This first vocational rehabilitation act provided limited services, and was restricted to those individuals who had some type of physical disability. The kinds of services provided were limited to vocational guidance and training, occupational adjustment, prosthesis, and placement services (Obermann, 1965).

The Vocational Rehabilitation Act of 1920 allowed for a partnership in which the individual states could choose (or not choose) to enter into an agreement with the federal government in which the federal government agreed to pay part of the costs of rehabilitation services for those people who qualified for services. This same type partnership continues to the current time (Obermann, 1965).

The vocational rehabilitation program became "permanent" as a result of the Social Security Act of 1935. With this legislation, vocational rehabilitation (VR) could be expected to continue unless Congress should determine that such a program was no longer needed.

With the passage and signing into law of the Bardon-LaFollette Act, mental disabilities were added as a new category of persons to be served. Vocational rehabilitation could now serve both the *physically disabled* and the *mentally disabled*. These continue to be the only disability categories served by the state-federal system of vocational rehabilitation. In addition to providing the vocational guidance, vocational training, prosthetics, and placement, the vocational rehabilitation program could now provide physical restoration services to its clients. It was critical that physical restoration services be added if the vocational rehabilitation program was to grow and meet the needs of people with disabilities (Obermann, 1965).

The emergence of the Vocational Rehabilitation Act of 1920 for the civilian population, had a close kinship with World War I. Similarly, the roots of the Vocational Rehabilitation Act of 1943 can be traced to needs identified in World War II. This act was passed during the period of war, and helped in identifying and preparing persons with disabilities to replace those in industry who were called to military duty. Although these persons with disability proved to be excellent workers, when the hostilities ended and the "able-bodied" returned, many of the persons with disabilities were replaced. Perhaps only by coincidence, each of these two major pieces of legislation (as well as the Social Security Act of 1935) was signed into law by a president who himself was, at the time of the signing of each respective act, a person with a disability, Woodrow Wilson, the Act of 1920, and Franklin D. Roosevelt (U. S. Dept. of HEW, SRS, RSA, 1970).

As vocational rehabilitation grew, the need for trained personnel became evident. Congress attended to this need with the passage of the VR Amendment Act of 1954. With the passage of this Act, university programs were provided funds to provide training for a wide array of professionals to meet the needs of the growing population of people with disabilities. Among the various professionals that could be trained as a result of this Act were rehabilitation counselors, rehabilitation psychologists, rehabilitation nurses, occupational therapists, physical therapists, rehabilitation social workers, and physicians (especially physiatrists). This is not an exhaustive listing of *rehabilitation specialists* for which training moneys were made available. Other special provisions of the Act allowed for more moneys to the basic rehabilitation program, as well as moneys for special projects, expansion and improvement of rehabilitation facilities, and research and demonstration projects. This major piece of legislation was signed into law by a president, Dwight D. Eisenhower, who had become disabled.

In addition to the VR Amendment Act of 1954, other rehabilitation-related legislation was enacted into law. The Hill-Burton Act for constructing hospitals was amended to authorize a special appropriation to help build rehabilitation facilities, primarily those of a medical nature. The Social Security Act was amended to protect the insurance benefits of people with disabilities. As a result of this legislation, a working relationship was established between rehabilitation and Social Security (U. S. Dept. of HEW, SRS, RSA, 1970).

In 1965 and 1968, rehabilitation legislation was passed which was intended to respond to some of the social ills of the time. The nation was experiencing civil unrest, which, in its extremes, included major "burning" within some cities. It was during this period that the nation saw a major welfare reform act. Rehabilitation was to become more sensitive to the social need, to evaluate and identify needs, and in those instances where the individual was found to have a disability, serve that individual in the normal manner. For those evaluated who did not meet the rehabilitation agency eligibility criteria, rehabilitation was to refer them to other social and employment programs to help meet the identified needs.

The Rehabilitation Act of 1973 was passed and signed into law by President Richard M. Nixon on September 26, 1973. Mr. Nixon had vetoed two attempts of the Congress to authorize a rehabilitation act to replace the Act of 1968, the authorization of which was due to expire June 30, 1972. In his two veto messages, President Nixon was concerned about the inflationary aspect of the proposed legislation, as well as the fact that Congress was opening the doors to rehabilitation of individuals with disabilities for whom there was no rehabilitation potential. Mr. Nixon was convinced that there currently existed programs to take care of these individuals. He believed that adding this provision to rehabilitation would destroy the purpose for which rehabilitation was created and grew (i.e., to prepare people with disabilities to enter employment and become self-sufficient).

Public Law 93-112 (U. S. Congress, House, 1973) was

> An Act to replace the Vocational Rehabilitation Act, to extend and
> revise the authorization of grants to states for vocational rehabili-
> tation services, with special emphasis on services to those with
> most severe handicaps, to expand special federal responsibilities
> and research and training programs with respect to handicapped
> individuals, to establish special responsibilities in the Secretary of
> Health, Education, and Welfare for coordination of all programs
> with respect to handicapped individuals within the Department of
> Health, Education, and Welfare, and for other purposes.

The Rehabilitation Act of 1973 opened the door to the person with a disability to become more of a partner in his or her rehabilitation. It required the development of the Individualized Written Rehabilitation Program (IWRP) which was to be developed jointly by the vocational rehabilitation counselor and the person with a disability (or, in appropriate cases, parents or guardians). The Act set specific guidelines relating to this IWRP development. The client had the right to request review and possible revisions of that IWRP. One must hasten to add that prior to 1973, the plan for rehabilitation was developed, and in the case of the knowing counselor, the plan was developed jointly with the client. The Rehabilitation Act, however, mandated this joint effort.

Under title V–Miscellaneous of the 1973 Act, special consideration was given to employment opportunities and accessibility. The federal government opened more doors to the employment of people with disabilities within governmental agencies. The Architectural and Transportation Barriers Compliance Board was established. Section 503 of the Act provided for affirmative action provisions for employment and advancement of people with disabilities in industries with federal contracts in excess of $2,500. Section 504 of the Act, a single sentence paragraph, prohibited discrimination under federal grants toward the individual with handicaps. Section 504 of P. L. 93-112 (U. S. Congress, House, 1973) states:

> No otherwise qualified handicapped individual in the United
> States, as defined in section 7(6), shall, solely by reason of his
> handicap, be excluded from the participation in, be denied the
> benefits of, or be subjected to discrimination under any program
> or activity receiving Federal financial assistance. (p. 39)

It was not until May 4, 1977, almost four years from the effective date of the law that the regulations implementing this single sentence were finally written and approved. Some 20 pages of *Federal Register*, three column print, was required to put into effect the intent of this one paragraph of the law.

The Rehabilitation Act Amendment of 1974 included a major amendment to the Randolph-Sheppard Act. This amendment provided more rights to the operators of vending stand programs developed under the authority of the Randolph-Sheppard Act. This amendment also provided for the profit of vending machines to revert to the vending stand operator in that building, or if there was no vending stand operator in that building, the profits of the vending machines would revert to the state agency.

Another major amendment to the Rehabilitation Act was passed in 1978. Included in that amendment was the establishment of the National Council on the Handicapped; Community Service Pilot Programs; and Projects with Industry, an effort to provide greater employment opportunities for individuals who had handicapping conditions.

The door for independent living rehabilitation was opened a crack as a result of the Rehabilitation Act of 1973. Through the 1978 amendments (U. S. Congress, House, 1978), comprehensive services for independent living were authorized. Title VII, Part A related to comprehensive services; Part B provided for centers for independent living; Part C authorized funding for independent living services for older, blind individuals; and Part D related to protection and advocacy of individual rights.

Major amendments to the Developmental Disabilities Services and Facility Construction Act were included in this amendment to the Rehabilitation Act. For federal participation, the Developmental Disabilities Services and Facility Construction Act defined the term *developmental disability* to be a severe, chronic disability, manifested before the person attains age 22, is likely to continue indefinitely, results in substantial functional limitations in three or more areas of major life activity, and reflects the person's needs for a combination and sequence of special, interdisciplinary, or generic care, treatment, or other services which are of lifelong or extended duration and are individually planned and coordinated (U. S. Congress, House, 1978, Title V, Section 503).

The Rehabilitation Act Amendment of 1986 established the qualifications for the Commissioner of the Rehabilitation Services Administration. Additionally, through this amendment, supported employment became a reality.

Purpose/Structure

The original purpose of the vocational rehabilitation program enacted in 1920 prescribed that persons, disabled in industry or otherwise, be provided vocational rehabilitation counseling, training, and job placement assistance toward the accomplishment of their return to self-sufficiency and employment activity in industry (Burress, 1980).

The rehabilitation system developed the rehabilitation process, an organized system for the delivery of prescribed services of a psychosocial, medical, and vocational nature to assist the rehabilitation counselor determine the need, eligibility, feasibility, and services necessary for a person with a disability to achieve a vocational goal. Prior to 1973, a rehabilitation plan was developed with, or for, the client. In the development of the plan, it was necessary to evaluate the client to determine the disabling conditions, and what services might reduce the effects of the disability. The rehabilitation counselor became the catalyst to effective rehabilitation. In the early days of rehabilitation, the resources were minimal. Medical services were not provided. The key was the vocational counseling, vocational training, and placement. Where needed, prosthetic devices could be procured and fitted.

In 1943, rehabilitation could serve the mentally ill and the mentally retarded. Although some states were making some progress with this group of individuals, it was not until after the 1954 VR amendments were implemented that this group became more accepted into rehabilitation counselors' caseloads. The training programs authorized under the 1954 amendments provided the knowledge and skills needed to work with this more severely disabled individual. The special projects allowed under the 1954 amendments made it possible for rehabilitation agencies to try new approaches. Increased funding and trained, competent rehabilitation counselors began to make progress in rehabilitating these individuals into employment.

Over the years, rehabilitation has changed the lives of the physically and mentally handicapped from a dependent status in society to one of social acceptance and economic independence. The people were able to enter the mainstream of American life.

Rehabilitation has been favorably treated by the United States Congress. This support has developed as a result of the success of the rehabilitation counselor in fulfilling the goal of Congress, that is, to rehabilitate people with disabilities into employment. It was not difficult to provide data that gave evidence that "rehabilitation pays." The taxes paid by rehabilitated clients far exceeded the cost of rehabilitation. As Congress provided increased funds and more favorable legislation, the numbers of people with disabilities successfully rehabilitated increased.

With the enactment of the Rehabilitation Act of 1973, Congress placed the emphasis on the rehabilitation of the severely disabled. As rehabilitation moves to fulfill its mandate, it is evident that the rehabilitation of clients with the more severe disabilities takes a longer period of time and the cost increases. Even so, when the various social service benefits that were paid to these clients are reduced or eliminated as the result of successful rehabilitation into employment, it can be shown that "rehabilitation pays." More importantly, the people with severe disabilities are entering the mainstream of American life. With the technology now available, people for whom there had been no potential, are being successfully rehabilitated into employment. Others, because of the severity of their disabilities, are being rehabilitated into independent living, with the hope that as technology increases, these individuals will have learned how to function independently and will also enter the mainstream of employment.

As medical technology, rehabilitation engineering, and other technologies advance, it will be the choice of the person with a disability not to be rehabilitated. It will no longer be a matter that technology is not able to take care of the needs of the individual.

UTILIZATION CRITERIA

The state-federal program of rehabilitation has very definite eligibility criteria. The program was not established to solve the problems of the world. The program was established to provide services to people who were physically disabled (and since 1943, mentally disabled), to prepare these individuals to enter the work force. Philosophically, rehabilitation is an effort to equalize the opportunity for employment of people with disabilities with their nondisabled counterpart.

To be eligible for rehabilitation services through the state-federal system (a) the individual must have a disability, physical or mental; (b) the disability must, for that individual, result in a substantial handicap to employment; and (c) there must be a reasonable expectation that identified rehabilitation services will make the individual more employable.

The first criteria can be established through medical and psychological examinations. This can be objectively determined. The second and third criteria are much more subjective, and it takes the expertise of the counselor with the interaction of the client to answer these. With the Rehabilitation Act of 1973, the client has, in fact, become a real partner in the determination of eligibility, as well in the determination of services that are needed.

The partnership of the counselor and client in no way diminishes the need for a trained, qualified counselor. To the contrary, it is even more important that the counselor has the knowledge and skills to translate technical information to the client in a way that can be used by the client. The partnership helps to ensure that the client has the opportunity to bring his or her expertise to the system.

Client Services

The vocational rehabilitation process is a sequence of rehabilitation services coordinated by a counselor with the understanding, agreement, cooperation, and coordination of the client. This case management approach, detailed in a previous chapter, involves specific "activities that facilitate the movement of each rehabilitant through the service process" (Wright, 1980). While an elaborate flow diagram/chart exists at the state-federal level to detail the particular steps, referred to as status codes, a generic description of client services is available from Bitter (1979) who outlines the vocational rehabilitation service paradigm as:
- Preliminary diagnostic study
- Thorough diagnostic study
- Extended vocational evaluations
- Individualized Written Rehabilitation Program

- Counseling and guidance
- Physical and mental restoration
- Training
- Job Placement
- Postemployment services

The focus of services is vocational preparation of the client for a return to work. To achieve this objective, considerable effort is expended to provide job-seeking skills training, direct placement interventions, trial employment, job development, and remediation of factors related to employer concerns. The end term services often lead to instruction in various recommended components (Rubin & Roessler, 1987) directed toward attainment and acceptable job maintenance behaviors. Specific training areas include: "(a) sources of good job leads, (b) employer expectations for prospective employees, (c) organization of the job search, (d) completion of job application blanks, (e) job interview training, and (f) supervised practice in job seeking." (p. 255)

Upon referral the vocational rehabilitation counselor seeks to assess:
- Personal demographic data
- Educational/training level
- Marital status/family status
- Primary source of support
- Sources of referral
- Major mental/physical disability and type
- Work status at referral
- Work history

During the rehabilitation process, questions which need to be answered concern:
- Psychological and vocational adjustment of the disabled
- Types of services provided
- Training/treatment services
- Time/cost of services

Work status/occupation at case closure

The Future of Rehabilitation

The future of the state-federal program of rehabilitation appears bright. The United States Congress continues to support the program. The funding level continues to grow even though the Congress seeks ways to reduce federal spending. The partnership with the states is intact. Rehabilitation has matured. Rehabilitation now recognizes that as it joins with others in solving problems related to disability, each entity becomes richer in aiding the person with a disability to become a true partner.

The American with Disabilities Act of 1990 has been passed by Congress and signed into law by President George Bush. President Bush has supported the passage of this Act and has used his good office in rallying support for the implementation. The Act is not a rehabilitation act. It is a Civil Rights Act for people with disabilities. This Act opens doors for people with disabilities. With the potential that this Act provides, the rehabilitation counselor should be able to make dramatic strides in improving job opportunities for people with disabilities. This will not be an easy job. Rehabilitation has never been an easy job. It is important for the counselor to become familiar with the act and its implementing regulations. People with disabilities have worked long and hard to get this legislation passed. It will be the rehabilitation counselor's responsibility to work with his or her client to be certain that the client's civil rights are protected, as well as aiding the client in becoming employable and employed.

References

Bitter, J. A. (1979). *Introduction to rehabilitation*. St. Louis: C. V. Mosby.

Burress, J. (1980). *Rehabilitation and legislation: Historical development of the vocational rehabilitation process*. Unpublished manuscript.

Obermann, C. E. (1965). *A history of vocational rehabilitation in America*. Minneapolis: T. S. Denison.

Rubin, S. E., & Roessler, R. T. (1987). *Foundations of the vocational rehabilitation process* (3rd ed.). Austin, TX: Pro-Ed.

U. S. Congress, House. (1973). *Public Law 93-112*. H. Report 8070, 93rd Congress.

U. S. Congress, House. (1978). *Public Law 95-602*. H. Report 12467, 95th Congress.

U. S. Department of Health, Education and Welfare, Social and Rehabilitation Service, Rehabilitation Services Administration. (1970). *50 years of vocational rehabilitation in the U.S.A. 1920-1970*. Washington, DC: U. S. Government Printing Office.

Wright, G. N. (1980). *Total rehabilitation*. Boston: Little, Brown.

Rehabilitation Facilities

Julie Kate O'Brien, Ph.D.

There are a variety of rehabilitation facilities in the United States that provide services for persons with disabilities. They may adhere to a vocational model, medical model, psychosocial model, or a combination of these models. The facility may provide a range of vocational opportunities or be specifically tailored to the avocational needs of persons with disabilities. Facilities are traditionally classified as sheltered workshops, work activity centers, transitional centers, or rehabilitation centers depending on their function.

A sheltered workshop involves piecework of a manufacturing nature in a segregated site. A segregated site implies that only persons with disabilities are employed in the actual work production. A work activity center provides services for persons who need to concentrate on work behavior development, rather than on earning a wage. Persons with disabilities who enter a transitional center can expect a relatively short term there. They receive evaluation and work adjustment development, and then move on to an appropriate employment opportunity. A rehabilitation center provides very comprehensive services, including medical restoration.

History/Legislation

The first program in the United States that resembled a rehabilitation facility was established in 1837. It was the Perkins Institution for the Blind and was located near Boston (Wright, 1980). During the beginning of the 1900s many programs developed by religious organizations began to emerge. Programs such as Goodwill Industries, St. Vincent de Paul, Volunteers of America, and the Salvation Army established sheltered workshops during the early 1900s (Bitter, 1979).

The development of facilities was greatly influenced by society's acceptance of persons with disabilities. The early programs provided services to veterans and persons with acquired disabilities, usually as a result of industrial accidents. Some societal members had difficulty moving past the archaic concepts that congenital disorders were random in their selection, not evidence of evil, and not just the individual family's responsibility. Providing services to persons with physical disabilities remained the status quo until the 1940s when programs for persons with mental retardation and mental illness emerged. Parents, advocacy groups, and legislative activity spurred the development of these services and eventually society moved in the direction of acceptance. Unfortunately, it is not until 1990, during the Bush administration, that a true civil rights act for persons with disabilities was signed into law (Americans with Disabilities Act, July 16, 1990).

Another influence on the history of facilities was the state and federal partnership vocational rehabilitation program. The state and federal program has been discussed in another chapter in this book in detail. It is interesting to note that the history of facility development is closely related to the expansion of the state and federal program. The original facilities supported by the state-federal program regrettably encouraged dependence of persons with disabilities on governmental programming and funding sources (e.g., sheltered workshops, Supplemental Security Income). Now, the trend is toward encouraging independence and programs which enhance life, that is, supported employment and the independent living movement. In summary, facilities have progressed from very segregated facilities to community-based programs which offer a continuum of options for persons with disabilities. They also have evolved from servicing specific disability groups, which society comfortably embraced, to persons with severe disabilities.

LEGISLATION

A review of legislation involving persons with disabilities further demonstrates the trends in facility development. The legislation review is presented in chronological order. Some landmark legal cases are also included due to their influence on service provision to persons with disabilities.

The Smith-Sears Rehabilitation Act of 1918 is often regarded as the parent of the vocational rehabilitation program, even though the focus was veterans and not civilians (Jenkins, 1987). It laid the premise that persons with disabilities needed societal help to reenter the world of work. The Smith-Fess Act of 1920 expanded rehabilitation services to the civilian population and developed the state and federal partnership program. The Social Security Act of 1935 provided stability to funding various programs and the lives of some persons with disabilities. The Social Security Disability Insurance (SSDI) program was initiated along with this Act. To be eligible for SSDI an individual had to:
- be under the age of 65;
- have a physical or mental condition that prevents substantial gainful work and is expected to last for 12 months, or is expected to result in death; and
- have a certain length of previous employment (Wright, 1980).

The Fair Labor Standards Act of 1938 authorized the Secretary of Labor to regulate subminimum wages earned by the handicapped (Matkin, 1983). The Randolph-Sheppard Act of 1938 provided an opportunity for persons with blindness to be gainfully employed, as it allowed for such persons to operate vending facilities on federal properties (Bitter, 1979). These programs are still in operation today, under the supervision of the state-federal partnership program. Rehabilitation services were extended to include persons with mental illness and mental retardation as a result of the Barden-LaFollette Act of 1943.

The Small Business Act of 1953 authorized a loan program for sheltered workshop expansion, and for persons with disabilities to operate their own businesses. The Vocational Rehabilitation Act of 1954 impacted directly on service delivery of facility programs. It authorized payment for vocational evaluation and work adjustment services (Wright, 1980). This act also provided for expansion and improvement programs of existing sheltered workshops and work activity centers.

During the 1960s, community-based and integrated service delivery systems emerged. The Mental Health Act of 1963 focused on developing community mental health centers. Deinstitutionalization, the movement of persons with disabilities out of large, state-funded institutions into a less restrictive environment in the community, began to occur (Fennessee, 1987). The Vocational Education Act of 1963 expanded and improved school-based vocational programs for students with disabilities.

The 1970s clearly demonstrated that persons with severe disabilities were being excluded from various programs, and that something had to be done. Much legal activity occurred during this period to begin to address this issue. In 1971, the *Griggs v. Duke Power Co.* case ruled employment procedures cannot be maintained if they cause discrimination. This opened the door for employment opportunities for persons with disabilities in the community. In 1972, the case of *Mills v. Board of Education* endorsed the rights of children with disabilities to educational placement in the least restrictive environment. In 1972, the landmark case of *Wyatt v. Stickney* endorsed the right to treatment and least restrictive environment for institutionalized persons. Also, in this year, *Pennhurst State School and Hospital v. Halderman* mandated that services to people with developmental disabilities must be served in the least restrictive environment (Flippo, 1980).

In 1973, the Architectural and Transportation Barriers Compliance Board, with the mission of ensuring that federally funded buildings and transportation systems were not discriminating against persons with disabilities, was developed. The needed physical access to the world of work for persons with disabilities was emerging. The Supplemental Security Income (SSI) program became effective in 1974. Persons with a total disability for one year or more and who did not qualify for SSDI were usually eligible for, and often received, medical insurance through the Medicaid program (Bitter, 1979).

The Education for All Handicapped Children Act passed in 1975. A continuum of educational options using the least restrictive concept was now required. The Carl Perkins Education Act of 1984 specified the inclusion of persons with disabilities, as well as other special interest groups, in vocational education programs. The Rehabilitation Amendments of 1986 demonstrated the concept of a continuum of options in vocational services. These amendments provided the supported employment program and emphasized service delivery to persons with severe disabilities.

FUNDING

There are a variety of funding sources available for rehabilitation facilities. This section presents four categories of funding sources. They are loosely classified as contractual, fee-for-service, fund-raising revenue, and donations/ private foundations.

Contractual funding involves a formalized intraagency agreement between the facility and another entity. The other entity might be a community-based agency in need of a specialized service offered by the facility. For example, most facilities have a contractual agreement with a major funding source such as a state's Department of Vocational Rehabilitation or Department of Mental Health and Developmental Disabilities. The contract will specify certain needed services, expected amount of clients to receive such services, possibly a specific eligible disability category, and assurances that the client's human and civil rights are protected. These contractual agreements may be called grant-in-aid programs.

Revenue is also generated by contractual production work. The sheltered workshop and supported employment participants complete work for which the facility receives reimbursement. The work may range from assembly and janitorial, to repetitive data entry tasks. Also, a facility may have a contract with the local school system for a service such as vocational assessment, job coaches, and work study placements for the district's special education students. Clarification of joint responsibilities (e.g., liability insurance, transportation) are usually included in the contractual agreement with a school district. The facility may be a subsidiary of a larger not-for-profit system (e.g., United Cerebral Palsy, Easter Seals) networks. Funds or advertising support from these national organizations are channeled to the local agency per a contractual agreement.

Progressive facilities are seeking new contractual opportunities. Facilities with bus fleets used on a limited time schedule may contract to provide senior citizen transportation. Seeking large research or innovative program grants may also provide additional funds to a facility. Also, contracting specific staff member's time and skills to other agencies in a consulting role may generate revenue. Fee-for-service involves the facility having a pricing structure for certain services. Two examples of purchasers of such services may be private insurance companies or workers' compensation attorneys. They would purchase needed services on an individualized basis. For example, an insurance company may need a situational assessment on a client who is adjusting to an acquired disability and, therefore, purchase these assessments on a fee-for-service basis.

Fund-raising efforts are usually an integral part of a facility's activities. Telethons, walkathons, and car washes not only generate funds, but provide community visibility for the facility and staff. Donations are often given to a facility by persons with an interest in persons with disabilities. A facility may have to diversify and establish a holding company if the facility receives many donations. The holding company permits more efficient handling of large donations which may produce interest. Donors may restrict funds to a certain agency function or allow the funds to remain unrestricted and, thus, used at the Board of Director's discretion.

These four funding sources are just a brief overview of possibilities. Facilities are always seeking alternative funding sources to decrease their dependence on state and federal fluctuating dollars. The future trend in funding is more collaboration with the private sector, rather than dependence on public monies.

UTILIZATION

Menz (1987) estimated that over 1.5 million individuals participate in services each year from over 5,500 sheltered workshops and 2,000 activity centers. Services will continue to increase as students with disabilities graduate from special education programs at the rate of 250,000 per year (Will, 1984). Due to medical advancements in treating persons with traumatic head injuries and their desire to return to the world of work, further expansion can be anticipated. The rehabilitation facility industry represents a $7.0 billion industry annually (Menz, 1987).

Greenleigh Associates (Wright, 1980) studied the types of disabilities people have who seek services from rehabilitation workshop programs. The primary disability (53%) was mental retardation, 19% of the persons had a diagnosis of mental illness, and 10% were persons with blindness. Also, approximately one-half of these persons had a secondary disability.

PERSONNEL

Job titles and descriptions for specific personnel vary due to a facility's mission, but certain generalities may be assumed. One can learn much about a facility's evolution towards community-based programming and its business orientation by the titles assigned to specific jobs.

Each facility will have a *Chairperson* or *President* of the Board of Directors. This person is elected to this volunteer position for a specified term. This person usually is a current board member, bringing to the position of chairperson experience with the facilities functions and needs. The chairperson interacts with the facility executive director or chief executive officer on a formal and informal basis and may or may not have a college degree. The qualifications for the position are usually community/business skills and interest in persons with disabilities. The board will also have *committee structure* responsible for certain functions, such as fiscal management, program direction, and personnel issues.

The *Executive Director* or *Chief Executive Officer* is the top management position in the facility. The person applying for this position usually has experience in the field of human services management, and is interviewed and hired by the Board of Directors. This person usually has a contractual agreement with the board. The executive director interacts with all personnel informally, but usually has a core management team. A bachelor's degree and more frequently a master's degree in a human service or business field are required for this level of management. The minimum skills for this job are fiscal management, grant writing/coordination abilities, knowledge of the needs of persons with disabilities, and personnel management.

The *Fiscal Manager* or *Accountant* reports to the executive director and supplies the fiscal management committee of the Board of Directors with needed information. Often, this person may have one or two specialized staff reporting to them whose responsibilities may be divided by accounts payable and accounts receivable. The fiscal manager usually has a bachelor's degree, although there are many fiscal managers whose years of experience with the facility are more valuable than a degree.

The *Operations Manager* or *Production Director* usually is a member of the management team or may have the management team reporting to them, thus giving this position direct access to the executive director. This person may or may not have college training, as years of business experience are often more critical than formalized education. The minimum skills for this position are business connections, sales, and knowledge about production work.

The *Client Services Director* or *Program Director* is a member of the management team and has a variety of staff members reporting to him or her. This position usually requires a bachelor's degree in a human service field and more frequently a master's degree is required. This person often has a staff of *program managers* or *case managers* reporting to them who are responsible for coordinating services for a specific number of persons with disabilities. The minimum skills for this position are knowledge of accreditation standards and behavior management, ability to develop and write reports/plans, and crisis counseling.

The *Vocational Evaluator* is responsible for the completion of vocational evaluation services. (The purpose of vocational evaluation is described in the *Client Services* section of this chapter.) This person usually has a master's degree and may be certified as a vocational evaluator by the Commission on Certification of Work Adjustment and Vocational Evaluation Specialists (CCWAVES National Office: Rolling Meadows, Illinois). The minimum skills needed for this position are knowledge of standardized assessments, work samples, psychometric interpretations, situational assessment, behavior management, and the ability to document behaviors and observations and present all information in a written report format.

The *work adjustment specialist* or *skills trainer* is responsible for developing a person's work behavior and skills to their optimal level of functioning, or modifying assigned work tasks based on the person's functional capacities. This specialist may be involved in an extended situational assessment program or an activity day program. Work adjustment specialists may have a master's degree and maintain certification with CCWAVES. The minimum skills for this position are behavior management techniques, knowledge of job modifications and task analysis, and incentives for employers to hire persons with disabilities.

The *employment specialist* or *job coach* is responsible for providing on-the-job support to a person in a community-based, integrated setting. These specialists may have a college degree, but often have demonstrated knowledge of modifying work tasks to maximize a person's functional capacities. The minimum skills for this position would be very similar to the work adjustment specialist.

The *employer development specialist, placement specialist,* or *procurement specialist* is responsible for identifying possible job sites and addressing the needs of potential employers. These specialists may have a high school degree and have demonstrated skills in sales, knowledge of tax incentives for employers who hire persons with disabilities, and job matching abilities. These specialists must be able to efficiently work with many of the staff members in the facility organizational structure. They must enjoy a nontraditional work schedule.

The traditional organization structure of a facility would have all client services personnel on one side of the organizational chart and the production personnel on the other side. Many facilities have found it beneficial to blend these roles to eliminate some of the territorial issues and demonstrate the flexibility to be responsive to employers, employees, and disabled persons needs in a timely manner.

Client Services

Rehabilitation facilities offer a variety of services with the most traditional being vocational evaluation, work adjustment, adult activities, a continuum of employment options, and referral assistance (Button, 1970). Additional services which may be provided are leisure activity development, job seeking club, job retention club, case management, transportation/residential coordination, crisis counseling, and adult basic education. Reviewing the primary purpose of each service will illustrate the versatile role a facility may play in the lives of persons with disabilities.

VOCATIONAL EVALUATION

The purpose of vocational evaluation services is to assist a person and the referral source in determining the person's vocational options, potential, and interests (Menchetti & Rusch, 1988). A variety of methods are utilized in this process. Standardized assessment tools are one method used to determine a person's aptitude and achievement levels. Most of these assessment tools are paper and pencil tests which may frequently need to be modified to accommodate a person's functional abilities and/or educational achievement levels.

Work samples are also used by vocational evaluators. This is a method of observing a person's current skill level in completing a task which is representative of a specific job or a cluster of jobs. For example, if a person expressed an interest in being a small engine mechanic, then they would be requested to complete a work sample involving assembling and disassembling an actual small engine. The evaluator rates the person's performance on time completion and demonstrated skill level. There are a variety of commercially available work samples representing many diverse work tasks. Work samples also allow a person the opportunity to experience hands-on an unfamiliar work task, and possibly discover additional vocational interest areas.

Situational assessment is the vocational evaluation method in which a person is placed in situations where specific behaviors are observed and documented. Such observations are used in further clarifying vocational potential. An example of this assessment would be if an evaluator placed a person in a situation where he or she had to find certain offices and to do so would involve successful use of an elevator. This situation would allow the evaluator to document the person's directionality skills. These three vocational evaluation methods are not all inclusive of all the tools available to the evaluator, but are presented to demonstrate the purpose of vocational evaluation services.

Referral questions which may be proposed to the vocational evaluator by the referring agency or the individual are:

- What are the person's vocational interests?
- What are viable vocational alternatives for this person in a competitive or supported employment placement?
- Does this person demonstrate proficiency with two-step, five-step, and twelve+-step directions?
- What is the person's preferred learning style?
- This person has expressed a strong interest in a specific vocation, in your opinion is such a vocation viable? Why or why not?

WORK ADJUSTMENT

The purpose of work adjustment "is to assist the vocational handicapped to improve their ability to function in work situations" (Pruitt, 1983). This service may be provided by many facility personnel ranging from a work adjustment specialist to a job coach.

Situational assessment methods are often used by work adjustment specialists in the manner that a job try-out is utilized. The person may be placed on a job task for a certain length of time. The time may range from one week to four weeks depending on the person's needs and funding agreements. Needed intervention strategies with respect to the person's ability to learn tasks, adjust to changes, interact with others, make decisions, and seek help when needed are observed and developed.

These services, though once tied to a facility-based, adult skills program format, are being integrated into community-based experiences. Once the concept was to train and then place a person in the job. Now it is understood that many persons with disabilities have difficulty generalizing a task from one environment to the next (Szymanski, Hanley-Maxwell, Hansen, & Meyers, 1988). Therefore, the model of placing a person in the actual work environment, and then providing the needed training and work adjustment, is more appropriate.

Examples of referral questions posed to a work adjustment specialist would be:

- What job modifications and/or job aids might this person need to maintain a regular work schedule?
- What verbal cues/prompts proved successful with this person in respect to work productivity?
- How should an employer successfully instruct this person in regards to a change in the assigned work tasks?
- Due to the person's functional capacities, how should the work environment be modified for safety issues?
- If a job coach is assigned to this person, what information would be helpful for this coach to know?

WORK ACTIVITIES

These services may involve a prevocational training class, but include a variety of additional activities. Persons with disabilities receiving this service would attend classes involving such activities as cooking, survival skills for the community, grooming/hygiene development, and vocational skill development. The participants in the work activities programs hopefully graduate into programs with more vocational training emphasis.

Examples of referral questions submitted to an adult activities specialist would be:

- What personal care assistance will this person need if they are to obtain independence in the residential environment?
- What level of residential placement appears appropriate for this person?
- Has this person obtain his or her maximum functional reading abilities, or would further training be of benefit?
- What level of money management skills is optimal for this person?
- What assistance will this person need to maneuver through the community transportation system?

EMPLOYMENT OPTIONS

Most facilities today offer a continuum of employment options or are striving to develop a continuum. Historically, a person referred to a facility would complete a vocational evaluation experience and work adjustment program with the majority of the outcomes being a work assignment in the shelter workshop program. Placement in this program would be based on the persons demonstrated productivity level, and work behaviors. If the person was more appropriate for a competitive job in the community, then the initial referring agency would resume the case or the facility may have had a placement specialist assume the placement responsibilities.

Today, the placement options provided by facilities have expanded. On one end of the continuum of options, may be a sheltered workshop program in a segregated site. Such a site would involve persons with disabilities completing the work tasks and payment would be based on a piece rate basis and sub-minimum wage. Another option may be an integrated work force of persons with and without disabilities completing assigned work in a building which once housed a segregated, traditional sheltered program. A third option may be a mobile work crew and/or enclave, which is typically a small group of persons working at a variety of sites throughout the community. This involves an employment situation where the person with the disability is placed on a job in the community, with a job coach providing support initially, with the goal of developing a natural support system for the person. Supported employment positions must involve at least 20 hours of work per week in an integrated setting. Of course, there is the option of a community-based job with competitive wages and no support other than placement assistance. This would represent the concept of least restrictive employment environment.

Examples of referral questions regarding placement would be:

- If you deem this person most appropriate for a segregated work site, why did you rule out supported and competitive employment?
- Does the selected job placement represent the person's expressed vocational interest, or was the area of interest not available locally or inappropriate?
- Do you see the person transitioning from the current suggested placement level to another level within the next 18 months?

REFERRAL ASSISTANCE

Many rehabilitation facilities find persons in the community engaging or contacting their community-based personnel regarding diverse social service needs. The facility personnel are aware of the other social service programs available in their area due to networking and advocacy work on behalf of person with disabilities in their own program. Referral assistance to other programs is provided by most facilities. In the advent of dwindling social service dollars, facility personnel use other agencies and programs to assist the facility's own program participants and provide specialized services. Agencies frequently referred to by many facility staff are:

- Social Security Administration
- Mental health centers
- Legal Aid
- Health programs
- Accessible transportation systems

OTHER SERVICES

Other services which may be provided by facility personnel are leisure activity development, job seeking club, job retention club, adult basic education, case management, transportation/residential coordination, and crisis counseling. Leisure activity development has become an identified need during the last decade of service delivery. Often persons with disabilities are returning from their vocational programs and have no evening/weekend activities planned. This lack of balance in their lifestyle will eventually threaten the success of the vocational placement. Assistance is given to develop other activities so the vocational placement is not in jeopardy.

Job seeking and retention clubs are group meetings of persons in which they have the opportunity to develop their skills in these specific areas, or share their experiences and feelings. Adult basic education is the opportunity for persons attending facilities to receive additional academic training to earn a general education diploma (GED). By obtaining this diploma, these persons have the opportunity to pursue certain community college and technical school programs which are currently not accessible with a special education certificate of completion.

Case management is a service where a professional helps coordinate all needed services for a person with a disabilities, and not just the vocational development issues. It may include transportation and residential needs, as well as mental health issues. Case management often involves issues such as financial planning and budgeting, as well as protection of the person's human and civil rights.

Crisis counseling is often needed by persons with disabilities on a short-term basis while awaiting services from the mental health system. Usually, a facility will have designated, rather informally, the staff person who has the appropriate degree or skill to handle such crisis issues. For example, a person may arrive at the work site and share that a close family member had died during the evening. This person's mental health status needs to be addressed and a determination made if a formalized intervention by mental health professionals is needed.

References

Bitter, J. A. (1979). *Introduction to rehabilitation*. St. Louis: C. V. Mosby.

Button, W. H. (1970). Sheltered workshops in the United States: An institutional overview. In *Rehabilitation sheltered workshops, and the disadvantaged: An exploration in manpower policy* (pp. 3-79). Ithaca, NY: Cornell University.

Fennessee, W. T. (1987). *Factors in the growth of rehabilitation facilities in America: 1945-1975*. Unpublished Doctoral Dissertation. Carbondale, IL: Southern Illinois University.

Flippo, E. B., Jr. (1980). *Personnel management*. New York: McGraw-Hill.

Jenkins, W. M. (1987). Rehabilitation history and legislation. In R. M. Parker (Ed.), *Rehabilitation counseling: Basics and beyond*. Austin, TX: Pro-Ed.

Matkin, R. J. (1983). The roles and functions of rehabilitation specialists in the private sector. *Journal of Applied Rehabilitation Counseling, 14*(1), 14-27.

Menchetti, B. M., & Rusch, F. (1987). Vocational evaluation and eligibility for rehabilitation services. In P. Wehman & M. S. Moon (Eds.), *Vocational rehabilitation and supported employment* (pp. 79-90). Baltimore: Paul H. Brookes.

Menz, F. (1987). An appraisal of trends in rehabilitation facilities: 1980 to 1984. *Vocational Evaluation and Work Adjustment Bulletin, 20*(2), 67-74.

Pruitt, W. A. (1983) *Work adjustment*. Menomonie, WI: Walt Pruitt Associates.

Szymanski, E., Hanley-Maxwell, C., Hansen, G., & Meyers, W. (1988). Work adjustment training, supported employment and time-limited transitional employment programs: Context and common principles. *Vocational Evaluation and Work Adjustment Bulletin, 21*(2), 41-45.

Will, M. (1984). *OSERS programming for transition of youth with severe disabilities: Bridges from school to working life*. Washington, DC: Office of Special Education and Rehabilitative Services, U. S. Department of Education.

Wright, G. N. (1980). *Total rehabilitation*. Boston: Little, Brown.

Private Rehabilitation

Ralph E. Matkin, Ph.D.

Working in the private sector offers some of the most exciting and challenging opportunities for rehabilitation service providers. It can be a source of financial reward and immense personal satisfaction, or it can be a hostile environment that overwhelms one's confidence. Although more and more rehabilitation practitioners (trained by programs with traditional curricula focused on public agency work activities) are seeking private employment opportunities, few seem to be aware of the demands placed on them by referral sources, clients, and professionals. Even fewer appear to be aware of the degree to which their rehabilitation knowledge and skills are transferable to diverse markets and practices.

The purpose of this chapter is to provide readers with an encapsulated foundation of practical information about private rehabilitation employment. Although the framework is based on a rehabilitation counseling perspective, the emphasis is on information about how the private sector operates, who are its significant "players," what to expect, and how to help consumers through the maze of insurance-based rehabilitation programs.

History/Legislation

HISTORY

The word *rehabilitation* means the act of restoring something or putting it back to a condition in which it should be. In sociological terms, it means restoring to a state of physical, mental, and moral health through treatment and training. Such definitions suggest that rehabilitative care has been provided to others long before there were identified programs systematically designed for that purpose. In current terms, however, a national movement towards increased private employment opportunities in the field of rehabilitation appears to have started on January 1, 1975 in California.

Private (for-profit) rehabilitation became a viable alternative to traditional public and private not-for-profit employment opportunities when California enacted section 139.5 of its labor code to mandate vocational rehabilitation services for eligible workers' compensation claimants. Colorado and Georgia passed similar laws the same year, as well as subsequently enacted in Alaska, Florida, Hawaii, Kansas, Louisiana, Maine, Massachusetts, Minnesota, New Mexico, and Washington. Among these states, however, Washington revoked its vocational rehabilitation component in 1985, followed by Colorado in 1987, while debated reexaminations continue in California, Florida, and Minnesota (LaFon, 1988).

Based on state initiatives since 1975, the phrase "private rehabilitation" today predominantly refers to assisting qualified *insurance* recipients to return to gainful employment. Without question, the largest volume of insurance-based referrals are workers' compensation claimants, followed distantly by related health coverages in government sponsored programs (e.g., Social Security Disability Insurance, Supplemental Security Income) and privately insured personal injury policies (e.g., medical coverage in automobile insurance). To understand the present context of private rehabilitation, it is important to be aware of the insurance-rehabilitation partnership roots.

The Compensation Principle

The compensation principle arose from employer-employee relationships that eventually were to shape modern worker benefit programs. Growing from the "common law rules" and employers' liability statutes (which were based on doctrines surrounding negligence), the workers' compensation principle abandoned the moral and legal concept of individual fault. In its place, emerged the idea that the hazards of work, and the employment relationship themselves, were reason enough for compensating job-related injuries. In other words, the concept of *liability without fault* served to relieve employers of liability from common law suits involving claims of negligence by attempting to achieve six basic objectives cited by the U. S. Chamber of Commerce (1990):

- Establishing predetermined, adequate, and prompt benefits for employees.
- Eliminating wasteful litigation and legal fees.
- Offering certainty of compensable payments.
- Promoting safety and health activities in the work place.
- Lowering the overhead expense ratios.
- Assuring medical and rehabilitative services.

LEGISLATIVE AUTHORITY AND FUNDING

The path between statements of principle and their translation into acceptable legislation often reveal many stumbling blocks and moments of uncertainty. The work of various state and federal commissions, investigating inequities of employers' liability laws, resulted in near unanimous condemnation of those systems. In their place, legislation was enacted which led to the current workers' compensation remedies. It is important to note, however, that workers' compensation statutes are found at both federal and state levels; the former applied to federal employees and other select groups, while the latter differs from state to state, as well as differs from federal acts.

Federal Statutes

Nearly 75% of all federal civilian employees are covered by a workers' compensation law. Of this number, nearly two-thirds are provided benefits by the Federal Employees' Compensation Act (FECA), while the other one-third are covered by the Longshore and Harbor Workers' Compensation Act. Employees of the remaining 25% under federal jurisdiction, generally, are covered by provisions contained in the Federal Employers' Liability Act (FELA), State Employers' Liability Acts, Jones Act, Railroad Retirement and Unemployment Insurance Acts, Social Security Act (covered in Section III of this book), Veterans Readjustment Act, Civilian Health and Medical Program of the United States (CHAMPUS), or related health and safety acts (NARPPS, undated).

1. FECA: Administered by the Division of Federal Employees' Compensation of the Office of Workers' Compensation, U. S. Department of Labor. Since its inception in 1949, the FECA remains one of the most liberal compensation laws in the country. FECA covers injuries which occur in the performance of one's job duties, as well as all diseases which are work related. There are only two classifications of disability; partial and total.

2. Longshore Act: Administered by the Division of Longshore and Harbor Workers' Compensation in the Office of Workers' Compensation, U. S. Department of Labor. The law covers injuries and all diseases arising from employment in U. S. maritime service. Both partial and total disability schedules are similar to FECA.

3. FELA: Employers are responsible for damages to employees for work-related injuries, but only for those injuries that occur as a result of employer negligence. Thus, the issue of comparative negligence (the extent to which the employer's negligence contributed to the injury) remains a relative matter in awarding compensation.

4. Jones Act (Merchant Marine Act of 1920): Injured seamen have three remedies: (a) maintenance and cure during any disability while one is on the ship's payroll; (b) suit for tort damages if negligence can be shown; and (c) suit for tort damages without proof of negligence, where there is evidence of an unseaworthy vessel or appliance.

5. Railroad Acts: Administered by the Railroad Retirement Board. Benefits begin immediately upon proof of a disability which is classified as either "permanent" (10 years of railroad service) or "occupational" (20 years of railroad

service or attainment of age 60 with 10 years of service and current employment with a railroad).

6. Armed Services Disability: Injury or disease incurred in, or aggravated by, active service in the line of duty.

7. Veterans Administration Disability: Available to veterans who were discharged or separated under conditions other than dishonorable discharge. Covers disability incurred in, or aggravated by, active service in the line of duty. Administered by the U. S. Department of Veterans Affairs (formerly the Veterans Administration).

8. Federal Coal Mine Health and Safety: Administered by the Division of Coal Mine Workers in the Office of Workers' Compensation Programs and Social Security Administration, U. S. Department of Labor. Provides benefits for total disability or death due to respiratory illnesses attributed to coal mining.

State Statutes

A basic, and often repeated, objective of workers' compensation on which there is broad agreement is that coverage under the acts should be universal. That is to say, compensation should be provided for all work-related injuries and diseases, as well as having a uniform statutory definition and eligibility criteria regardless of jurisdiction. For various historical, political, economic, or administrative reasons, however, no state law covers all forms of employment, although a fairly uniform statutory definition exists which extends benefits to personal injury caused by accidents arising from, or directly related to, employment (U.S. Chamber of Commerce, 1990). Although nearly nine out of every 10 American workers who are potentially eligible for work-injury compensation come under the jurisdiction of state laws, the remaining 12% must depend on state employers' liability legislation or tort law as their basic remedies.

1. Workers' Compensation: Three basic eligibility criteria are involved: (a) an injured worker must be employed in an occupation defined by the state's compensation laws; (b) the disability must be compensable in nature; and (c) there must be a causal relationship between employment (e.g., work activities performed) and the disability (Matkin, 1985). State workers' compensation programs are administered through the court system, a special state commission or board (usually part of the state office of labor), or a combination of both. Unlike federal statutes, there are generally five classifications of disability: (a) *temporary-total*—the injured employee is totally incapacitated for work beyond the day of the accident, but is subsequently able to return to work without permanent impairment; (b) *permanent-total*—the injured worker is injured permanently, which totally incapacitates him or her from carrying on a gainful occupation; (c) *temporary-partial*—the injured worker is partially incapacitated the day of the accident, but is able to continue working the same day, and is subsequently able to work without permanent impairment; (d) *permanent-partial* disability occurs

when there is a permanent loss of a member of the body; and (e) *fatality* covers an injury or illness that results in the employee's death.

2. Employers' Liability Acts and Tort Law: Both forms are designed to ensure that employees who are not protected by other compensation statutes have the right to sue for damages on the grounds of employer negligence, as well as prevent employers from using the three common law defenses (i.e., fellow-servant doctrine, assumption of risk doctrine, contributory negligence doctrine).

Employer-, Union-, Association-Sponsored, and Individually Purchased Compensation Systems

At least 23 different programs are available through one's employer, union, affiliation with a professional organization, and through individual purchase (NARPPS, undated). In each case, the worker pays either a portion or all of the cost for coverage. Among the most noteworthy disability compensatory programs are:

- Group Life: Provides coverage for total and permanent disability for full-time employees or members of an association or union who are covered by group life insurance.
- Travel Accident: Provides coverage for death or dismemberment resulting from an accident while traveling on company business for full-time employees or members of an association or union.
- Group Long- and Short-term Disability: Short-term plans are usually limited to nonoccupational disabilities that result in an inability to perform one's own occupation. Long-term plans usually define disability as an inability to perform one's own occupation for two years and any reasonably suitable occupation thereafter. Both plans are available to full-time employees.
- Group Life Insurance Total and Permanent Disability: Covers total and permanent disabilities of full-time employees who are covered by group life insurance benefits.
- Deferred Compensation: Provides compensation for termination from employment due to a disability.
- Association Disability Income: Provides compensation for the inability to perform one's occupation (with or without additional stipulations) to members of sponsoring associations.
- Individual Disability Income: Same as above, but purchased entirely by the individual seeking coverage.
- No-Fault Automobile Disability Insurance: Currently 26 states require all licensed drivers to carry this plan which provides compensation for disability due to an automobile accident.
- Automobile Insurance (other than no-fault): Coverage is similar to above for automobile owners/licensed drivers living in states that do not require no-fault coverage.
- Credit Disability Insurance: Coverage is available to those with outstanding debts through credit card use.

- Mortgage Disability Insurance: Coverage is available through the lending institution underwriting the cost of home or office purchase.
- Business Overhead Expense: Covers business costs while disabled for self-employed individuals.
- General Liability Insurance: Available to everyone and although the benefits are determined on a case-by-case basis, compensation may be related to loss of future earnings capacity, disfigurement, pain and suffering, medical expenses, and so on, based on an injury contributed to by fault or negligence of another party.

Finally, the cost of funding the compensation benefits cited is derived from the source of each program. For example, tax dollars may be the source of revenues for publicly sponsored compensation plans, while private enterprise generally is the source of funding for plans offered to unions, associations, employers, and individual policy holders. Rehabilitation practitioners generally have their fees paid by the group which administers the compensation program (e.g., Office of Workers' Compensation Programs in federal coverage, private insurance companies in state and individual cases). It is also important to note that each program may have "fee schedules" that affix a ceiling reimbursement for services rendered. California, for example, enacted legislation in 1991 which limits the fees that rehabilitation professionals can charge for various services provided to eligible workers' compensation claimants. At the federal level, the Social Security Administration pays a fixed amount per case for vocational expert testimony in disability hearings.

PERSONNEL

It is unlikely that an absolute number of professionals working in private rehabilitation can be defined accurately. Among the reasons for this uncertainty are: (a) *rehabilitation* is a term that is not solely confined to human service professions (e.g., urban rehabilitation, home rehabilitation; there was even a job announcement for a "rehabilitation counselor" in the Detroit Free Press in 1985 that called for expertise in building renovation and city planning!); (b) the term rehabilitation connotes an occupational field composed of many human service professions; and (c) practitioners tend to identify with their respective professions (e.g., counselor, nurse, occupational therapist, physical therapist, physician) rather than as a more generic *rehabilitationist*. In 1988, for example, the Office of Employment Services (OES) reported over 707,000 "vocational rehabilitation consultants" working in such standard industrial classification (SIC) codes as public and private education, job training and related services, amusement and recreation services, bowling and billiard establishments, beauty shops, and museums-zoos-botanical gardens to name a few (Vertek, 1990)!

Specializations

During the development of the Certified Insurance Rehabilitation Specialist (CIRS) national examination by the Board for Rehabilitation, over 3,400 practitioners participated in its initial validation (Matkin, 1987). Data from that project revealed perhaps the most comprehensive description of those who perceive themselves as working in private rehabilitation: administrators, job development/ placement specialists, nurses, occupational therapists, physical therapists, psychologists, rehabilitation counselors, rehabilitation educators, supervisors of rehabilitation personnel, vocational evaluators, and work adjustment specialists.

The variety of job titles CIRS practitioners noted above represent educational training commensurate with their professional affiliations ranging from three-year registered nursing programs to doctorates. In that regard, entry into private rehabilitation may be further restricted by state licensing, certification, and registry requirements necessary to practice one's chosen occupation. In 1991, for example, 33 states require counselors in the private sector to be licensed or otherwise registered in their jurisdictions of practice. CIRS practitioners primarily work for private rehabilitation firms that specialize in serving workers' compensation claimants, in insurance companies overseeing cases referred to direct service providers, and in private practice (Matkin, 1987).

TRAINING

First and foremost, practitioners who work in the private sector must be trained and skilled in the academic disciplines they represent as professionals. Assuming that private rehabilitation professionals are skilled administrators, counselors, nurses, psychologists, physicians, and so forth, they must also learn to adapt their professional abilities to the accountability, regulatory, and economic demands of the insurance industry, which is the principal fee payer for clients who are referred for services. Five content areas have been identified by the CIRS examination (Matkin, 1991) as the contextual knowledge base composed of:

- Disability Legislation: Content covers areas of federal legislation pertaining to issues about accessibility, equal employment opportunities, rights of people with disabilities, regulations and criteria of federal programs of insurance compensation (e.g., FECA, Social Security), and other statutes affecting provision of rehabilitative human services.
- Rehabilitation Service and Care: Content covers basic areas of rehabilitation services provided to people with disabling conditions, treatment and practice required to care for a variety of physical and emotional conditions, and vocational aspects of disabling conditions.
- Vocational Assessment and Job Placement: Content covers identification of functional impairments, the relationship of disabling conditions to the functional requirements of a variety of work activities, methods and techniques used to analyze, modify, or restructure jobs and work environ-

ments, information required to perform labor market surveys, and techniques used to develop job openings and secure employment for people with disabilities.

- Forensic Rehabilitation: Content covers the activities involved in preparing for, and delivering, expert testimony in legal and quasilegal arenas such as administrative law hearings, depositions, and court cases.
- Case Management of Human Disabilities: Content covers activities involved in managing the case of one client, as well as managing many client cases simultaneously.

Purpose/Intent

Is there a need for rehabilitation to exist in the private sector? First, private rehabilitation offers an alternative to an otherwise public service monopoly. Second, consumers have more opportunity to select providers who can tailor their services to unique consumer needs and desires. Third, privatization offers more potential employment opportunities for trained human service providers, particularly for those entering and graduating from rehabilitation counselor training programs. Fourth, the variety of, and ever-changing, work demands placed on private rehabilitation practitioners compel training programs to assess the content of their curricula more frequently. Fifth, privatization compels practitioners to maintain and upgrade their knowledge and skills as new technologies develop in order to remain professionally competent and competitive. Sixth, the emergence of private rehabilitation has spurred professional organizations to develop more comprehensive guidelines of acceptable conduct for their memberships. Seventh, privatization has increased the emergence of professional "credentialing" and occupational status among the newer human service disciplines (e.g., rehabilitation counseling). Eighth, state-required and issued credentials can potentially increase state revenues. Finally, privatization provides greater opportunities for information about rehabilitation to be circulated to the public in order for people to make more informed decisions about service selection and qualifications of care givers.

How has private rehabilitation continued to exist, and what are its chances for survival? Rehabilitative services provided in the private sector have survived because of public demand, practitioner competence, and legislative lobbying by professional disciplinary organizations. Needless to say, survival of private rehabilitation, first and foremost, depends on the quality of the practitioners' skills who decide to enter this arena. In the absence of such skills, not only would public confidence decline and demand decrease, but political support would erode despite lobbying efforts by organizations to influence legislators favorably on behalf of their members.

GOAL

Based on the fact that approximately 80% of all private rehabilitation practitioners deal with workers' compensation recipients referred by insurance companies and self-insured employers (Matkin, 1985), the primary goal of individualized client planning is *return to work*. The following hierarchy reported by Matkin (1985) punctuates this philosophy:
1. Return the client to work performing the same job with the same employer.
2. Return the client to work performing the same (but modified) job with the same employer.
3. Return the client to work performing a different job, that capitalizes on transferable skills, with the same employer.
4. Return the client to work performing the same or modified job with a different employer.
5. Return the client to work performing a different job, that capitalizes on transferable skills, with a different employer.
6. Return the client to work performing a different job, that requires extensive or prolonged retraining, with the same or different employer.
7. As a last resort, return the client to work in a self-employed capacity. (pp. 73-74)

The *return-to-work* philosophy and goal of private rehabilitation has a direct bearing on the nature and duration of services offered by the majority of practitioners contained in the next section.

Client Services

DESCRIPTION OF SERVICES

To meet the challenge of returning disabled clients to competitive employment, a sequential set of services are set in motion that outwardly resemble those performed in the public rehabilitation sector: evaluation, treatment, training, job placement, and follow-up monitoring. In addition to these primary service categories, important subcategories include medical case management, vocational counseling, job analysis, labor market surveying, and vocational-oriented testimony. Finally, as private sector practice expands, a handful of rehabilitation professionals are using their vocationally oriented knowledge to offer specialized services in areas such as employer-based employee assistance programs, functional capacity assessment, work hardening, pain management, medical care cost containment research and consultation, life care planning, estimating future lost earnings, consultation with organized labor, career guidance and counseling, employment agency consultation, architectural and transportation barrier assessment consultation, health care planning, child and family services, substance abuse treatment, orientation and mobility training, supported employment services, client assistance programs, special education, independent living programming, and program evaluation.

Medical Case Management

The goals of this service are: (a) to minimize the recovery period without jeopardizing medical stability; (b) to assure proper medical treatment and other restorative services in a timely and sequential manner; and (c) to assist in medical cost containment (Matkin, 1985). The function of the medical case coordinator is to establish treatment goals in concert with participating medical personnel, planning discharge from the medical/ treatment facility, and monitoring the recovery process.

Vocational Counseling

This service is difficult to perform without a formal (i.e., testing) or informal (i.e., background information processing) assessment of vocational strengths and weaknesses. The activities of vocational counseling involve: (a) gathering and assessing past work history and other work-related (e.g., hobbies, avocational interests) activities in relation to future vocational choices; (b) assessing the significance of the presenting disability in terms of functional capacity for similar and related jobs; (c) exploring (with the client's active participation) feasible alternative career choices; (d) reviewing materials and reports concerned with medical, educational, and training issues; (e) discussing factors related to acceptable work adjustment; (f) assessing the consistency of a client's vocational choices with personality, medical condition, and other significant vocational factors; (g) interpreting test results to clients in a vocational choice context; and (h) consulting with experts in related areas to determine the likelihood of job placement before recommending a specific vocational goal.

Job Analysis

The purpose of job analysis is to determine what jobs are and to define their limits; that is, where job activities begin and end. To accomplish this purpose in the most meaningful and useful manner, jobs should be analyzed as they exist, in the setting where they exist, and at the time they exist. These activities require: (a) becoming familiar with the technologies and terminology associated with the job to be studied; (b) arranging with the employer for the analysis to occur; (c) performing the job analysis; (d) reviewing the results with all concerned parties; (e) noting additional, omitted, or modified activities; and (f) reporting the results.

Labor Market Surveying

Before recommending a vocational goal or implementing job search strategies, conducting a labor market survey is essential. Labor market information indicates what jobs exist, estimates their frequency in the economy of a given region, and forecasts their growth or decline in the future. Activities involved in performing such a survey include: (a) acquiring current employment statistics from a local office of the U. S. Department of Labor (an excellent source is the local regional office of a state's Employment Development Department); (b) using the U. S. Department of Labor's biannually published *Occupational Outlook Handbook* to find organizations to contact in specific job fields; (c) contacting local training sites and employers to learn their specific job requirements and application criteria; and (d) reporting findings about estimated long-range and short-term openings, upward or lateral career opportunities within the job, entry level and ceiling earnings, and specific employee qualifications that are required (e.g., physical capacity, education, experience, job temperament).

Vocational-Oriented Testimony

Providing expert witness testimony requires much more than a passing familiarity with legal and quasilegal (administrative) systems. First, it is essential to have the recognized credentials of one's profession. Second, it is essential to have a "track record" of training and experience in the area in which one is offering expert opinion. One must be thoroughly familiar with methods of legal inquiry (i.e., subpoenas, depositions, direct examination, cross examination, redirect and recross examinations, hypothetical questions). Third, it is essential to know the difference between the allowable parameters constituting "expert opinion" and "(common) opinion." Finally, it is essential to know one's legal limits of confidentiality, and other issues pertaining to one's professional ethical standards.

TYPICAL REFERRAL QUESTIONS

The information requested from private sector rehabilitation professionals depends on the nature of the referral source (e.g., state workers' compensation board, federal workers' compensation system, insurance representative, applicant attorney, defense attorney, hearing office/judge), the reason for referral (e.g., medical, psychological, and vocational evaluation, future lost earning capacity), and the service offered by virtue of the practitioner's training. Some typical referral questions to expect include:

- What is the nature and extent of the client's disability?
- Can the client return to his or her usual and customary occupation? If not, what residual functional capacity does the client have that can be used to qualify for other substantial gainful employment?

- What are the jobs the client can perform without additional training? What are the jobs the client can perform with minimal (on-the-job) training?
- How many jobs are currently available in the client's immediate residential area that he or she is qualified to perform with little or no training? What do they pay?
- What is the long-range and short-term outlook for jobs in a given field in the client's immediate area of residence?
- How long will it take for the client to resume competitive employment?
- Is it possible for an employer to modify a job to accommodate the client's disability? If yes, what modifications are necessary, will modifications restrict able-bodied employees from performing the job if the client is absent, and how much will the modification(s) cost?
- What are the client's vocational interests, aptitudes, and abilities? What are transferable to other jobs?
- How cooperative and motivated is the client?
- What are *your* fees? How long have you been practicing? What professional credentials do you have? How many similar cases have you had in the past year? How long have you been located in this area? How soon can you deliver a report?

References

LaFon, R. H. (1988). The past, the present and future: How can we avoid the pitfalls and realize the potential of vocational rehabilitation. *Journal of Private Sector Rehabilitation, 3,* 75-84.

Matkin, R. E. (1985). *Insurance rehabilitation: Service applications in disability compensation systems.* Austin, TX: Pro-Ed.

Matkin, R. E. (1987). Insurance rehabilitation job tasks, associated knowledges, and recommended training sites. *Journal of Private Sector Rehabilitation, 2*(1), 3-54.

Matkin, R. E. (1991). *Revalidated content areas of the certified insurance rehabilitation specialist (CIRS) national examination.* Unpublished report to the Certification of Insurance Rehabilitation Specialist Commission, Rolling Meadows, IL.

NARPPS. (undated). *Disability compensation systems.* Blue Jay, CA: National Association of Rehabilitation Professionals in the Private Sector.

U. S. Chamber of Commerce. (1990). *Analysis of workers' compensation laws.* Washington, DC: Author.

Vertek, Inc. (1990). *Occupational access system: Job match* (ver. 1.1) [Computer program]. Bellevue, WA: Author.

Work-hardening Programs

V. Robert May III, Rh.D.

Work hardening has evolved from the early 1980s into a dominant, highly structured work evaluation and treatment protocol originally tailored for the private vocational and industrial rehabilitation sectors (Matheson, 1988; May, 1988a). State rehabilitation agencies quickly noticed how effective work hardening was in resolving disability issues presented by injured workers who were managed by private sector case managers. The subsequent state agency response was to modify and adapt work-hardening program models in state vocational evaluation centers, thus allowing the work-hardening movement to have a pronounced influence in both rehabilitation sectors.

The rapid growth and prominence of this vocational evaluation and therapeutic treatment program lends itself to the cost-containment efforts of the private health insurance sector during the early to mid-1980s (May, 1986). In an attempt to curtail medical insurance costs and expenses, health care benefit providers devised innovative but controversial payment systems (i.e., the Diagnostic Related Groups [DRG], Medicare freeze of physician fees). Under the current DRG system, funding is predicated on the type of illness, rather than on the actual patient need (May & Reifsteck, 1986). Thus, patient exposure to medical and rehabilitation treatments is greatly reduced, and with medicare payments providing approximately 40% of an average hospital's income, public and private hospitals' revenue bases have experienced significant cuts. To counter decreased revenues, hospitals, private physician groups, and independent health care centers have had to focus on attracting markets with guarantee payment systems which are protected by state law (i.e., workers' compensation insurance payment systems). By the nature of its program design and funding appeal, work-hardening program development "exploded"; its position of prominence has become unparalleled, and work hardening has become a "buzzword" in rehabilitation, industrial medicine, labor law, and the nation's media (Matheson, 1988).

DEFINITION

Work hardening is a combined evaluative and treatment process originally designed to resolve disability or dysfunctional issues confronting industrially injured workers. The early, developmental stages of work hardening limited the scope of this definition to suggest that it is a work-oriented treatment program that has as an outcome which is measured in terms of improvement in the client's productivity (Matheson, Ogden, Violette, & Schultz, 1985). However, as work-hardening development progressed, its seemingly simplistic definition became more diversified and complex. Matheson (1988) upgraded his definition such that this process is now defined as a prescriptive, individually structured productivity development program that uses conditioning tasks and simulated work activities that are graded to present to the disabled worker increased work demands to improve work tolerances and facilitate a return-to-work status. A more practical interpretation suggests that work hardening combines job simulation, physical and emotional conditioning with that of physical work capacity evaluation to achieve a return-to-work outcome (May, 1988a).

History/Legislation

Work hardening has many different forms depending on the specific influence of the discipline managing the outpatient, industrial rehabilitation program. For example, industrial rehabilitation programs with work-hardening components managed by physical therapists will have a strong physical therapy influence in its program goals/objectives, as well as in its delivery of services. Similarly, programs managed by occupational therapists will have that discipline's influence in service delivery and program goals/objectives, and the state agency vocational evaluation centers which offer work-hardening services will demonstrate a strong vocational evaluation/case management influence. However, regardless of what discipline manages the work-hardening program, the present form of work hardening, as practiced across the United States, Canada, and Australia, was developed at Rancho Los Amigos Hospital in Downey, California, by Matheson (Matheson et al., 1985). Programs modeling Matheson's concepts have been described by practitioners including Bettencourt, Carlstrom, Brown, Lindau, and Long (1986), Matheson (1984), Matheson and Ogden (1983), Matheson et al. (1985), May (1985, 1986, 1988a, 1988b), May and Reifsteck (1986), May, Stewart, and Barnes (1986), Stewart, Peacock, Parsons, and Johnson (1985), and White (1986).

Matheson et al. (1985) and May (1988a) traced work-hardening program evolution to the early professional developmental efforts of occupational therapy leaders, beginning with the *work cure* movement for World War I veterans by *reconstruction workers* (as the first occupational therapists were called), and culminating with the profession's focus on industrial work-therapeutic programming in the 1980s (May, 1988a). Matheson et al. (1985) traced the occupational therapy influence to its development of industrial therapy programs in mental hospitals. These programs were well developed by the late 1930s, and were defined as the prescribed use of activities inherent to the hospital operation, planned for the mutual benefit of the patient and the institution. Occupational therapy programs originally adopted craft activities which provided bedside occupations for patients and assisted in the selection of appropriate types of vocational training for the patients (May, 1988a). However, as the industrial programs evolved within the hospitals, various jobs were analyzed within the institution and assigned to patients according to skill level, physical demands, and mental demands (Matheson et al., 1985). The occupational therapists coordinated work assignments insuring that proper patient/job matches were achieved (i.e., patient's worker trait profile met aptitudes, interests, experiences, and therapeutic goals).

The craft approach to simulated work, as cited in May (1988a), fell into discord with the medical profession in the early 1950s due to the medical community's increasingly scientific approach to disease and treatment, thus claiming that craft therapy lacked scientific rationale. Therefore, the medical profession proved to be the influential body that compelled the occupational therapy profession to accept and apply *work* therapy as it is regarded in private sector industry (i.e., specific work skill development, remuneration for work performed, work conditioning).

Certain legislation, combined with the medical profession's endorsement, facilitated the occupational therapy profession's prominence in work-hardening program development. The passage of the Vocational Rehabilitation Act of 1920 provided funding for states to develop vocational rehabilitation programs for disabled persons (May, 1988a). This Act provided occupational therapy administrators the justification to include in their program goals, the development of vocational evaluation components with the focus being to return the patient to gainful employment (May, 1988a). Hospital program expansion for occupational therapists was perpetuated by subsequent amendments to the 1920 Act in 1943 and 1954 (Barden-LaFolette Act, P. L. 113; Vocational Rehabilitation Amendments of 1954, P. L. 565). This legislative activity expanded the populations eligible to receive vocational rehabilitation services to include patients with psychogenic illnesses and those in need of physical restoration (May, 1988a). Occupational therapy programs based in hospital settings were ideally structured to service these new eligible populations.

As opportunities for occupational therapists regarding vocational rehabilitation program development became abundant in the late 1940s and early 1950s, curative workshops evolved (Matheson et al., 1985). The primary function of these workshops was to restore the impaired body part to as normal function as possible, with return to work as the eventual goal. These workshops used graded activities to improve function, and were often planned in accordance with the patient's physical demands of his or her job (May, 1988a). Thus, the first *work-hardening* programs were put into practice, paving the way for the more sophisticated models practiced today.

The vocational evaluation component of the work-hardening process evolved during this period with the aide of the occupational therapy professional movement. Prior to this period, occupational therapists used work samples they had developed from their earlier days in the work cure movement. The early 1950s period lacked appropriate evaluation tools, or tools which lacked validation criteria and normative data (May, 1988a). This void was filled by the efforts of the Institute for the Crippled and Disabled Rehabilitation and Research Center in New York City (May, 1988a). This research facility developed the *Tower* evaluation work-sample system, which was the first effort towards establishing normative data for individual performances for specific work tasks (May, 1988a). As a result, occupational therapists employed in the curative workshops and other work-hardening industrial rehabilitation settings were sent for training in the *Tower* system.

The occupational therapy movement underwent a change in its therapeutic focus beginning in the late 1950s and early 1960s. During this period, occupational therapists returned to medical/physical rehabilitation centers in an attempt to develop a stronger professional identity (Matheson et al., 1985). However, by the late 1960s, occupational therapists had made the transition back into vocational rehabilitation centers, but with an emphasis on prevocational and work-adjustment programs. It would not be until the 1980s that the occupational therapeutic movement reached the status in industrial rehabilitation settings that it enjoys today. The emphasis in work hardening is on task analysis (simulated work activity with repeated measurement of the participant's progress) that evolved from the occupational therapy curative workshop movement, and the work sample developmental efforts of this professional body.

STAFF CONSIDERATIONS

Work-hardening program staff typically include a physical therapist and/or an occupational therapist. More recent program development literature has incorporated the expertise of the vocational evaluator (May, 1987). Additional staff members may include psychologists, the respective attending physician, program medical director, rehabilitation nurse, social worker, or vocational rehabilitation case manager. The exact team-member composite is contingent on the organizational structure of the facility (i.e., free-standing physical therapy/occupational therapy clinic, hospital, independent medical clinic, public rehabilitation facility).

What determines the constitution and complexity of the program, as well as the comprehensiveness of the team, is not so much what the facility administration prefers, but rather what funding in terms of insurance reimbursements are required to maintain solvency. It is well known that psychological services and vocational services have difficulty with reimbursement from third party insurance benefit providers. Workers' compensation benefit providers will not authorize payment for such services if preauthorization is not obtained. Thus, program administrators have a tendency to utilize the professionals who third party benefit providers recognize and accept for such funding (i.e., physical therapists, occupational therapists).

As noted above, program solvency supersedes staff composition considerations. More often than not, solvency is determined by the ability of the organization to secure patient-referral sources, either through various financial arrangements/ incentives with physicians or through securing contracts with local industry. Such contracts specify to the respective referral source which work-hardening programs will be financially accepted and supported. Thus, staff composition, expertise, or service delivery quality may have little bearing on whether or not an injured worker is referred to a particular program.

Purpose/Intent

The goal of industrial rehabilitation is to return injured workers to work (May et al., 1986). Thus, the primary work-hardening goal is to assist the injured worker in achieving a level of productivity (within the confines of a clinically controlled setting) that is acceptable in the competitive labor market (May, 1986). This process incorporates graded work activities as conditioning tools, and assists the injured worker in reaching selected critical demands (i.e., those demands that are more likely to produce symptoms that limit work tolerances) and developing worker traits (Holmes, 1985; Matheson & Ogden, 1983). Thus, work hardening assists a person with developing a sufficient amount of physical stamina such that an eight-hour workday can be achieved with minimal discomfort.

Although appearing simplistic in scope, the work-hardening process is rather complex and conceptually involved. The *true* work-hardening program is based on the *Stage Model of Industrial Rehabilitation* developed by Matheson (1984). This model is presented in Table 1.

Pathology is defined as an injury or disease process (Matheson, 1988). This stage is where the injured worker's pathological findings are explored. The physician is the key team member at this stage, but other members may play a significant role in determining the decree of pathology.

Impairment is defined as the measurable consequence of pathology taken as a disruption of physical or mental integrity (Matheson, 1988). Again, physicians are responsible for this rating procedure.

Functional limitations are measured in terms of general tasks that are not specifically tied to any one role, but are found in many of the roles associated with each respective injured worker during the course of his or her daily activities. The injured worker's reports of symptoms and limitations are corroborated through behavioral observations of function.

Disability reflects the effects of functional limitations on one's daily roles, and is defined as the social consequence of the injured worker's functional limitations. The degree of disability is noted in the manner in which these functional limitations affect the injured worker's customary roles. The team member most associated with this assessment is the occupational therapist.

Table I. Stage Model of Industrial Evaluation*

Stage	Area Assessed	Measured By or In Terms Of
One	Pathology	Physicians, Psychiatrists, Psychologists
Two	Impairment	Physicians, Psychiatrists, Psychologists, Physical Therapists, Exercise Physiologists, Occupational Therapists
Three	Functional Limitations	Physicians, Psychiatrists, Psychologists, Physical Therapists, Exercise Physiologists, Occupational Therapists
Four	Disability	Occupational Therapists, Vocational Evaluators, Physical Therapists, Psychologists
Five	Feasibility	Occupational Therapists, Vocational Evaluators, Rehabilitation Counselors, Case Managers
Six	Employability	Occupational Therapists, Vocational Evaluators, Rehabilitation Counselors, Case Managers
Seven	Vocational Handicap	Occupational Therapists, Vocational Evaluators, Rehabilitation Counselors, Case Managers
Eight	Earning Capacity	Economists, Vocational Experts

*Adapted from Matheson, 1984.

Feasibility for competitive employment (vocational feasibility is defined as the acceptability of the injured worker as an employee to the employer). This stage is where the "patient" or "client" is first regarded as an "employee" in the industrial rehabilitation process, and specific work behaviors are assessed. The occupational therapist and the vocational evaluator are best suited for this stage, and work characteristics involving safety, productivity, and interpersonal behavior are assessed.

Employability, or the individual's ability to become employed within a certain labor market, is best reviewed by the occupational therapist, the vocational evaluator, and the rehabilitation case manager as a team. This stage is unique from feasibility in that while feasibility addresses the general acceptability of a person as an employee, employability addresses the ability for an individual to become employed within a particular labor market.

The *Vocational Handicap* concerns the individual's ability to become employed within a particular occupation. How the individual functions within the demands of a specific occupation is assessed, and the occupational therapist, vocational evaluator, and the rehabilitation engineer are the key team members to make this assessment.

The final stage, *Earning Capacity*, is best determined by the economist and labor market analyst, with support provided by the vocational evaluator and vocational expert. Earning capacity is measure in terms of work-generated income over the worker's life.

Applying the above stage model to a typical work-hardening program, the consumer will find that *Pathology* and *Impairment* have, or should have, been identified prior to the injured worker's admission to the program. The final stage, *Earning Capacity*, is a service which is typically reserved for litigation purposes, since one's change in earning capacity should have no bearing on that individual's functional potential to work. Attorneys will request this information to build a plaintiff's case for damages, or from a defense counsel's perspective, attempt to minimize damages if earning capacity can be shown to have been minimally influenced by the injured worker's post-work-hardening disability status.

Client Services

The true work-hardening program involves the injured worker in a simulated work environment, complete with similar work time schedules which include breaks and lunch periods. The injured worker is expected to spend between four and eight hours in the daily program, which may involve a consecutive day period totalling between one and six weeks. The program is designed to simulate the individual's customary work in terms of environment and tasks. The hourly work day, as well as task complexities, may be graduated with the goal being to achieve the worker's current job's physical exertional demands, environmental demands, and productivity criteria.

The admission's procedure to a work-hardening program is as complex as the actual treatment program. Before any individual is admitted to work hardening, it must be determined that the individual can benefit from the prescribed therapeutic regimen. This is best determined through one of several evaluation procedures.

WORK TOLERANCE SCREENING

This procedure is designed to address the physical capacity forms often submitted to physicians by case managers or insurance adjustors when questioning the physician about a worker's specific work-functioning parameters. Early development of this procedure was documented by Reuss, Rawe, and Sunquist (1958), and modification of their evaluation techniques was researched by Harrand (1986) who redesigned the procedure to fit in today's work hardening models.

Work tolerance screening is a three- to six-hour intensive evaluation procedure that measures the physical work performance factors that are basic to work output (Matheson & Ogden, 1983). More specifically, it assesses the worker's total functional work tolerances involving trunk and extremity strength and flexibility, maximum lifting capacity, general mobility, and tolerances for repetitive work capacity (May & Reifsteck, 1986). It also measures the worker's critical work demands, which are simulated in the controlled, clinical setting.

Work tolerance screening has two basic applications in work hardening. First, it can be used as a diagnostic tool with which to determine the need for further medical intervention versus proceeding with work-hardening treatment. Secondly, it can be used as a "benchmark" for determining the worker's progress during the therapeutic treatment program; it allows the rehabilitation team to pace the worker's program based on the physical limitations identified in the initial tolerance screening (Crewe, 1986; Reuss et al., 1958).

WORK CAPACITY EVALUATION

Work capacity evaluation (WCE) is defined as a comprehensive vocational evaluation process that usually takes place over three to five consecutive days, and assesses the person's vocational work tolerances, aptitudes, temperament, and attitudes, as well as work feasibility (i.e., safety, productivity, interpersonal work behaviors) (May, 1988a, 1988b). It also measures a person's ability to dependably sustain work performance in response to broadly defined work demands.

WCE is a multicomponent evaluation process, consisting of the work-tolerance screening procedure, vocational evaluation work samples and pencil/paper tests, and simulated work activities. This process may also utilize actual work equipment required of the employee to perform his or her job. It is this procedure which determines the injured worker's potential to benefit from work hardening, an essential criteria by which one is either accepted or rejected from the therapeutic program.

Today's programs may offer both evaluation procedures, but the WCE is the most popular of the two procedures. This is due to the evaluative comprehensiveness and the wealth of information that can be assimilated and processed before admitting the injured worker to the program. The Work Tolerance Screening is best applied in situations where time is a factor, or where the referral source desires to have a WCE form completed and no work-hardening program has been authorized or scheduled.

STANDARDIZATION CRITERIA

When an injured worker first enters a work-hardening program, that person should see an industrial appearing complex with many different types of industrial tools, standardized work samples, building supplies, treatment rooms, and staff offices. Programs offering physical therapy services in conjunction with the hardening procedures will include the treatment rooms, either separated by curtains or enclosed by walls. The square footage of the hardening floor may range between 500 to 10,000 sq. ft. The injured worker should begin the program with a clinical intake interview, followed by a work-capacity evaluation which includes a musculoskeletal screening and physical therapy assessment, and then a functional analysis provided by either the occupational therapist or the vocational evaluator. If a vocational evaluator is involved, then an occupational therapist will also be utilized for the functional study, but the inverse is not necessarily applied.

There is no guarantee that the above scenario will occur when an injured worker enters any work-hardening program, and there is no guarantee that services offered will be beneficial to the injured worker. However, efforts have been made to standardize work-hardening program policy, protocol, and organizational structure through the development of program standards. The California Vocational Evaluation and Work Adjustment Association (C-VEWAA) attempted to establish guidelines for all programs in California in 1984, supported by the State Division of Industrial Accidents and by workers' compensation benefit providers (Edgcomb, 1987). The Commission on Accreditation of Rehabilitation Facilities (CARF) soon followed suit, and assembled a professionally representative steering committee, in 1988, to establish specific clinical standards of practice in work hardening. These standards were disseminated to clinical and therapeutic personnel for comment and revisions. The first year for facility accreditation under the CARF guidelines was 1989. Since this first accrediting year, Florida and Ohio have established that only facilities meeting CARF accrediting standards for work hardening will be reimbursed for services rendered to injured workers. It is anticipated that several more states will adopt similar policy within the next five years, and by the year 2000, only CARF-accredited programs will be reimbursed for services in all 50 states.

Accreditation does not guarantee quality. It only assures the consumer that the program has met a set of standards determined to be necessary to minimize risk or harm to the injured worker and to maximize his or her therapeutic benefit. Accreditation applies only to the facility, and not to the individual clinicians administering the services. However, there are several clinical standards worth noting that the reader may consider when selecting a work-hardening program in the client's local community. Several such CARF standards are summarized as follows:

- Program goals should be identified and documented during the admission stage of the program. *Application*: This is best accomplished at the onset with the submission of specific referral questions. Once the team understands what the referral source desires from the program, then specific goals and objectives can be delineated.
- Program time frames should be documented at the admission stage of the program. *Application*: The exact length of the program should be documented in writing by the evaluating team at the conclusion of the work capacity evaluation. The referral source is encouraged not to accept an indefinite time period. Often, evaluation teams will conclude that more time is needed before a definite discharge date can be determined. This is not acceptable, as the discharge date is easily determined by a well-experienced industrial rehabilitation team.
- The evaluation process should take place within the context of the demands of competitive employment. The process should document a benchmark from which to establish the initial plan or the person's functional/vocational disposition and should include, but not be limited to, one or more of the following functional capacity evaluations: baseline evaluation, job capacity evaluation, occupational capacity evaluation, and work capacity evaluation.

- Assessment, coordinated program planning, and direct services should be provided on a regular and continuing basis by the interdisciplinary team, which should be made up of the following professionals: occupational therapist, physical therapist, psychologist, and vocational specialist.
- The exit/discharge criteria should include, but not be limited to, the following issues concerning the person served:

    Returning to Work–Will the client return to work at the time of discharge from the program?

    Meeting Program Goals–Were all goals met, and if not, which ones were not, and why.

    Declining Further Services–Why were services declined by the injured worker? Referral source?

    Noncompliance with Organizational Policies–Which policies were violated and why?

    Limited Potential to Benefit–Has the injured worker peaked in his or her performance? Has this person reached maximum medical improvement (MMI)?

    Requiring Further Health Care Interventions–Did other problems surface which suggest additional medical interpretation and diagnostics are warranted?
- The exit/discharge summary should delineate the following:

    The person's present functioning status and potential.

    The functional status related to the targeted job, alternative occupations, or the competitive labor market.
- The exit/discharge summary should be prepared and disseminated within seven working days of the exit/discharge date. *Application*: The consumer should expect to receive a full and detailed report of the injured worker's experience in the work-hardening program within a seven-day period post-discharge.

REFERRAL CONSIDERATIONS

Work-hardening programs have evolved into sophisticated evaluation and treatment programs designed specifically to assist injured workers with returning to the competitive labor market. Programs have experienced a phenomenal growth over the last 11 years, though their roots can be traced back to the early occupational therapy movement in the 1930s. Today's programs reflect a comprehensive structured program with multidisciplined evaluation and treatment staff. The more sophisticated programs may consist of physical therapists, occupational therapists, vocational evaluators, vocational rehabilitation counselors/case managers, social workers, psychologists, rehabilitation nurses, and physicians. Those with lesser budgets may include only a physical therapist and one or more team members.

When choosing a work-hardening program, the consumer may wish to consider the following:

- Goal Structuring: Are specific program goals structured at the onset of the program, and monitored to ensure specified time frames for goal attainment are met? Are time frames for predicting goal attainment established at the onset of the program?
- Accessibility: How accessible are the therapists, program manager, and medical director (if there is one) for questions regarding client progress? Are phone calls immediately returned? Does the facility allow the rehabilitation specialist on-site access to the client and staff for periodic follow-up conferences? Are weekly staffings open to family members and/or case managers?
- Report Dissemination: Is the final report of the client's performance disseminated within a seven-day period? Does it address the specific referral questions submitted at the time of referral? If program goals are not met and the client fails, are recommendations provided in writing to address the next rehabilitation step in the individual's health care?

The referral source should be aware that work-hardening programs make no guarantees of returning injured workers to work, nor guarantee that program goals will be met within the specified time frames. The injured worker may demonstrate an ability to benefit from the program, but may not achieve the program goals to qualify for placement in the competitive labor market. If program goals are not met, and the program has demonstrated good goal structuring, planning, and delivery of service, at the least, the referral source should know which is the best direction to pursue for the injured worker in terms of continuing rehabilitation efforts if at all appropriate.

Work hardening is still in its developmental stages, and research in such programs is still in its infancy. The consumer plays a significant role in the development and maintenance of quality standards for work-hardening programs through his or her choice of programs. With such influence potential, the consumer can provide the necessary input and influence to ensure established standards of practice are met, and modifications to existing standards, as well as new standard development, remains ongoing.

References

Bettencourt, C., Carlstrom, P., Brown, S., Lindau, K., & Long, C. (1986). Using job simulation to treat adults with back injuries. The *American Journal of Occupational Therapy, 40*, 12-20.

Crewe, N. (1986). Assessment of physical functioning. In B. Bolton (Ed.), *Handbook of measurement and evaluation in rehabilitation* (pp. 235-247). Baltimore: Paul H. Brookes.

Edgcomb, J. (1987). Work hardening guidelines 1984: As proposed by California V.E.W.A.A. *Vocational Evaluation and Work Adjustment Bulletin, 20*, 133-134.

Harrand, G. (1986). *The Harrand guide for developing physical capacity evaluation.* (Available from the Career Development Center, 1515 Ball Street, Box 600, Eau Claire, Wisconsin 54702).

Holmes, D. (1985). The role of the occupational therapist-work evaluator. *The American Journal of Occupational Therapy, 39*, 308-313.

Matheson, L. (1984). *Work capacity evaluation: An interdisciplinary approach to industrial rehabilitation.* Anaheim, CA: Employment and Rehabilitation Institute of California.

Matheson, L. (1988). Integrated work hardening in vocational rehabilitation: An emerging model. *Vocational Evaluation and Work Adjustment Bulletin, 21,* 71-76.

Matheson, L., & Ogden, L. (1983). *Work tolerance screening.* Anaheim, CA: Employment and Rehabilitation Institute of California.

Matheson, L., Ogden, L., Violette, K., & Schultz, K. (1985). Work hardening: Occupational therapy in industrial rehabilitation. *American Journal of Occupational Therapy, 39,* 314-321.

May, V. R. (1985). Physical capacity evaluation and work hardening programming: The Carle Clinic Association model. In C. Smith & R. Fry (Eds.), *The national forum on issues in vocational assessment: Issues papers* (pp. 233-239). Materials Development Center, Stout Vocational Rehabilitation Institute, School of Education and Human Services, University of Wisconsin–Stout, Menomonie, WI.

May, V. R. (1986). Integrating vocational rehabilitation in medical settings. *American Archives of Rehabilitation Therapy, 34,* 1-8.

May, V. R. (1987). Work hardening: A multidisciplinary team approach. *West Work Newsletter, 4*(1), 1.

May, V. R. (1988a). Work hardening and work capacity evaluation: Definition and process. *Vocational Evaluation and Work Adjustment Bulletin, 21,* 61-66.

May, V. R. (1988b). Work capacity evaluation and work hardening: Process and applications in private sector rehabilitation. In P. Deutsch & H. Sawyer (Eds.), *A guide to rehabilitation* (pp. 6A-1 – 6A-46). New York: Matthew Bender.

May, V. R., & Reifsteck, S. (1986). Surviving the crunch: Developing and marketing an industrial rehabilitation program. *Journal of the Medical Management Association, 33*(5), 50-56.

May, V. R., Stewart, R., & Barnes, L. (1986). Industrial rehabilitation: A physical capacity evaluation and work hardening model. *Carle Selected Papers, 38*(2), 39-43.

Reuss, E., Rawe, D., & Sunquist, A. (1958). Development of a physical capacities evaluation. *American Journal of Occupational Therapy, 12*(1), 1-8, 14.

Stewart, W., Peacock, C., Parsons, D., & Johnson, P. (1985). A triadic approach to the vocational assessment of the industrially injured. In C. Smith & R. Fry (Eds.), The issue papers: *National forum on issues in vocational assessment* (pp. 185-189). Materials Development Center, Stout Vocational Rehabilitation institute, University of Wisconsin–Stout, Menomonie, WI.

White, G. (1986). Work hardening. *The Claimsman, 10*(1), 17.

Rehabilitation Engineering/Technology Services

Frank D. Puckett, Rh.D.

Rehabilitation engineering is the application of science and technology to increase the personal independence and enhance the functional capability of persons with disabilities. It is a part of how individuals deal with, and are compensated for, their physical or sensory impairment. The use of a cane is an early application of an assistive device to address the needs of someone with a mobility impairment. Worksite and tool modifications have historically been a part of one's adjustment to a functional limitation.

Whether one is working in the medically related area of sensory aids and artificial limbs, or working with individuals to remove architectural/physical barriers, the goal of rehabilitation engineering is the solving of problems faced by persons who are disabled. Often the problems are simple, occasionally they are complex, but the focus of the engineer's effort is the person or persons who are impaired in their pursuit of basic life goals due to their disability.

History/Legislation

The 1986 Amendments to the Rehabilitation Act defined rehabilitation engineering as "the systematic application of technologies, engineering methodologies, or scientific principles to meet the needs of and address the barriers confronted by individuals with handicaps in areas which include education, rehabilitation, employment, transportation, independent living, and recreation" (House of Representatives, 1986, pp. 4-5). The Act required that state vocational rehabilitation agencies ensure that rehabilitation plans include "where appropriate, the provision of rehabilitation engineering services to any individual with a handicap to assess and develop the individual's capacities to perform adequately in a work environment." Section 103(a)(1) of the Act states that determination of eligibility for services should include "evaluation by personnel skilled in rehabilitation engineering technology," where appropriate.

Another legislative initiative which impacts the provision of rehabilitative and assistive technologies is the Technology-Related Assistance for Individuals with Disabilities Act of 1988. Under this Act, grants are awarded "to provide financial assistance to the States to help each State to develop and implement a consumer-responsive statewide program of technology-related assistance for individuals of all ages with disabilities . . . " (Technology-Related Assistance for Individuals with Disabilities Act of 1988, p. 102 STAT 1045). This Act promotes the same access to assistive technologies as was provided to rehabilitation clients through the 1986 Amendments to the Rehabilitation Act, and to children with disabilities through the Education for All Handicapped Children Act of 1974.

Clarification of terminology was provided through the Technology Assistance Act namely, "What is an assistive device?" and "What are assistive technology services?" Under the Act, an assistive technology device is "any item, piece of equipment, or product system, whether acquired commercially off the shelf, modified, or customized, that is used to increase, maintain, or improve functional capabilities of individuals with disabilities." And, assistive technology services are "any service that directly assists an individual with a disability in the selection, acquisition, or use of an assistive technology device" (Technology-Related Assistance for Individuals with Disabilities Act of 1988, p. 102 STAT 1046).

Through these legislative initiatives, it seems clear that Congress intended that persons with disabilities have full access to the benefits of rehabilitation technology in various settings to include work, school, and leisure activities.

PERSONNEL

With all the developments in the field of rehabilitation technology in the last 10 years, an easy consensus has been reached regarding definitions for assistive devices and assistive technology services. Less definitive is the issue of who is qualified to render these services, and who should carry the title *Rehabilitation Engineer*. One distinction which is being made in the various job classifications is that rehabilitation engineer would be a classification reserved for an individual who holds a degree in engineering (Scheck, 1990). Most other professionals in this field would use the terms rehabilitation technologist, adaptive equipment specialist, or assistive devices specialist. More important than one's title is the training and professional competence the individual has in assistive technology.

Purpose/Intent

The Rehabilitation Engineering Society of North America (RESNA), a national association for the advancement of rehabilitation and assistive technologies, classified rehabilitation engineering services in the following manner:
- Personal vehicles and driving aids
- Prosthetics and orthotics

- Home modifications
- Worksite and vocational equipment modifications
- Communications and controls
- Computer applications
- Quantification and diagnosis of human performance (OSERS Task Force, 1988)

Another classification which relates more specifically to the types of client services which counselors or caseworkers would attempt to secure for their clients is the following:

- Adaptive devices for independent living and activities of daily living
- Sensory aids for individuals with hearing or visual impairments
- Adaptive driving controls and modified vehicles for transportation
- Wheelchairs and other mobility devices
- Custom seating and corrective postural positioning
- Augmentative communication devices
- Adapted worksites and tool modification
- Adapted computer systems

ADAPTIVE DEVICES FOR INDEPENDENT LIVING AND ACTIVITIES OF DAILY LIVING

Activities of daily living (ADL) are those tasks performed routinely to meet one's basic daily needs (e.g., dressing, eating, bathing, grooming, personal hygiene, cooking, pursuit of leisure activities). Specifically, ADL tasks are separated from work-related activities such as employment and education. Most individuals, young and old, disabled or nondisabled prefer to do these tasks as independently as possible. Through the appropriate use of assistive devices, a person with a physical or sensory impairment can often regain lost capability for one or more of these ADL tasks. Occupational therapists (OT) are specifically trained to perform this type of assessment. The guideline used by most therapists for this type of assessment is the following: recommendation of a device or devices which will restore independence for the task or assist the individual in performing the task in a more timely fashion, or with a greater degree of safety. The types of devices prescribed for ADL range from simple eating utensils, to often expensive and complex electronic environmental control units that control lights, appliances, television, telephone, and temperature setting.

SENSORY AIDS FOR INDIVIDUALS WITH HEARING AND VISUAL IMPAIRMENTS

For individuals with a significant hearing loss, communication and signaling often rely on visual input and to a lesser degree tactile sensation (vibrations). Simple solutions, such as flashing lights for a doorbell ring or alarm clock, are quite easily accomplished. Electronic teletype communication devices allow deaf and hearing-impaired persons to use the telephone. Speech to text conversion devices are being developed for word processing, and may have application for hearing-impaired persons in the future. And, basic research is on-going to convert "deaf speech," which is often difficult to understand, to a printed output (Abdelhamied, Waldron, & Fox, 1990). In the area of medical research, cochlear implants have been successful in restoring "perception of sound" for formerly deaf persons but are limited in their usefulness for understanding speech.

For persons with a severe visual loss, the opposite approach is taken, that is, signals and messages are converted to auditory or tactile signals. Talking books and voice output from computers are typical adaptations to meet this need. Text to speech conversion programs/equipment are available (Kurzweil reading machine) and have created a more direct access to information for person with visual or reading disorders. Sonic or sonar aids to assist individuals with mobility have been developed and tested in various locations, but, as yet, are not widely used by persons with visual impairments.

ADAPTIVE DRIVING CONTROLS AND
MODIFIED VEHICLES FOR TRANSPORTATION

The application of technology to allow persons with disabilities to access private and public transportation (e.g., bus, plane, train) has significantly increased the personal mobility and ease with which disabled persons can travel. Although not always convenient, these services are becoming more accessible. This trend is increasing even more with the implementation of the Americans with Disabilities Act. Wheelchair lifts for buses and vans, and loading ramps for trains and airplanes have reduced, though not eliminated, many transportation barriers for mobility-impaired persons.

In the area of personal transportation, new technologies such as reduced effort acceleration/braking and steering systems allow persons with limited strength to operate a personal vehicle (typically a van). The latest technology in adaptive driving controls is a joystick-controlled system for individuals who have functional use of only one extremity. Except for the traditional automotive hand controls, most control systems are quite costly, and require that careful assessments be conducted in order to assure safety in vehicle operation. Personal wheelchair restraint systems are an often overlooked issue. Whether the individual is driving or riding as a passenger, separate restraints for the individual and the wheelchair are critical for ensuring safety. A number of wheelchair restraint systems have been crash tested, and should be the system of choice for most applications. Given the new technologies, more individuals with severe disabilities can achieve the goal of driving a personal vehicle. The question remains, are they able to accomplish this in a safe manner.

WHEELCHAIRS AND OTHER MOBILITY DEVICES

New designs and materials have radically changed the appearance of wheelchairs and other equipment for mobility-impaired persons. The choice for mobility aids ranges from versatile motorized scooters for individuals who can ambulate, but not for long distances, to full-size, power-base wheelchairs which can accept a number of specialized seating units. Various control systems exist for individuals to operate powered wheelchairs including joystick, chin control, head control, foot control, and sip-n-puff (breath control). Physically gaining control over a powered wheelchair is secondary to determining that the individual has the reasoning, visual perception, and judgement to operate the wheelchair. With proper training and support, children as young as five years old have successfully used powered mobility. Many options and features exist, and the assessment to determine the optimal mobility system for an individual should include "trying out" as many of these features as possible.

CUSTOM SEATING AND CORRECTIVE POSTURAL POSITIONING

It is often the case that the standard seating system in a wheelchair or motorized scooter is not adequate or optimal for the person, often due to the individual's physical deformity, problems with decubiti, and so on. In these circumstances, a specialized seating system is required which offers corrective postural positioning to address problems of scoliosis or other spinal deformity, and offer some degree of protection against the development of pressure sores or decubiti. Materials utilized in these systems take several forms (i.e., plywood, foam, and vinyl; custom formed plastics; mold injection foam products). For less severe cases, commercial products, such as Roho® or Jay® cushions will occasionally meet the individual's needs. This area of custom seating and positioning is highly specialized, requiring the services of trained and experienced clinicians. A typical clinical team for specialized seating would include physical therapy, occupational therapy, and rehabilitation technology. Improper position-ing in a wheelchair or other seating unit adversely affects one's health and comfort. Satisfying the client's needs for proper wheelchair seating and position-ing, can result in improved comfort, work tolerance, and functional capability of the upper extremities.

AUGMENTATIVE COMMUNICATION DEVICES

When individuals cannot utilize speech to fully meet their needs for communication, they are potential candidates for some type of augmentative or assistive communication aid. Conditions such as cerebral palsy, stroke, brain injury, and various types of neuromuscular diseases often result in diminished communication ability. Despite the severity of the disability, almost anyone who has a desire to communicate can realize some benefit from properly prescribed augmentative communication assistance. The range of devices used in augmentative communication vary from simple letter boards, to electronic computerized communication systems. The assessment strategy in augmentative communication focuses on cognitive ability, level of language development, and physical ability to access a keyboard, electronic switch, and so on. A speech pathologist is usually the key clinician for this type of evaluation.

ADAPTIVE WORKSITES AND TOOL MODIFICATION

The goal of worksite modification is to maximize the individual's functional capability and independence, in the safest and most cost-efficient manner possible. Simply gaining entrance into buildings can present obstacles. Accessibility to restrooms and food service areas are also frequent problems in work environments. A rehabilitation engineer and an occupational therapist would be an excellent team to address workplace modifications. If the company or industry employs building engineers, these individuals could also assist with this activity. Worksite and tool modification projects typically follow a systematic protocol. If the individual cannot adequately perform the task, then a rehabilitation technologist would examine the job or task in the following manner: change what is done, change the way it is done, or change who does it. Reasonable solutions might include use of assistive devices and adapted tools, changing the process by which the task is performed (choosing a more ergonomically efficient approach for the individual), or exploring a job sharing option whereby the target individual shares/swaps some of the tasks with another co-worker.

ADAPTED COMPUTER SYSTEMS

The emergence of microcomputers has revolutionized employment and educational opportunities for persons with disabilities. If one has the cognitive ability to work with computers, there is virtually no one so physically disabled that they cannot gain access to a microcomputer. Input to a microcomputer can be gained by voice, or any voluntary physical trait to include simple eye movements. Computer output can be converted to speech, print, braille, or raised dots for tactile sensing by deaf-blind persons. Accessing a computer is a matter of gaining control over input of data/commands to the system, and converting output into a form which is readily accessible to the user. One simple guideline for choosing a computer system is the following: identify the task to be performed, choose the software programs which will best handle the task, then select the computer and adaptive peripherals required to meet the client's needs. Choosing the computer first, and trying to make it fit the client's needs, can often lead to frustration and less than optimal results.

Client Services

Usually, one of the first questions asked by counselors and caseworkers is "How can I determine if my client will benefit from assistive devices or specialized equipment?" When planning assistive technology services, it is important to obtain assistance from personnel skilled in rehabilitation technology. Use of technological devices should be guided by the following considerations:

- The ability of the individual to comprehend and benefit from the technology;
- The financial resources needed to purchase and maintain the devices or equipment;
- Availability of a sufficient support system for training and continuing maintenance of the technology (Corthell & Thayer, 1986).

With careful consideration to these issues, one can hopefully avoid improper prescriptions and mismatch of technology. The approach least likely to succeed is to simply purchase devices and let the client and family determine how best to use them. "Good rehabilitation practice" applies to applications of assistive technology, as it would for more traditional services, where careful planning and competent assessment services are more likely to lead to a successful outcome.

To assess an individual's potential benefit from assistive devices, one could begin by evaluating the person's level of independence for various activities of daily living. The potential benefit of assistive devices in ADL generalizes rather well to other areas such as work, education, and leisure. The rating procedure illustrated in Table 1 provides some indication of the level of need for technological assistance.

Table 1. Rating Scale

A. Independent, no assistance needed; no other concerns noted
B. Independent, but uses an assistive device; necessary effort and level of safety are acceptable
C. Partially dependent on another person, or task is difficult and too time consuming, or task is not performed in a safe manner
D. Totally dependent on other person(s)

Use the above scale (A - D) to rate the person's level of independence for the following self-care and other daily living activities.

_____	Bathing	_____	Eating, food preparation
_____	Grooming	_____	Dressing, undressing
_____	Toileting	_____	Transferring to/from a wheelchair
_____	Ambulation	_____	Propelling a wheelchair
_____	Use of phone	_____	Use of public/private transportation
_____	Social activities	_____	Handling crisis/emergency situations

While not exhaustive, this scale represents a sufficient sample of tasks to obtain a baseline for determining level of need for assistive technology. For all items rated "A" or "B," the individual appears to be meeting his or her needs in a reasonable fashion. However, for those items classified as "C" or "D," an evaluation should be conducted to determine the client's potential benefit from adaptive and assistive devices. A key consideration is how easily or safely individuals meet basic daily needs. Assistive devices are often appropriate in situations where an individual can perform a task independently, but the task requires an unusually long time, the required effort is exhausting, or the task is performed in a way that places the person at risk of injury.

This rating scale focuses primarily on daily living tasks, and not specific work activities. Work related tasks are highly variable. It can be argued that if one is sufficiently independent in most or all daily living tasks, it is reasonable to expect those skills and compensatory strategies to be applicable in an employment or educational setting.

OBTAINING COMPETENT EVALUATION FOR ASSISTIVE DEVICES

A comprehensive rehabilitation center which has rehabilitation engineers/technologists on staff would likely be able to address this need. Other potential sources of help include the following:
- Durable medical equipment (DME) dealers
- Technology-based service center in a university
- Rehabilitation technology specialists working in state vocational rehabilitation programs
- Private rehabilitation technology companies
- National disability organizations
- Information/referral centers on disability issues
- State programs funded under the Technology Assistance Act

RESNA maintains a nationwide list of over 200 specialists in assistive technology. Each state rehabilitation agency has information on facilities which provide these types of services. States which have on-going Technology Assistance grants are excellent sources of information on assistive device specialists. If the same person or facility was recommended by more than one of these resources, it would suggest that the individual or facility has attained a certain reputation for this area of technology. Resource manuals and guidebooks on rehabilitation technology are also helpful in this regard (Corthell & Thayer, 1986; Hale, 1990).

There are no fool-proof methods for selecting a competent consultant in assistive devices. Some indicators of knowledge and experience are the following:
- Member of RESNA
- Member of the National Special Education Alliance
- Attendance at rehabilitation technology conferences
- Knowledge of appropriate resources in assistive technology

Contacting a national organization, such as United Cerebral Palsy, can provide an objective resource to determine knowledge potential consultants should have for a specific area of assistive technology. These resources should be able to provide guidance with regard to the following: "What questions should I ask of a potential vendor or assistive technology service consultant?" For example, questions which could be asked of a potential consultant for adaptive computer controls include:

- Are you familiar with the Trace Center in Madison, Wisconsin?
- What technology conferences have you attended in the last two years?
- What is the function of the Adaptive Firmware Card? (This unit permits persons with physical limitations alternate input modes to the computer.)

A person who cannot answer these questions satisfactorily, is less well informed in the area of adaptive computer interfaces, and, therefore, his or her chances of prescribing an appropriate solution are somewhat diminished. A similar set of questions could be developed for other areas of assistive technology, such as augmentative communication and adaptive driving. Obviously, a person could be well informed on adaptive computers and still not arrive at the optimal solution for a specific individual.

WHEN SEVERAL OPTIONS EXIST, WHO DECIDES WHICH DEVICE IS BEST?

Input can be obtained from several sources, however, the decision should be made jointly by the individual, his or her family, and the funding source. If any one of these individuals is opposed to the choice, then the chances of success are compromised. Clinical input can be obtained from a variety of sources, such as occupational therapists, physical therapists, speech pathologists, physicians, and rehabilitation technologists. These clinicians make recommendations and provide options, but the decision rests with the individual, his or her family, and the funding source representative (e.g., counselor, caseworker).

OTHER ISSUES TO CONSIDER WHEN PURCHASING ASSISTIVE DEVICES

When "shopping" for assistive devices, you want to be an informed consumer, as you would for any other type of purchase. Some key issues are the performance characteristics of the device, and the ease and availability of repairs and maintenance.

- Evaluate the performance characteristics of the device. How well does the device meet the requirements of the individual? Does the device have extra functions, capabilities that are of no value in this situation? For the same performance characteristics, is the device substantially more expensive than other units?
- Consider the durability and reliability of the unit. How does it perform in various environmental settings, such as excessive heat or cold? What data exist to describe the reliability of this unit verses others of the same type?

- With respect to repairs and maintenance, will these be obtained locally? A problem for the client and the counselor exists when arrangements for repairs and maintenance are not clarified before the device is delivered.

THE IMPACT OF REHABILITATION TECHNOLOGY

Some caseworkers/counselors consider waiting until a client has completed a certain phase of rehabilitation or training before considering a complete assessment for adaptive equipment. A point to consider, the individual's progress in the rehabilitation or training program may have been compromised in that he or she did not have the proper equipment to perform optimally. An experienced clinician/technologist can guide the individual and his or her caseworker as to what equipment should be considered at various points in the client's rehabilitation program. Also, technology is constantly changing, and necessitates periodic reassessment of the need for, and potential benefit of, assistive technologies.

Rehabilitation technology is a relatively new discipline in rehabilitation practice; policy, procedures, and expected outcome are still evolving. Also, for some counselors and caseworkers, there is limited knowledge and confidence when prescribing assistive devices. Certainly, there are examples where this effort went awry and the device/equipment failed to meet expectations, or perhaps proved useless. However, more numerous are situations where competent assessment and careful delivery of assistive technology services resulted in the person accomplishing a task which was felt to be impossible. When applied in a cautious and careful manner, adaptive technologies can have tremendous impact on the quality of life and rehabilitation potential of persons with disabilities.

References

Abdelhamied, K., Waldron, M., & Fox, R. A. (1990). Automatic recognition of deaf speech. *Volta Review*, *92*(3), 121-130.

Corthell, D. W., & Thayer, T. (1986). *Rehabilitation technologies*. Thirteenth Institute on Rehabilitation Issues. Menomonie, WI: Stout Vocational Rehabilitation Institute.

Hale, P. N. (Ed.). (1990). *Rehabilitation technology services: A guide for the rehabilitation counselor*. Ruston, LA: Center for Rehabilitation Science and Biomedical Engineering, Louisiana Tech University.

House of Representatives. (1986). *Rehabilitation Act Amendments of 1986*. (Conference Report 99-955 to accompany H. R. 4021). Washington, DC: U. S. Congress.

OSERS Task Force. (1988, May). *Rehabilitation engineering services in the state-federal vocational rehabilitation system*. Report from OSERS Task Force on Rehabilitation Engineering. Washington, DC: Office of Special Education and Rehabilitative Services.

Technology-Related Assistance for Individuals with Disabilities Act of 1988, U. S. C. § 2201.

Scheck, A. (1990). Rehab engineers vote for two certification levels. *Team Rehab, 1*(2), 30-31.

V. Vocational and Employment Services

Employment Security—Job Service

Timothy P. Janikowski, Ph.D., C.R.C.

History/Legislation

The depression and massive unemployment experienced in the late 1920s and early 1930s gave impetus to the Wagner-Peyser Act of 1933 which created the United States Employment Service as a permanent, federally based bureau. At the time, it was funded by federal grants to be matched on a 50-50 basis by each state in the union. The local employment offices, created by the Act, were to be administered by the states but were compelled to meet federal grant criteria. The aim of the U. S. Employment Service was to: (a) promote and develop a nationwide system of employment offices; (b) set-up and coordinate a system of interstate clearance of information and of labor between offices; (c) maintain a veterans' and a farmers' placement service; and (d) take extraordinary steps to meet the then existing unemployment crisis, and to ensure that every state was provided with a public employment service (Atkinson, Odencrantz, & Deming, 1938).

In 1939, the United States Employment Service was combined with Unemployment Compensation in a Bureau of Employment Security. Hence, today the State Employment Security agencies have two primary responsibilities. The first is to assist in the job placement of those seeking employment (through the auspices of the Employment or Job Service). The second function is to administer and deliver benefits of the Unemployment Insurance programs.

The more than 2,000 United States Employment Security agencies and approximately 18,000 agency personnel currently in the United States, are funded from both federal and state taxes. Federal taxes stem from the Federal Unemployment Tax Act (FUTA), passed to generate funds to administer the National Employment Security System; FUTA funds are based on taxable wages paid to employees. The tax is collected from employers by the Internal Revenue Service, and revenues are distributed to each state by the federal government.

FUTA funds provide the moneys for the staff used to screen job applicants, find jobs for the unemployed, process claims for unemployment benefits, and collect the state unemployment tax. State taxes are collected to pay unemployment insurance benefits to qualified unemployed workers, and are collected by the Employment Service. Unemployment Insurance program eligibility requirements are determined by each state's legislature.

Employers support the bulk of the U. S. Employment Security System by paying two separate payroll taxes, a federal (FUTA) tax to staff and operate the state-federal system, and a state (Unemployment Insurance) tax to pay benefits to sustain unemployed workers. Both state and federal moneys are maintained on deposit in the U. S. Treasury in a unified, federal trust fund which is administered by the federal government.

In the 1970s, national Employment Service staffing numbers stood at a stable level of about 30,000. The current level of staffing, however, has been reduced through staffing cuts and office closures to approximately 18,000. Because of these reductions and related problems regarding access to funding, many state governments wish to alter the access and allocation of moneys targeted for Employment Service use. The National Governors' Association (NGA) is a consortium of 48 state governors that is attempting to address Employment Service funding issues. In 1989, the NGA State Employment Security Service Act was passed with the intent to legislate core services for the Employment Service and Unemployment Insurance programs, the two programs which constitute the Employment Security System. The bill also delineates funding levels and specifies how the dollars are to be distributed. The implementation of this Act has yet to be realized, however, and the future funding status of the Employment Security System remains unclear.

Purpose and Structure

The thousands of offices that constitute the federal-state Employment Security System are physically divided into four levels and locations. First, the federal bureau is housed in Washington, DC, and serves as the umbrella organization for the national system, organizationally as part of the Department of Labor. Second, federal field operations are located in 11 regional offices geographically distributed throughout the United States. Third, the 54 state and territory offices each have a central headquarters, usually housed in the state's capital. Finally, there is the network of local employment security offices in each jurisdiction, these offices are located in a manner as to minimize the traveling time of the job seekers using the agency.

As alluded to earlier, United States Employment Security System has two primary functions. The first is to assist with the job placement of unemployed workers, which it accomplishes through the Employment or Job Service (for sake of consistency, the latter term will be used throughout the rest of the chapter). The second function is to administer and deliver unemployment insurance benefits, which is done through Unemployment Insurance programs. Although Job Service and Unemployment Insurance are two separate programs, agency personnel often fill dual roles, performing job functions related to both programs. Because of the focus of this book on utilizing community resources, the discussion below will be restricted to the Job Service.

Job Service Programs and Services

Each Job Service office is a creation of its parent state's legislature and is under the jurisdiction of the state government, however, it must conform to federal laws. Although state agencies conform to federal legislation, there is wide variation among states in respect to state laws, administration practices and procedures, and agency organizations. Because of this variation, the Job Service personnel, programs, and services will be presented generically. Occasionally, a specific program or service will be presented for purposes of illustration. The reader is strongly encouraged to contact his or her local Job Service in order to obtain information regarding specific programs and services available. Job Service personnel are very receptive to working with community agencies and professionals, and a close working relationship between referral sources and the Job Service will produce the best results for clients seeking Job Service assistance.

The funding for the Job Service comes from state and federal taxes, hence, all programs and services are extended to job seekers and employers *free of charge*. With the exception of certain programs and services, clients need not meet any criteria to utilize the Job Service. In short, everyone is eligible to seek and obtain free assistance from the Job Service.

The programs and services offered by the Job Service to job seekers include: job placement, vocational counseling, vocational assessment, job seeking skills instruction, special population programs, and registration for special programs. In addition to assistance to job seekers, the Job Service also provides services of benefit to employers, these include: posting job orders, applicant screening and referral, new or expanding business assistance, collection and dissemination of labor market information, and employment-related informational programs. The remainder of the chapter will entail a discussion of these services. Again, the reader is encouraged to contact his or her local Job Service agency to take full advantage of the particular programs and services offered.

JOB PLACEMENT

Job placement assistance is probably the most utilized Job Service program. The Job Service actively solicits job orders from potentially every employer in its area, state, and region. These job orders are compiled into a list which is made available to job seekers. Until recently, maintaining and using a listing of current job openings was a laborious, time-consuming process which required the assistance of Job Service personnel. Today, the process of maintaining and accessing a current listing of, literally, thousands of job openings has been enhanced through the use of computers, often eliminating the need for assistance from Job Service personnel. Minnesota, for instance, developed and implemented a computer-based, self-service job search system, listing job openings immediately after employers placed the job orders. This on-line, statewide system allows the job seeker to directly access a computer terminal, without assistance from Job Service personnel, and respond to "user-friendly" directions via a keyboard. The job seeker selects one of nine occupational areas which is subsequently divided into sub-categories. When a sub-category is selected, the computer screen displays more specific information about job titles, wages, location, and employer selection criteria. The job seeker may then select jobs in which he or she is interested and the computer will provide information regarding steps necessary to apply and interview for the jobs (Minnesota Department of Jobs and Training, undated). This type of computer-based job search system is becoming commonplace throughout the United States Job Service agencies, and allows for a stream-lined, individualized search of current job openings, obviating the need for assistance from Job Service personnel.

VOCATIONAL COUNSELING

Vocational counseling through the Job Service agencies is offered to: (a) those who are entering the work-force for the first time, (b) those who wish to change their current occupations, and (c) individuals experiencing difficulty obtaining suitable employment due to personal or economic conditions. The traditional approach to vocational counseling has its roots in the Vocational Bureau of Boston (1908), and typically entails a three-step process where first, job seekers are given assistance in understanding their interests, personalities, abilities, and limitations; second, they are provided with information on the demands and rewards of various types of work; and third, they are helped to develop a clear conception of how these two sets of data are inter-related (Parsons, 1909). In short, the vocational counselor, through individualized interviews, testing, and information gathered from other sources, assists the job seeker in understanding his or her strengths, limitations, and preferences, and how they relate to the world of work. The outcome of this process is the identification of an appropriate vocational goal(s) and development of a concomitant vocational plan(s). This service is typically available to job seekers regardless of levels of education, skill, or experience.

VOCATIONAL ASSESSMENT

The Job Service is equipped to administer, score, and interpret a variety of occupational tests, such as vocational aptitude, clerical skills, interest, and educational achievement tests. Although a number of tests are available, two are routinely administered: the General Aptitude Test Battery (GATB; U. S. Department of Labor, 1970) and the United States Employment Service (USES) Interest Inventory (U. S. Department of Labor, 1981). These tests constitute the

Counselee Assessment/Occupational Exploration System developed expressly for the United States Employment Service.

The GATB has been referred to as the best validated aptitude test battery ever developed (Droege, 1983) and is designed to measure nine aptitude areas which are part of the Worker Qualification Profiles (WQPs): intelligence or general learning, verbal, numerical, spatial, form perception, clerical perception, motor coordination, finger dexterity, and manual dexterity. The GATB has been normed on many groups of employees, applicants, and trainees in different kinds of jobs, hence score patterns have been established which show the critical aptitudes and minimum scores required for thousands of occupations (Anastasi, 1988). Some Job Services maintain local norms which validate the GATB against jobs offered by local employers, who in turn use GATB test scores as one of their selection criteria.

In 1990, the U. S. Department of Labor restricted the use of the GATB to voluntary vocational counseling only. According to *Labor News* ("Dole suspends," 1990), the use of the GATB as an employment referral and selection criterion has been suspended because of "...concerns over whether the test adequately serves all individuals including minorities, veterans, those with disabilities, and older workers ... The Labor Department will conduct a two-year study to sharpen the employment aptitude measure in the job selection and referral process" (p. 1). After the GATB has been re-normed and its reliability and validity re-established, it will probably be used once more as a referral and selection criterion by the Job Service and employers.

The USES Interest Inventory is designed to measure interests in 12 areas: Artistic, Scientific, Plants and Animals, Protective, Mechanical, Industrial, Business Detail, Selling, Accommodating, Humanitarian, Leading-Influencing, and Physical Performing. The goal of research and development concerning the USES Interest Inventory was to

> ... work toward a closely coordinated system which would permit counselors to measure the counselee's occupational interests and then help these counselees to explore occupations in line with their strongest interests...the USES Interest Inventory can now be used to measure occupational interests in direct relation to the Interest Areas of the Guide for Occupational Exploration (U. S. Department of Labor, 1981, p. 16).

An important advantage of the GATB and USES Interest Inventory is that they are used in conjunction with publications which are related to the world of work, such as the Dictionary of Occupational Titles (D.O.T.; U. S. Department of Labor, 1991), Guide for Occupational Exploration (G.O.E; U. S. Department of Labor, 1979), and the Occupational Outlook Handbook (O.O.H; U. S. Department of Labor, 1976), to facilitate the process of matching the job seeker with an appropriate job.

JOB-SEEKING SKILLS

Job-seeking skills instruction may be provided through written materials, individual and group instruction, and audiovisual presentations. Instruction and advice is given in such areas as completion of job application forms, developing a resumé, writing cover letters, interviewing, and critical vocational behaviors necessary for maintaining employment (e.g., grooming, attendance, punctuality). Regardless of the nature and extent of the job seekers' work-related skills, job-seeking skills instruction can make the job search process more efficient and effective. One of the outcomes of job-seeking skills instruction is that the job seeker learns skills which will assist him or her both now, and in future job searches.

SPECIAL POPULATION PROGRAMS

A number of special population programs are offered to provide additional assistance to job seekers in special groups: veterans, people with disabilities, minorities, welfare recipients, and young people. As mandated by federal law, priority is given to veterans (over nonveterans) in job referrals and training, and every Job Service has at least one staff member responsible for directing services for veterans. Further, the Job Service works directly with the Veterans Administration to promote veterans' on-the-job training programs which entail wage subsidies to employers hiring veterans.

People with disabilities, who are job ready, are given special attention. Each Job Service has a Handicapped Specialist who works closely with the state public rehabilitation office to provide additional assistance with counseling, testing, referral, and job development and placement.

The Job Service promotes employment opportunities for minority-group applicants regardless of race, color, creed, sex, national origin, religion, or political affiliation. For instance, Hispanic and Indo-Chinese job seekers may receive special job placement assistance from bilingual Job Service staff, who are trained in the cultural needs of these groups. In addition, the staff will cooperate with other social service agencies to provide assistance with employment related problems. Most larger Native American (Indian) reservations are serviced by special Job Service staff who perform job development activities and make employer contacts. Special mobile branch offices, often referred to as Job-mobiles, serve areas economically depressed or experiencing critical employment problems. Migrant and seasonal farm workers may be afforded help with finding farm work. Farm workers seeking nonfarm work may receive support from bilingual Job Service counselors who can refer them to training or supportive services or conduct specialized job searches.

Young people, aged 16 to 22, may benefit from special Job Service programs such as temporary summer employment, allowing youth to gain valuable work experience. Further, the Job Corps, a federally funded residential job training program, provides counseling, classroom training, and hands-on experience in a variety of occupations. Another program designed for young people is the

Cooperative School Program which provides counseling, testing, and job information to high school students and those who have dropped out of school.

Those receiving welfare may qualify for special Job Service programs as well. For instance, the Work Incentive Program (WIN) gives persons receiving Aid to Families with Dependent Children (AFDC) specialized training and job finding assistance. WIN legislation requires all AFDC recipients, except those legally exempt, to register for its services.

SPECIAL PROGRAMS

Depending upon the particular state and location of the Job Service, a number of special programs may be available to the job seeker. Special programs include: bonding, Targeted Jobs Tax Credit (TJTC), Job Training Partnership Act (JTPA), and programs for professionals.

The Job Service offers fidelity bond coverage for persons who require bonding to secure a job, but who are unable to do so in the usual manner because of prison records or credit ratings. This federally funded program, is supplied without cost to either employer or employee, for up to 18 months. The bond is normally issued two weeks after request, and bonding may range from $500 to $10,000. After an 18-month period, if the employee's work performance has been satisfactory, the employer will then assume responsibility for bonding arrangements.

The Targeted Jobs Tax Credit (TJTC) program offers tax incentives to employers if they hire individuals who belong to a targeted group. For every eligible person hired, the employer will receive a wage credit equal to 40% of wages paid, up to $6,000—or a maximum of $2,400. The job seeker must register with the Job Service and demonstrate membership in a targeted group such as: (a) handicapped persons who are enrolled in, or have completed, state or veteran's vocational rehabilitation programs (some workers' compensation recipients may also qualify); (b) young people, ages 18 to 22 who are from low-income families; (c) persons who have received general welfare assistance for 30 or more days; (d) those receiving AFDC, or who are participating in WIN programs; (e) low-income, Vietnam-era veterans; (f) low-income persons who have been convicted of a felony; and (g) recipients of Supplemental Security Income (SSI) payments.

The Job Training Partnership Act (JTPA), enacted in 1982, evolved out of the Manpower Development and Training Act (MDTA) of 1962 and the Comprehensive Employment and Training Act (CETA) of 1973. The goals of JTPA are to increase earnings and employment of the unemployed and to decrease welfare dependency (Bresnick, 1986). JTPA emphasizes the involvement of private industry and is managed, in part, by Private Industry Councils (PICs), which are comprised of local citizens, a majority of whom must be private business leaders. JTPA programs are designed to increase the skills and employability of job seekers by providing them with classroom training, on-the-job training, and related services.

Because of its emphasis on assisting the unemployed and disadvantaged, the Job Service has gained a reputation for primarily working with those interested in unskilled or semiskilled occupations. Although a majority of job openings posted by the Job Service may be unskilled or semiskilled, a wide variety of job openings are posted on professional, technical, managerial, and sales occupations as well. An example of a Job Service program designed to meet the needs more highly skilled job seekers is the Job Service Resumé System, a multistate bank of applicant records maintained on a single mainframe computer file. Assistance is offered to job seekers in preparing a one-page resumé which outlines their qualifications and job goals. These resumés are then placed on file in the mainframe computer. Participating states in this system are Illinois, Indiana, Michigan, Minnesota, Ohio, and Wisconsin. Using remote terminals, each state submits applications to this file and searches for resumés meeting specifications of professional-level job openings listed by employers. Upon finding an applicant's resumé which meets the requirements of the job, the computer prints a confidential copy of the one-page resumé for the employer's consideration. The employer then notifies the local Job Service of the candidates he or she wishes to contact.

PROGRAMS AND SERVICES FOR EMPLOYERS

Job Service programs and services of benefit to employers include posting job orders, applicant screening and referral, new or expanding business assistance, collection of labor market information, and employment-related informational programs. A brief discussion of these programs and services follows.

The Job Service serves as a clearinghouse, bringing job seekers and employers together. Employers, at no cost, are able to post job openings and related information in a place accessible to a wide range of job seekers. Job Service personnel are available to assist employers in developing accurate and concise job orders, saving the employer time and money in recruitment and interviewing. As indicated earlier, the advent of computers has created a fast, efficient medium for listing current or anticipated job openings.

In addition to posting job openings, Job Service personnel specialists will perform screening interviews using employer selection criteria, and refer selected applicants for employer consideration. In each state, the Job Service is the single largest source of job-ready applicants. Again, the Job Service's intent is to save the employer time and effort in identifying qualified applicants.

Upon request, the Job Service conducts special recruitment for new or expanding businesses, aiding with advertisement and increased interviewing assistance. Employers, if requested, may be provided with office space at the Job Service to interview job applicants.

The Job Service remains abreast of labor market conditions by collecting and maintaining local, state, regional, and national labor market information. The Job Service collects, analyzes, and publishes comprehensive data regarding estimates of labor force, wage surveys, employment projections by selected occupations and industries, and population and labor force data with ethnic and gender classifications to aid with employer short- and long-range planning needs.

Lastly, the Job Service provides informational or education programming in a variety of employment-related domains. Information may be obtained informally, through seminars, workshops, and audio-visual presentations. Typical informational programs include—but are not limited to—employee recruitment and interviewing, the management of work, unemployment compensation, labor law, affirmative action and Equal Employment Opportunity, and other legislative information.

References

Anastasi, A. (1988). *Psychological testing* (6th ed.). New York: Macmillan.

Atkinson, R. C., Odencrantz, L. C., & Deming, B. (1938). *Public employment service in the United States.* Chicago: Public Administration Service.

Bresnick, D. (1986). *Managing employment & training programs: Making J.T.P.A. work.* New York: Human Services Press.

Dole suspends use of job aptitude test. (1990, July 10). *Labor News*, p. 1.

Droege, R. C. (1983). U. S. Employment Service aptitude and interest testing for occupational exploration. *Journal of Employment Counseling, 20*, 179-185.

Minnesota Department of Jobs and Training. (undated). *Minnesota job search . . . The first step.* Pamphlet.

Parsons, F. (1909). *Choosing a vocation.* New York: Houghton Mifflin.

U. S. Department of Labor. (1970). *Manual for the USES General Aptitude Test Battery. Section III: Development.* Washington, DC: U. S. Government Printing Office.

U. S. Department of Labor. (1976). *Occupational outlook handbook* (1976-77 ed.). Washington, DC: Government Printing Office

U. S. Department of Labor. (1979). *Guide for occupational exploration.* Washington, DC: Government Printing Office.

U. S. Department of Labor. (1981). *Manual for the USES Interest Inventory.* Minneapolis: Intran.

U. S. Department of Labor. (1991). *Dictionary of occupational titles* (4th ed). Washington, DC: Government Printing Office.

Job Training Partnership

Susan M. Viranyi

Job training and education are essential in the rehabilitation of individuals toward more competitive employment. Through work experience, on-the-job training, and classroom instruction, individuals are prepared to meet employer demands and perform job responsibilities with more confidence and individual motivation. The Job Training Partnership Act (JTPA) works to train individuals of all ages for more competitive, permanent positions in the work force who, otherwise, are unable to obtain employment due to economic and social barriers (U. S. Congress, 1982).

History/Legislation

The JTPA has its beginning in four different job training acts, dating back 30 years. The Manpower Development and Training Act, enacted in 1962, was the first major legislation concerned with retraining heads of families unemployed due to technical changes on the job. It worked toward institutionalized and on-the-job training, and was administered by state employment services in coordination with vocational education agencies (Smith, 1985). In response to the changing needs of specific groups of workers, the Economic Opportunity Act of 1964 established a number of target programs designed to meet the training requirements of displaced and economically disadvantaged workers for a changing labor market. This act was administered through the Office of Economic Opportunity, local community action agencies, and school systems, but program standards and guidelines were enforced by the federal government. In 1971, the Emergency Employment Act was mandated in response to a constant rise in the rate of unemployment. It worked to aid in the placement of unemployed and underemployed people, especially in high rate areas in the nation. Finally, in 1973, the Comprehensive Employment and Training Act (CETA) replaced all previous training acts in an effort to decentralize authority and bring more programming and operation responsibility to the state and local government level. The premise was that local officials were in the best position to plan and monitor training programs, as they could best determine the needs of their own populations (Smith, 1985). CETA was enforced as the major legislation for employment training until 1978, at which time the mismanagement and misappropriation of funds became evident, and fraud was suspected at all levels. Attempts were made to amend the act through the reallocation of funding, however, support for CETA was diminishing as it did not prove to be overly effective in serving the needs of those at the lowest poverty levels. CETA was amended in 1978 and reauthorized until September 30, 1982. Congress was then faced with the task of replacing legislation for job training, as well as reestablishing credibility with the people of the United States, to set forth a plan to provide jobs for the neediest populations using available funds in the most equitable manner (Smith, 1985).

The goal of the 97th Congress was to continue the state and local involvement in job training, and expand service delivery and monitoring of training programs to the local business level. The fundamental principles used in the development of the Job Training Partnership Act encompassed the following:

- To strengthen the involvement of the private sector
- To increase the role of the state government and decrease that of the federal government
- To concentrate resources on training persons for jobs and to avoid income maintenance programs under the guise of a training program
- To concentrate on training those who cannot compete in the labor market without additional help
- To concentrate on results, rather than on details of how those results were achieved, by applying and enforcing meaningful performance standards (Quayle, 1982).

Both parties of Congress worked toward these principles in their development of legislation. Through joint hearings of the House and Senate, which included state and local authority as witness on employment and training, two bills were introduced in Congressional conference in September, 1982. Each claimed to improve the delivery of job training and education to the most economically deprived, through a partnership effort with the state and local industries (Smith, 1985). On September 30, 1982, Congress reached a bipartisan agreement on the Senate's bill, the Training for Jobs Act, and the bill from the House of Representatives, the Job Training Partnership Act. Both bills were revised to clarify program delivery and funding allotment issues, and put together to comprise the Job Training Partnership Act of 1982. President Ronald Reagan signed the bill into law on October 13, 1982, to become effective on October 1, 1983 (Smith, 1985). At the time of signing, President Reagan (1982) commented on the Act: "This program will train more than one million Americans every year in skills they can market where they live. We've eliminated the bureaucratic and administrative waste that has marked so many so-called job bills in the past." The structure of the JTPA, in itself, explains the delivery system and program objectives that work to enforce the job training partnership between private industry and individuals in need of marketable, skilled training.

STRUCTURE AND FUNDING

For fiscal year 1990, about $3 billion federally funded dollars were appropriated to participating states for JTPA programs (Starobin, 1989). Currently, all states are participating. The allotment of funds to individual states follows a prescribed formula:

33-1/3% allocated on the related number of unemployed individuals;

33-1/3% on the basis of unemployed individuals in the state in excess of 4.5% of the civilian labor force; and,

33-1/3% on the basis of the related number of economically disadvantaged individuals in the state (Smith, 1985).

Accordingly, the monies are distributed by the U. S. Department of Labor directly to the governor's office of each state and further redistributed to the various programs listed under the Act. An understanding of the state breakdown of authority required by the JTPA helps to clarify the appropriation of state funds.

Under the JTPA, the governor of the state is responsible for developing several groups to aid in the service delivery of the program. First, a State Job Training Coordinating Council (SJTCC) must be appointed to represent the population of the state. Members of the SJTCC include representatives of state agencies and organizations directly involved in employment and training and human resource utilization within the state, representatives of local governments, local businesses and industry, and other eligible members of the general public, organized labor, community-based organizations, and local educational agencies (U. S. Congress, 1982). The SJTCC will aid the governor by reviewing job training plans and making annual reports of all state agencies providing employment and training, namely, the programs set forth by state Service Delivery Areas.

Service Delivery Areas (SDAs) are the functional service units for programming under the JTPA. The governor is responsible for dividing the state into SDAs, each consisting of a local government with a population of 200,000 or more, or any consortium of contiguous units of general local government with an aggregate of 200,000 or more (U. S. Congress, 1982).

Finally, each SDA is managed by an appointed Private Industry Council (PIC) comprised of representatives of the private sector, educational agencies, organized labor, rehabilitation agencies, community-based organizations, economic development agencies, and public employment services (U. S. Congress, 1982). It is responsible for developing an implementation plan in the SDA for the disbursal of JTPA funds. Depending on state and SDA size, the regional PIC can either develop JTPA programming directly with private businesses in the SDA, or contract an independent agency within the SDA to coordinate JTPA programs. In choosing an independent SDA service provider, primary consideration is given to those agencies or organizations that have proven to be effective in the delivery of comparable or related training services. Funding to those agencies cannot duplicate state or locally funded services or programs already available in the SDA. Also, educational agencies and institutions will be given the opportunity to provide educational services unless programming under the Act can be more effective in enhancing the occupational growth of participants. Finally, no occupational skills training programs developed by independent agencies will be funded unless the level of skill meets the guidelines established by the PIC (U. S. Congress, 1982). Ultimately, the PIC is responsible for reviewing and overseeing programs to ensure that funds are used appropriately and performance standards are being met (Tindall, 1986).

Overall funding under the JTPA calls for at least 70% of state allotted funds to be used for direct training and programming, and the remaining 30% to be used for support services required by program participants. Program funds are further appropriated according to the specific titles of the Act. Title IIA of the JTPA allows for the funding of youth and adult training programs at the SDA regional level. PICs receive 78% of all state program funds, 60% to be used for adults and 40% for youths in training. Up to 10% of these funds can be used for handicapped and hard to serve populations from both age groups. This title also allots funds (the remaining 22% of state funds) for programming through State Education Agencies (matched at the local level), incentive grants, and programs for the elderly, all of which are coordinated directly through the governor's office (U. S. Congress, 1982).

Summer Youth Employment and Training Programs are made possible under title IIB of the JTPA. Federal funding under this title is separate from state allotment moneys, and is appropriated as deemed necessary by the governor. These additional funds are distributed by PICs at the local level of the SDA, however, SDAs are encouraged to coordinate the 40% title IIA funding with the summer funding, so that youths can receive continuous support throughout the year (Tindall, 1986).

The governor's office is also allowed funding, as necessary, for Employment and Training Assistance for dislocated workers, under title III of the Act. Additionally, the U. S. Department of Labor directly funds federal programs at the state level under title IV of the Act. Approximately $618 million are allocated annually for the Job Corps program in each state, under title IVB (Smith, 1985). The Job Corps program provides funding for residential centers where basic educational training, counseling, health care, and similar services are offered to help disadvantaged individuals prepare for jobs and responsible citizenship ("Major job," 1985). Other federal programs funded under title IV include programming for native Americans and migrants (Part A), Veterans (Part C), and other National Activities (Part D). All federal programs, aside from the Job Corps, equate to 7% of the total funds allotted under title IIA of the Act (Smith, 1985).

As is evident through the major allotment of funding, training programs developed for adult and youth populations in local SDAs are the main action of the JTPA. It is the programming under titles IIA and B between PICs and SDAs that actually provides for individualized on-the-job training and classroom instruction toward job readiness, and, thus, will be the focus for most counselors seeking to assist clients.

Purpose/Intent

"This act provides funding for job training for economically disadvantaged individuals and others who are in special need of training to begin employment" (U. S. Congress, 1982, p. 1322). By examination of the eligibility and performance standards, it is evident that the JTPA works to fulfill its stated purpose for individuals to achieve results and, ultimately, increase their level of living.

To participate in JTPA-funded programs, individuals usually fall into one of, or a combination of, the following age groups: youth, aged 14-21; adults, of any age, who are unemployed, underemployed, or faced with employment dislocation due to a business closure; or, any older individual, aged 55 or older, experiencing a specific barrier to employment (U. S. Congress, 1982). Primary consideration is given to applicants found to be economically disadvantaged. Economic status is determined through application, but disadvantaged individuals generally include any one of the following: welfare or food stamp recipients, foster children, or the homeless. Types of welfare or economic aid that are considered include: General Assistance, Refugee Assistance, Social Security Insurance, and Aid to Families with Dependent Children (U. S. Congress, 1982). Individuals who receive, or are blood-related to an individual receiving, any of the above types of aid are automatically eligible for training services under JTPA. Additionally, the following barriers to employment are considered, in conjunction with economic status, and usually qualify individuals for acceptance:

- School drop-out, or at risk of dropping out
- Limited English proficiency
- Pregnant/parenting teen
- Handicapped (Department of Rehabilitation clients automatically accepted)
- Older worker
- Veteran
- Vietnam-era Veteran
- Criminal offender
- Substance abuser
- Single head of household with dependent children (Illinois Department of Commerce and Community Affairs, 1990).

Each applicant is considered individually, and acceptance is affected by the size and available funds of the particular SDA. Generally, if some form of economic, educational, or employment deficiency is evident and directly, negatively affecting employment status, an individual may be eligible for JTPA sponsorship (U. S. Congress, 1982).

Specific performance standards have been established by the Secretary of Labor for the effective evaluation of all JTPA programs. For adult training programs, an overall increase of employment earnings, and a reduction in welfare dependency must be evident. Appropriate factors for participants include: placement in unsubsidized employment, retention in unsubsidized employment, and/or an increase in earnings. Generally, the number of individuals and families receiving cash welfare payments and the amount of payments should be reduced. The standard for youth programs includes: individual attainment of recognized employment competencies as determined by the Private Industry Council; elementary, secondary, post-secondary completion, or the equivalent thereof; enrollment in other training programs; or apprenticeship or enlistment in the armed forces. Variations in the performance standards are developed by the

Secretary of Labor, depending on varying state populations and unemployment rates (U. S. Congress, 1982).

By setting performance guidelines, local SDA programs are challenged by their PIC to produce results or risk contract loss. SDA programs can ensure positive results by constant promotion of JTPA programs through their local job service agency and other human service agents, and consistent delivery of client services.

Client Services

The client service delivery model for JTPA programming is authorized through the regional PIC and individual SDA agency offices. As outlined earlier, the PIC is responsible for the distribution of funding under titles IIA and B, as well as the monitoring, reviewing, and setting of performance standards of evaluation for the programs set forth by the independent SDA agency. Generally, agencies that would normally provide training services (e.g., a local union training organization) are chosen by PICs to administer and monitor JTPA programming using the funding provided. Personnel for the JTPA program, therefore, are carried over from the existing staff of the SDA agency contracted through the PIC. Personnel experience ranges from high school graduates to degreed business persons, usually without prior experience in JTPA programming. Once an agency is contracted, internal changes to the staff include the assignment of various program coordinators, employability assessors, bookkeepers, fiscal clerks, and follow-up personnel. Education in the legislation and programming of the JTPA occurs on-the-job and through state and regional seminars and programming meetings held by the state and the regional PICs. SDA agency contracts are enacted for two years, and are subject to review and termination by the PIC pending performance and outcome of programming (W. Felts, personal communication, February 21, 1991).

Client services can begin in a number of different places associated with the SDA regional office. Outreach offices run by SDA personnel are located in select areas of the SDA region, perhaps, one in each county. Clients can be referred to the outreach offices for JTPA eligibility assessment by a variety of human service agencies, including the local employment service, Department of Rehabilitation, school districts, and the local public aid office. Once eligibility for services has been confirmed, the client may undergo further vocational or academic evaluation to determine program placement, needs, and interests. Outreach counselors work with individuals by informing them of the programs currently available through JTPA and helping them decide which will be of most benefit (Illinois Farmers Union-Training, Inc. [IFU-T], 1990a).

Following the funding allotments provided in titles IIA and B and the guidelines listed above, a typical SDA JTPA agency might include programming in three separate areas: classroom training, on-the-job training, and youth programs.

CLASSROOM TRAINING

The JTPA provides for remedial education, basic literacy skills, and bilingual training, as well as pre-apprenticeship programs, institutional skill training, and support services under title IIA (U. S. Congress, 1982). These programs are not limited, and may also include two-year or certificate programs through local community colleges or universities. Courses and programs for classroom training are offered based on employable skills evident in current regional labor markets (W. Felts, personal communication, February 21, 1991). Educational programs funded through JTPA include services, fees, and tuition payments associated with successful completion of the program (IFU-T, 1990b).

Individuals involved in educational JTPA programming are followed-up on their progress regularly, and client service centers located on campuses of colleges involved in programming are available for student assistance and counseling on a daily basis. Upon completion of programming or certification, clients are referred to college placement centers for job seeking assistance and career planning. If a client completes a remedial or basic skills program, he or she may be eligible for further JTPA programming through on-the-job training.

ON-THE-JOB TRAINING

Individuals can also benefit from an applied educational experience with on-the-job training. JTPA program coordinators will assist individuals in finding meaningful employment or enable them to learn a skill or trade while working. Regional SDA coordinators of on-the-job training programs are responsible for procuring and enforcing contracts with local private industry and businesses, and providing workers to fulfill those contracts. Employers participating in JTPA programs are reimbursed for their training efforts with 50% of the trainees' entry level wages (IFU-T, 1990a). Additionally, after the trainee has completed his contracted training time through JTPA, on-the-job training personnel follow-up to monitor the employee's progress and maintenance of job function. On-the-job training contracts with private industry are variable in time, depending on the skill being taught and the needs of the trainee (W. Felts, personal communication, February 21, 1991).

YOUTH PROGRAMS

Title IIA provides funding for the employment and educational training of youths aged 14-21. Title IIB is specifically designed to aid, as necessary, youths in summer employment and training programs, to continue training and support throughout the year. Funds may be used for basic and remedial education, institutional and on-the-job training, work experience, counseling, out-reach activities, job referral and placement, job search, and job clubs (U. S. Congress, 1982). Youth programs are targeted for at-risk youths, including school drop-outs, remedial students, and economically disadvantaged individuals. JTPA programming hopes to assist youths in preparing for future work environments by maintaining and improving academic and work experience skills. A competency system of pre-employment/work maturity skills awareness and basic education skills training works to instill a work ethic and sense of worker responsibility to youths who are uninterested or uninvolved with their future employment status (IFU-T, 1990c).

Over the years it has been enforced, the Job Training Partnership Act has worked to improve the lives of those most economically disadvantaged and most in need. Legislation in 1986 amended the JTPA by extending funding to various federal programs and shifting allotment formulas to favor areas in the country with highest unemployment and economic instability (Starobin, 1989). As legislation keeps changing and congressional leaders work to provide for the most underprivileged in the United States, the premise enacted through the JTPA of partnerships through local governments and private industry should stay intact. In this way, state and local governments can maintain control over the needs of their people, and a more effective method of training individuals toward economic and employment independence can endure.

References

Illinois Department of Commerce and Community Affairs. (1990). *JTPA–II Standard Application–All Titles*. (Available from IFU-T, Inc., Zeigler, Illinois.)

Illinois Farmers Union-Training, Inc. (IFU-T) (1990a). *Create a job for yourself*. JTPA newsletter. (Available from IFU-T, Inc., Zeigler, Illinois.)

Illinois Farmers Union-Training, Inc. (1990b). *Newsletter on college programs and certification through JTPA*. (Available from IFU-T, Inc., Zeigler, Illinois.)

Illinois Farmers Union-Training, Inc. (1990c). *Newsletter on JTPA youth programs*. (Available from IFU-T, Inc., Zeigler, Illinois.)

Major job and training programs. (1985). *Congressional Digest, 64*, 102-3.

Quayle, D. (1982). Introduction to 52184: Job Training Act of 1982. *Congressional Record, 128*(3), 3652.

Reagan, R. (1982). Remarks on signing the Job Training Partnership Act: October 13, 1982. *Public papers of the President of the United States, Book II*. Washington, DC: Government Printing Office.

Smith, W. E. (1985). *A history of the initial development of the 1982 Job Training Partnership Act*. Unpublished doctoral dissertation, Southern Illinois University, Carbondale, Illinois.

Starobin, P. (1989). Job act rewrite favors cities over suburban areas. *Congressional Quarterly Weekly Report, 47*, 1952.

Tindall, L. W. (1986). Understanding the Job Training Partnership Act. In L. W. Tindall, J. Gugerty, & B. Dougherty (Eds.), *Partnerships in business and education: Helping handicapped students become a part of the Job Training Partnership Act* (pp. 1-14). Madison, WI: University of Wisconsin-Madison.

U. S. Congress. (1982). Public Law 97-300: Job Training Partnership Act. *U. S. Statutes at Large*, 97th Congress, 2nd Session: Vol. 96 (pp. 1322-1399). Washington, DC: U. S. Government Printing Office.

Private Employment Services

James T. Herbert, Ph.D., C.R.C.

When discussing vocational and employment services within the private sector, it is important to distinguish between the two services. Although these service terms are often used interchangeably, they represent different processes. Vocational services, as used in this chapter, describe a planned sequence of vocational assessment techniques and career information that culminates in an identified occupational goal consistent with client interests, skills, and abilities. These services require careful evaluation, discussion, planning, and coordination so that clients have a greater self-awareness and appreciation of selecting and reaching an appropriate vocational goal. Employment services, as described here, represent the culmination of the vocational preparation process. These services may involve, but are not limited to, assisting clients in developing placeability skills such as locating job leads, demonstrating appropriate job interview and job keeping behaviors, and understanding how to effectively use written sources of information when applying for employment (e.g., resumé, application form). In essence, vocational services facilitate client self-understanding as it relates to choosing a job or career path; whereas, employment services are directed toward realizing this path once it is deemed that the client is, in fact, "job ready." Consequently, while private companies, agencies, or firms have the same goal—to secure employment for an individual; the methods, process, and skills of the placement specialist and client seeking employment are dramatically different. In simplest terms, private employment services can be categorized by clientele who are either interested in temporary employment, permanent employment, executive recruitment services, or personnel consulting services. The former two categories serve as the focus of this chapter.

TEMPORARY SERVICE COMPANIES

This industry consists of businesses that supply workers for a specific time period to other employers on a fee or contractual basis. Temporary workers usually substitute for other regular full-time workers who may be absent because of illness, vacation, union strikes, or other reasons for which regular employees can not perform their jobs. These transitional workers will also be employed during high seasonal demand periods or special projects with limited duration. Consequently, work orders for temporary employees need to be filled almost immediately. If the employer can not be served quickly and effectively, the temporary service company will soon be out of business. In most situations, the employee will start within one or two days after the employer has placed a work order with the company. There are, however, many situations in which the employer must have workers on the same day the request is made.

In order to identify employment skills, persons interested in working for temporary service companies must be screened by the company representative, tested in various skill areas, and undergo employment reference checks. In some cases, temporary service companies will provide limited technical training such as text (word) processing, telemarketing, or basic accounting. Depending upon the individual company, the job seeker may be required to absorb part, all, or none of the training fee. Most temporary service companies tend to specialize in one of four major occupational areas: office/clerical, industrial, medical, or technical/professional fields. While the majority of temporary service companies tend to be local business entrepreneurs, others are affiliated with national companies (e.g., Accountemps Inc., Career Blazers, Kelly Services, Inc., Manpower Inc., and The Olsten Corporation). According to the National Association of Temporary Services, there are 3,500 national, regional, and independent companies operating over 10,000 offices throughout the United States (National Association of Temporary Services [NATS], 1988).

EMPLOYMENT AGENCIES

These businesses also serve employers by identifying a pool of qualified job applicants, but are different from temporary service companies in several respects. Most notably, instead of seeking temporary jobs, clients from employment agencies are placed in permanent full- or part-time positions. Employment agencies attempt to match employer needs with job seekers registered with the agency. An agency representative meets with prospective employees to assist them in identifying their job skills. Typically, this process results in an employee resumé which the agency later distributes to appropriate employers. Likewise, the potential job seeker also has an opportunity to review positions that are listed with the agency. In essence, the employment agency serves as a retailer or broker that maintains an inventory of resumés and job listings. Unlike the temporary service industry, once an employee obtains the job, he or she becomes a member of the employer's permanent work force. In return for finding the individual a job, the employment agency charges a prescribed fee which may be paid by either the job seeker, which is termed an applicant paid fee, or the employer. If the fee is paid by the employer, it can be either on a contingency basis, where the fee is collected only after a candidate is hired by the employer, or on a retainer basis in which payment is not contingent upon hiring the referred candidate. Finally, it should be noted that some employment agencies also offer temporary services to employers. These agencies are sometimes described in the industry as "full-service employment agencies."

History/Legislation

The history of private employment services was partially founded on a very simple concept—employees and employers often found it easier if someone else assumed the responsibility for locating employment prospects. Rather than relying upon word of mouth or advertising, both the job seeker and the job provider, would prefer to have someone else conduct a job search and recruit appropriate personnel. Private employment services also proliferated because of special employment situations whereby the employer did not necessarily wish to increase its permanent work force and traditional methods in identifying qualified workers were not successful.

Temporary help companies emerged after World War II because of existing labor shortages (Rudney, 1978). Since this beginning, temporary help companies have evolved over "three generations" (NATS, 1988). The first generation was characterized by temporary workers who were assigned to perform routine work during emergency situations, such as a regular worker absence or a sudden upsurge in work production. The second generation emerged during the 1960s in response to businesses desiring to cut fixed costs. Cost overruns, such as overtime pay to permanent employees during peak production periods or layoffs during slack periods, and unemployment claims during employee layoffs were major reasons why temporary workers were used to supplement the permanent work force. The current and third generation of temporary services have diversified to include such other industries as health care services, marketing, professional, and technical fields. In addition, many companies currently use temporary help services on long-term special projects as well as routine jobs where turnover is problematic. As a result, temporary help companies in today's market represent a fundamental aspect of corporate life. Nearly 90% of companies with more than 500 employees use temporary services (Grossman & Magnus, 1989). While the majority of temporary jobs have historically involved office/clerical positions, considerable growth has been noted in other areas as well. For example, a national survey of companies who are members of the National Association of Temporary Services (NATS) revealed that 52% of jobs were in accounting/finance, 30% in data processing, 14% in engineering, 12% in factory work, 9% in consulting, 9% in health care, and 7% in administrative work (Halcrow, 1988). Although the temporary service industry has not experienced significant growth during the past several years, it is anticipated that the industry will experience moderate growth during the next decade (Silverman & Dennis, 1990). This anticipated growth is expected because, just as in the past, employers will continue to seek workers with specialized training while wanting to reduce costs as much as possible; certain labor markets will experience hiring peaks and cutbacks; and a sizeable work force will desire flexible work schedules to accommodate personal needs and lifestyles (Halcrow, 1988).

Private employment agencies started in the United States around 1820 (Martinez, 1969). Their beginnings were, in some ways, very similar to today's business practices. Whereas personnel consultants today specialize in various employment disciplines, early pioneers specialized according to salary levels (National Association of Personnel Consultants [NAPC], 1990). Private employment agencies continued to operate as the "only business in town" until the Great Depression occurred. At that time, the United States Employment Service was created to provide a public employment service (*see* Employment Security-Job Service chapter). As the effects of the Depression abated with the expansion of the economy brought on by World War II, employment agencies eventually specialized by employment fields. Consequently, a shift from filling employer orders for unskilled positions to a new placement emphasis which addressed professional, technical, and managerial jobs resulted. Today, more than 20,000 full-time placement firms exist and employ over 80,000 persons in the industry (NAPC, 1990).

With regard to legislation as it relates to the private employment service industry, a primary issue concerns the license requirement of private employment agencies. Currently, 27 states have no licensure requirement with regard to employment agencies that charge fees to employers and, of these, 11 states do not require licensure of agencies that charge fees to individuals (i.e., client applicant fee).[1] This licensure requirement is essentially intended to protect the consumer from unfair business practices.

The same applicant fee laws required of permanent placement agencies in designated states are not applicable to the temporary help industry and executive recruitment firms, however. In fact, the National Association of Temporary Services (NATS) has argued that their industry is different because the same laws and regulations applicable to any employer must be followed as well by temporary employment companies; for example, those laws prohibiting discrimination on the basis of age, disability, gender, race, and religion. As such, NATS contends that no basis for imposing additional regulations are required of temporary employment service companies (B. Steinberg, personal communication, January 8, 1991).

FUNDING

There are two considerations when examining funding sources of private placement services, "Who pays the fee for finding employment for the individual?" and "How much will it cost?" In the case of temporary service companies, the fee

---

[1] Employer charged fees are as follows: *Maine, New Hampshire, Vermont*, Massachusetts, *Rhode Island*, Connecticut, New York, Pennsylvania, Maryland, Virginia, North Carolina, Georgia, *Florida, Alabama, Mississippi*, Ohio, Minnesota, Texas, Kansas, Nebraska, *South Dakota, North Dakota*, Colorado, Utah, Arizona, *New Mexico*, and California. States in italics do not require a license to charge fees to individuals.

is paid by the employer according to an hourly rate. In general, the service charge ranges between 35% and 60% markup for services provided by the temporary employee. Temporary service companies justify this fee because the employer does not have to invest in recruitment costs, fringe benefits, unemployment and medical insurance, overtime, or severance pay (Lewis & Schuman, 1988). Employment agencies, on the other hand, may charge either the employer or the individual a set fee or percentage of the annual salary. These fees are usually set at around 30% of the employee's first year of income. In some instances, such as repeat corporate clients, the fee may be reduced somewhat. Of course, if the agency has a contingency fee arrangement, and does not provide any job applicant which the company hires, then no fee can be collected. If, on the other hand, the agency has a retainer fee arrangement, then payment is guaranteed no matter what the outcome. Consequently, these fees can easily range from several to many thousands of dollars. Executive search and recruitment firms, as expected, charge even higher fees. Typically, these fees approximate one-third of the first year's compensation including salary and bonus, and an additional 10% to 20% for incurred expenses. Since this industry concentrates on high-level professional, managerial, and technical positions, the fees can be quite lucrative.

PERSONNEL

There is a host of professionals who are willing to assist other persons in resolving employment problems which may be associated with getting a new job or becoming more effective in the existing job. Within the realm of vocational concerns, psychologists, counselors, social workers, and paraprofessionals often assist clients in resolving work-related problems that are personal and social in nature. There also exists a host of specialists who deliver vocational, as well as employment services, but, because of their expertise, provide such services to particular clientele. For example, rehabilitation counselors, mental health specialists, social workers, gerontologists, and secondary guidance counselors typify this group. Further, recognizing the extensive body of knowledge that has accumulated in vocational and placement training, career/employment counselors have historically played a critical role in facilitating client career paths. Last, and perhaps not as recognized by human service workers as making an important contribution in helping others resolve employment problems, are those private employment professionals with business, marketing, and personnel management training.

Although some individuals would contend that private service personnel do not comprise a profession (Byrne, 1986), it is clear that professional associations exist to address the needs of each type of private employment service. Within the industry, several organizations such as the National Association of Temporary Services (NATS), National Association of Personnel Consultants (NAPC), and Association of Executive Search Consultants (AESC) are available. These associations have developed prescribed ethical codes and professional practice guidelines to promote quality service. To become a member of each organization, generally, requires the person to pay a prescribed membership fee and complete a signed statement to follow the ethical codes and professional practices, a process very similar to procedures found in many human service associations as well.

Within the private employment services industry, there are two types of certification currently available. The first, Certified Personnel Consultant (CPC) requires the individual to work at least two years (full-time) as a consultant, and sign a written statement attesting that the person will comply with the NAPC ethical code and professional practice guidelines. The second, and most recent type, Certified Temporary Staffing-Specialist (CTS) requires one year full-time experience and an agreement to comply with the professional ethical code and practices. If these conditions are fulfilled, persons are eligible to sit for the national certification exam in their respective areas. Applicants may repeat the exam until a passing score has been obtained.

Purpose/Intent

Given the information presented in this chapter and the chapter describing the Job Service program, the human service worker might wonder whether duplicity exists in private and public employment services. Or, stated in more direct terms, "Why is there a need for a private employment service which charges a considerable fee-for-service, if the public employment service provides placement that is already free?" This question is one that has caused considerable debate between the two major employment systems. The private employment system contends that the public system or Job Service is wasting tax dollars to find employment of persons who are already employed. Accordingly, the private employment industry believes that state/federal monies should only be directed to unemployed persons, and not subsidizing employed workers looking to change careers or assisting large corporations in finding suitable employees thereby reducing hiring costs (Luman, 1987). Given that the number of Job Service counselors has declined by almost half since 1981 (Morgan, 1989), it would seem that efforts to find more job applicants would not be necessary. However, these two systems, while providing the same essential service, have markedly different clientele and occupational outcomes. A review of placements by public and private employment agencies as noted by Clark (1988) revealed that, " . . . public agencies [were] relatively more specialized in the placement of domestic, nondomestic service, clerical, and unskilled workers, while private agencies concentrate[d] on the placement of clerical, professional, technical, managerial, and nondomestic service workers" (p. 385). This finding emphasizes an essential difference between the two service systems. In addition, as Clark contends, while the public employment service has historically served as a broker for employers and employees, the private system has always maintained that job placement is the most critical performance criterion. The final and perhaps critical difference between the systems is that not all clients who seek public employment services intend to seek employment. Some clients register with the employment service in order to secure other secondary benefits such as food stamps and unemployment insurance benefits as opposed to seeking employment (Clark, 1988).

With regard to private employment services, the major reason that explains their success is they have, in essence, effectively served both employer and employee in recruiting, finding, and hiring efforts. While employment agencies and executive recruitment firms take the hassle out of hiring, temporary service companies go one step further to the point where employers do not assume any of the responsibilities for finding appropriate workers. Employers who use temporary service companies do not have to worry about employee turnover, absenteeism, supervision, or administrative costs. All employee wages, benefits, unemployment and workers' compensation, social security, and related taxes are assumed by the temporary service company. In return, the company charges an agreed upon hourly bill rate for these services. The benefits for employees who work for temporary service companies are varied. Many individuals choose temporary work because it provides work schedule flexibility, opportunities to improve work skills and explore new career fields, an additional income source, and a mechanism to obtain full-time, permanent work (Carey & Hazelbaker, 1986). These advantages can be particularly important for single parents, high school and college students, retirees, and persons wanting to re-enter the work force after some period of not working competitively. Consequently, while recent economic slowdowns indicate that the temporary employment industry has not experienced growth during the past several years, it is believed that this industry will expand toward the year 2000 as companies deal with tighter labor markets, higher labor costs, and the continuing demand to improve productivity levels (Silverman & Dennis, 1990).

As the composition of American workers changes over the next several decades, private employment agencies must diversify and seek new potential workers if they are to continue to realize their purpose in finding qualified workers for employers. This awareness has led the industry to market services to traditionally disenfranchised groups who have not had the same types of employment opportunities as other workers. Two examples of traditionally disenfranchised groups that have recently received greater attention in the private employment industry are older workers and persons with disabilities (LaPerch, 1990; Stoller, 1990). This diversification will play an important role for the private employment industry, especially since the actual number of available workers will continue to decrease as the next century approaches.

Client Services

Regardless of which type of employment service is used, the primary service is essentially the same—to place suitable workers in appropriate jobs. As such, private employment services have an obligation to both the company client and the job applicant. Perhaps what differentiates these services, as noted earlier, is the type of clientele each placement service attempts to assist. The primary service which temporary placement companies provide is to have available workers who can meet employer needs on a very short notice. To accomplish this task, the private company must conduct formal testing, check employment and personal references, and interview each prospective employee before assigning work. If done properly, employers will have some assurance that the temporary worker has been appropriately matched according to the job demands. This process is certainly more effective than a job interview which is the primary method used by employers. In addition, many temporary employment companies also provide insurance protection so that the company client is protected against loss and liability. These benefits serve as major incentives to company clients.

There are also several benefits to clients seeking temporary work. Perhaps one major benefit is that individuals have the flexibility to determine which jobs they are interested in working and on what basis. Temporary service companies also offer immediate employment at competitive wages to supplement income, an opportunity to establish a work history and develop specific skills, and provide the worker with a variety of work settings and experiences which can be useful when making career choices for later permanent employment if so desired.

Private employment agencies and executive recruitment and search firms also provide the benefit of identifying an available pool of qualified workers. The difference though has to do with the complexity in identifying skilled employees. Employment agencies have the majority of client (job applicant) referrals as a result of self-initiated contacts whereas the executive recruitment firm initiates all contacts in identifying potential workers. Executive recruitment firms do all of the work in order to secure a list of job candidates.

REFERRAL CONSIDERATIONS

When preparing clients for private employment services, the first consideration must be which service is most appropriate given individual client needs. Although there are specific questions that human service workers should have their clients address, there are a number of generic issues that are important. Certainly, the reputation of the private employment service is crucial. Clients may wish to speak with other persons that are currently using, or have recently used, the service in order to evaluate service quality. For persons with particular career/job interests and skills, the private employment service specialist should have familiarity with the industry of interest in terms of employer requirements and job openings. Although professional competence is sometimes hard to evaluate, recognition of professional certification serves as one indicator. Clients may wish to inquire whether the professional has obtained a certification in a particular employment service area. As noted earlier, two types of certification exist, depending upon the services provided and clientele served. Membership in a professional association such as those identified earlier may also serve as another indication of one's professional commitment. Finally, before deciding upon one type of company, agency, or firm, it is in the client's best interest to visit several similar placement services so that a more informed choice can be made. The relationship between the placement service specialist and the job seeker is unique. Therefore, it is in the client's best interest to work with an employment specialist who can establish client rapport and mutual trust, and demonstrates the ability to implement an effective job search.

There are, however, specific concerns with respect to each type of private placement service that human service workers may wish to review with their clients before a referral is initiated:

Temporary Employment Companies

1. Investigate whether any training opportunities to improve skills are available. If available, is training free, or is there some type of employment commitment (i.e., amount of hours) to be eligible for training?
2. Have all employment documentation available when visiting the temporary employment service. Examples include a state-issued driver's license or photo identification, social security card, birth certificate, or alien registration card. Written information specifically detailing previous employment including job title, place of employment, supervisor's name and telephone number, job duties, and dates of employment should also be done prior to the visit.
3. Clients should be prepared for an interview and possible testing to document employment skills. In some instances, clients should also be prepared to undergo alcohol/drug testing. Recent hiring trends have suggested that an increasing number of employers are requiring drug testing of all employees, including temporary workers.
4. Assist clients in becoming informed consumers of private employment services by identifying a written list of questions prior to the interview. Some important areas may include types and length of typical work assignments, employee benefits (e.g., vacation, sick, merit raises, bonuses), policy and level of contribution required by employee or temporary service to accrue benefits (i.e., accumulated over consecutive or cumulative work periods), and consequences if employer wishes to hire the temporary worker as a regular employee. Having a clear idea as to what employment restrictions apply such as time and length of employment available, transportation problems, and type of employment being sought also need to be examined prior to the interview.
5. If obtaining immediate employment is critical, many temporary service personnel will indicate that the best time to visit is Monday mid-morning or mid-afternoon Friday. These two times seem to be the busiest periods when job orders are filled and workers are needed to fulfill employer demands.
6. Clients should be told of any special employment situations that may be detrimental (e.g., an overly demanding supervisor, potential or existing union strike or lockout, racist or sexist work environment).

Employment Agency

Although many of the same recommendations noted previously are also
applicable, there are some specific issues if it is an applicant (client) fee paid
arrangement:
1. Always obtain a written statement as to what fee and reimbursable expenses,
   if any, are included. If there are any concerns with regard to the client's
   reading and comprehension skills, the client should never sign any contracts
   until reviewed by some other competent and trusted individual.
2. Job applicants should be told of any questionable business practices of
   employers whom they are interested in considering before conducting on-site
   job interviews.
3. Distribution of client resumés should not be given unless written permission
   outlining under what conditions is first obtained. Clients must have control
   as to which employers review resumés to avert any instances that may
   jeopardize employment status of applicants who are presently working.
4. Clients should receive a detailed, written job description outlining duties,
   salary, and terms of employment before making any final decision.
5. Agencies that only spend five to 10 minutes with prospective clients should
   be avoided, since this time seems insufficient in assessing one's work skills
   and employment interests. Current professional practice indicates that at
   least 30 minutes to an hour is required (M. K. Hamm, personal communication, January 28,1991).
These aforementioned questions and concerns may assist human service
workers in helping clients become informed consumers of private employment
services. Certainly, the private employment industry can be a valuable resource
to many clients. While not discussed, perhaps the central question is whether
clients would be better off in developing their own resources in learning how to
obtain employment. In some cases, this alternative may be the clear choice. The
human service worker may either decide to teach these skills to clients or, perhaps,
use the services of a personnel consulting firm. In other instances, using the vast
array of services to facilitate employment, including those within the private
employment industry, may constitute a second option.

A FINAL CAVEAT IN USING PRIVATE EMPLOYMENT SERVICES

Recognizing that the major purpose of private employment services is to recruit
and place individuals in suitable employment, there have been a number of
criticisms against the industry. To present a balanced view, these criticisms should
be articulated so that both human service workers and the clients they serve may
become more fully aware of them.
One basic criticism is that the private employment industry seems more driven
by a profit motive, than a human service motive. Certainly, private employment

services are in the business to make money, but there are some who contend that the amount of work expended seems more concerned with quantity vs. quality. For example, Levenson (1988) believed applicant charged fees were quite inconsistent with the actual amount of work that was performed by employment agencies. One might also question the extent of employment screening on the basis of a job interview lasting approximately 30 to 45 minutes. There has been a consistent body of literature to indicate that personnel interviews to evaluate one's job potential is quite dubious despite its continuing practice (Arvey & Campion, 1982).

A second criticism against the private employment industry is that it serves in continuing hiring discrimination practices. This criticism has been particularly levied against employment agencies (CBS News, 1990; Martinez, 1969). This allegation is not particularly surprising given that the primary client of employment agencies is the client who pays the recruitment fee. In most cases, this means company clients who have retainer or contingency search fee arrangements. As such, it becomes incumbent upon the private employment agency/executive recruitment firm to provide the kind of worker the employer desires. Consequently, the employment agency or firm is an extension of the company client. In order to fulfill the expectations desired by the company client, certain subjective characteristics that are unrelated to job performance may also be desired by the employer. These hiring preferences may have to do with one's age, ethnicity, gender, marital and religious status, or physical appearance. Although federal and state laws prohibit employment discrimination, lawsuits initiated by the job seeker who perceive discrimination are quite rare. Certainly, the costs in terms of time and expense may be one disincentive but, as Freedman (1986) indicated, a lawsuit by someone using an executive search firm would indicate that the executive was considering another job. If known by the present employer, this fact may severely jeopardize current employment. This same predicament would also apply for the person who uses an employment agency who is currently employed, but is privately exploring or being recruited for other career/job opportunities. Parenthetically, it should be noted that while allegations of discrimination have also been directed toward the private employment industry, there is a specific clause in the professional ethical code by members of the National Association of Personnel Consultants that indicates that consultants should not violate equal employment laws with regard to race, sex, color, age, religion, national origin, and handicap. No such specific clause is included by the Association of Executive Search Consultants. In the case of temporary service companies, discrimination should not be an issue since, like all employers, they are required to follow federal and state law regulations.

A third criticism of the industry that is specifically levied against temporary employment service companies is that these workers do not seem to obtain the same types of benefits as permanent employees doing comparable work. For example, a recent congressional hearing found that temporary workers, on average, received lower wages, fewer health care benefits, inadequate pensions, and limited skill upgrading and retooling than their full-time, permanent employee counterparts (Committee on Government Operations, 1988). Reasons to account for fewer benefits and lower salaries among temporary workers are directly related to employer attempts to reduce costs. These findings, of course, should not characterize the entire temporary employment service industry. However, it seems clear that human service workers should at least review these potential liabilities before clients enlist the services of a temporary employment company.

With these caveats in mind, it is hoped that human service workers will consider the potential benefits and liabilities with every client before engaging any private employment service. Certainly, this industry has much to offer our clientele.

References

Arvey, R. D., & Campion, J. E. (1982). The employment interview: A summary and review of recent research. *Personnel Psychology, 35*, 281-322.

Byrne, J. A. (1986). *The headhunters*. New York: Macmillan.

Carey, M. L., & Hazelbaker, K. L. (1986). Temporary jobs. *Occupational Outlook Quarterly, 30*(3), 21-25.

CBS News [Sixty Minutes]. (1990, February). *All-American*. (Journal Graphics No. 2221), New York, NY: Author.

Clark, W. (1988). Production costs and output qualities in public and private employment agencies. *The Journal of Law and Economics, 31*, 379-393.

Committee on Government Operations. (1988). *Rising use of part-time and temporary workers: Who benefits and who loses?* Washington, DC: U. S. Government Printing Office.

Freedman, H. S. (1986). *How to get a headhunter to call*. New York: John Wiley & Sons.

Grossman, M. E., & Magnus, M. (1989). Temporary services: A permanent way of life. *Personnel Journal, 68*(1), 38.

Halcrow, A. (1988). Temporary services warm to the business climate. *Personnel Journal, 67*(10), 84-89.

LaPerch, W. J. (1990). Employment agencies and persons with disabilities. *Personnel Consultant, 13*(6), 23-24.

Levenson, D. A. (1988). Needed: Revamped recruiting services. *Personnel, 65*(7), 50-52.

Lewis, W., & Schuman, N. (1988). *The temp worker's handbook*. New York: AMACOM.

Luman, J. (1987). Maybe they shouldn't get their money's worth. *Personnel Consultant, 10*(1), 39-40.

Martinez, T. M. (1969). *Past and present counseling and placement procedures in private employment agencies—An empirical study*. Washington, DC: Department of Labor, Manpower Administration, Office of Manpower Research (ERIC Document Reproduction Service No. ED 054 300).

Morgan, R. H. (1989, October). *Written testimony concerning the public employment service*. Presented before the Subcommittee on Employment Opportunities of the Committee on Education and Labor House of Representatives, Washington, DC.

National Association of Temporary Services. (1988). *Temporary help meets businesses' changing demands*. Alexandria, VA: Author.

National Association of Personnel Consultants. (1990). *National directory of personnel consultants*. Alexandria, VA: Author.

Rudney, S. (1978). Is temporary work for you? *Occupational Outlook Quarterly, 22*(4), 12-14.

Silverman, L., & Dennis, S. J. (1990). The temporary help industry annual update. *Contemporary Times, 9*(3), 10-14.

Stoller, W. H. (1990). Older workers benefit from "over-qualified" stigma. *Personnel Consultant, 13*(6), 15-17.

Supported Employment

Paula K. Davis, Ph.D.
Cheryl Hanley-Maxwell, Ph.D.
Edna Mora Szymanski, Ph.D.

Human service workers often are required to look outside their own agency to find resources to assist their clients in obtaining and maintaining a job. Supported employment is a relatively new vocational rehabilitation service (Szymanski & Parker, 1988), and, thus, many community service providers have limited or no knowledge about it.

Supported employment is a service option for people with severe disabilities. It is based on a philosophical foundation that includes such principles as: normalization (Wolfensberger, 1972), dignity of risk (Perske, 1972), least restrictive environment, zero exclusion (Wehman, 1988), and the right to self-determination (Wolfensberger, 1972). The essence of these principles is that people, no matter how severe their disability, should be enabled to work in integrated environments; and that, as much as possible, they should control all decisions about their lives. These principles, when taken together form the foundation for supported employment practices.

The purpose of this chapter is to provide an overview of supported employment. Topics that will be covered include: (a) a definition of supported employment and its characteristics, (b) a description of the models of supported employment, and (c) a summary of the components of the supported employment process.

Legislative Definition

Supported employment is defined by the Rehabilitation Act Amendments of 1986 as:

> ...competitive work in integrated settings (a) for individuals with severe handicaps for whom competitive employment has not traditionally occurred, or (b) for individuals for whom competitive employment has been interrupted or intermittent as a result of a

severe disability and who, because of their handicap, need on-going
support services to perform such work.

Four components of this definition are critical and can be viewed as defining
characteristics of supported employment: (a) competitive work, (b) integrated
settings, (c) severe disabilities, and (d) on-going support. Each of these components
must be present to label a service as "supported employment." Each will be defined
and frequent misapplications will be discussed.

COMPETITIVE WORK

The term competitive work, as used in the definition of supported employment,
is "work that is performed on a full-time basis or on a part-time basis, averaging
at least 20 hours per week for each pay period, for which an individual is
compensated in accordance with the Fair Labor Standards Act" (Federal Register,
May 12, 1988). This definition does not address benefits, level of earnings, and
advancement potential. These issues, however, are critical factors in determining
whether or not there has been improvement in the consumer's quality of life (e.g.,
enhanced physical and social integration, improved financial well-being, increased
self-determination), which is an intended result of community integration in
general, and supported employment in particular (Rusch, Chadsey-Rusch, &
Johnson, 1991).

Target jobs that provide income that is just enough to disqualify the individual
from social security benefits and do not replace lost benefits with employer-
provided benefits, do little to enhance the quality of life for the individual. Neither
do jobs that provide little or no opportunity for advancement in terms of hours,
wages, benefits, or position. Service providers who see the securing of a job as "the
placement" rather than a part in the development of an employment history also
do little to enhance the quality of life for the supported employee (Whitehead,
1989). While these jobs may meet the literal requirement of competitive work, they
do not meet the spirit of supported employment. Supported employment is intended
to be a vehicle that expands opportunities for previously unserved or unsuccessful
individuals and improves their quality of life, not a restrictive community-based
placement that may result in more isolation and more restrictions than those
encountered in other service options.

INTEGRATED WORK SETTINGS

The requirement for integrated work settings is met if supported employees
have regular contact with nondisabled persons (other than support personnel) at
the work site. Integration is further defined by Shafer and Nisbet (1988) as "the
participation of a worker in the operation of the work culture at both the
environment's required level and the worker's desired level" (p. 57). This definition
indicates the critical need for an adequate match between the needs and resources
of the supported employee, and the physical and social aspects of the job. Success

in integration is measured by: (a) the level of acceptance of the supported employee by co-workers, (b) the degree of interdependence in work tasks between supported employees and their co-workers, (c) the type and amount of interaction between co-workers and the target employee (in relation to the norm for that setting), (d) the degree to which interaction is fostered by physical proximity, and (e) the level of participation of the supported employee in the decision-making process at the work site (Shafer & Nisbet, 1988).

The integration component requirement is violated if workers are not provided with regular and consistent opportunities for interaction with nondisabled co-workers (Shafer & Nisbet, 1988). Mobile work crews that operate only at night or in isolated settings, that have no members (other than the supervisor) who are not disabled, or that have no contact with persons who are nondisabled blatantly violate the integration requirement. More subtly, sites where supported employees are not provided with training in social survival skills, where co-workers are never targets for behavior change, or where unilateral decisions are made for workers rather than with workers violate the integration requirement (Shafer & Nisbet, 1988).

SEVERE DISABILITIES

The definition of supported employment specifies that it is a service for persons with severe disabilities who would otherwise be unable to obtain or maintain competitive work. The presence of a severe handicap means that an individual has a:

> ...disability that seriously limits one or more functional capacities (mobility, communication, self-care, self-direction, interpersonal skills, work tolerance, or work skills) in terms of employability, and whose vocational rehabilitation can be expected to require multiple vocational rehabilitation services over an extended period of time... (Federal Register, May 12, 1988).

The handicap may be the result of a single disability "or a combination of disabilities determined on the basis of an evaluation of rehabilitation potential to cause comparable substantial functional limitation" (Federal Register, May 12, 1988).

Although this definition of the target population appears clear, data indicates that many persons targeted for supported employment are individuals for whom this option is unduly restrictive (e.g., persons with mild handicaps) (Lagomarcino & Rusch, 1989). Persons who are appropriate for supported employment must meet not only the definition of severe disabilities, but they must also meet the qualifying employment criteria listed in the federal definition of supported employment. That is, supported employees must be persons who not only need support to acquire critical employment skills, but also need on-going support to maintain or generalize those skills (or acquire new skills) throughout the duration of their employment (Wehman, 1988). Persons who need short-term, intensive services to acquire new skills are more appropriately served by other service options (e.g., time-limited transitional employment, on-the-job training). If persons receiving time-limited services need retraining after a period of successful placement or periodic follow-up to assist in skill or job maintenance, post-employment, rather than on-going support services, may be used to provide this intervention.

ON-GOING SUPPORT SERVICES

> On-going support services, as used in the definition of supported employment, is: continuous or periodic job skill training services provided at least twice monthly at the work site throughout the term of employment to enable the individual to perform the work. The term also includes other support services provided at or away from the work site, such as transportation, personal care services, and counseling to family members, if skill training services are also needed by, and provided to, that individual at the work site (Federal Register, May 12, 1988).

For persons with psychiatric disabilities, on-going support does not have to meet the previous criterion but does have to be available as worker needs arise (Federal Register, May 12, 1988). Thus, support may be provided less often, based on frequency and intensity of need, and the service can still be considered supported employment.

The appropriateness of on-going support must be evaluated based on its effect on the work performance of supported employees. Support that does not enhance the autonomy and adaptability of the target individual due to errors in timing, intensity, or style of delivery are interventions that often lead to excessive dependence on the job coach for cues and reinforcers. These interventions are not considered quality services (Rusch & Hughes, 1989), and are the result of a misunderstanding of the philosophies, values, and technologies that underlie the concept of supported employment.

Each of the four characteristics described above are necessary components of supported employment. An employment program can be evaluated on each of these components to determine the degree to which it is in compliance with the definition of supported employment. These common features, however, do not mean that all supported employment programs will be identical.

Service Delivery Models

Supported employment allows for varying types of intervention models. The type of model used is usually determined by consumer need and service provider creativity. The most frequently seen model of supported employment is the job coach model, used in both individual and group placements. These job coaching variations include: (a) mobile work crews, (b) enclaves, and (c) individual placements (Moon & Griffin, 1988; Rhodes & Valenta, 1985). In each of these variations, the job coach or employment specialist provides assessment, place-ment, training, and follow-up services.

INDIVIDUAL MODEL

The individual placement model is considered by many professionals to be the least restrictive of all the supported employment models (U. S. Department of Education, 1988). This model allows for one-to-one instruction at the targeted job site, systematic fading of the employment specialist, and regular follow-along through on-site visits for the duration of the consumer's employment (Moon & Griffin, 1988). While the service delivery format enhances the probability that integration will occur on the physical level, service personnel must ensure that social or interpersonal integration also occurs across the course of the working day.

Other individual placement models, such as those suggested by Nisbet and Hagner (1988), enhance integration potential by utilizing: "(a) the informal support that is available within work environments...(and) (b) the formal support that is part of the natural business world such as employee training or employee assistance..." (p. 263). These models are listed at the end of this section.

GROUP MODELS

The enclave and mobile crew approaches are known as *group models*. In order to meet federal standards regarding integration, each "group" must not exceed eight disabled individuals (Federal Register, August 14, 1987). The mobile crew contracts with businesses to perform a service and generally moves from business to business performing this service (e.g., janitorial, lawn care). The enclave also contracts with a company for work, however, the enclave typically performs all work on one employer's premises (Mank, Rhodes, & Bellamy, 1986; President's Committee on Employment of People with Disabilities [PCEPD], 1987; Szymanski, Hanley-Maxwell, & Parker, 1987).

Generally, the group models are used for persons with the most severe handicaps for whom an individual placement is not appropriate. The group models offer more intense, continuous support than the individual placement, and are considered to be more restrictive. In addition, the limitations on integration opportunities with nondisabled workers add to the restrictiveness of these options. Special care must be taken to ensure that consumers served in the group models are integrated with nondisabled persons during coffee breaks, lunches, and during working hours at the various job sites (Bellamy, Rhodes, & Albin, 1986; PCEPD, 1987; Szymanski et al., 1987). Employment of nondisabled co-workers as model workers, working alongside consumers with disabilities, is one method to achieve increased integration. Scheduling mobile work crew hours during typical work hours (8:00-5:00) and physically integrating enclave members throughout the host site's work spaces, will also assist in achieving increased integration.

Because individualization of service is an important feature of supported employment, variations of these three models will exist (Hanley-Maxwell, Griffin, Szymanski, & Godley, 1990). Variations that match the particular consumer being served, the employment site constraints, the community, and the community's economic base are appropriate, as long as the essential core features of supported employment are retained (Bellamy, Rhodes, Mank, & Albin, 1988). Some of these variations include: (a) mentors, (b) training consultants, and (c) attendant services (Nisbet & Hagner, 1988).

Model Components

The three supported employment models mentioned have several commonalities. All three models basically adhere to a five component structure consisting of (a) job development, (b) assessment, (c) job placement, (d) job-site training and adaptation, and (e) on-going assessment and follow-along. The manner in which each component is performed, however, may change from model to model, from one job site to the next, and even across supported employees.

JOB DEVELOPMENT

Job development, an integral part of supported employment, is a continuous process that occurs throughout all components of service delivery. Feedback obtained during each component provides further refinement of available job options, as well as identification of future placement possibilities (Szymanski et al., 1987). Job development for some supported employment options (e.g., mobile work crew, enclave) may be different than job development for individual placements because sites for group placements must be able to physically accommodate small groups of consumers, or accept the structural and ideological changes that often accompany enclaves (e.g., job sharing) (Szymanski et al., 1987).

ASSESSMENT

In supported employment, assessments are ecologically based and involve the evaluation of the environment, the employee, and the congruence between the two (Parker, Szymanski, & Hanley-Maxwell, 1989). The environment is evaluated through a job analysis, similar to job analysis as it has been done traditionally in rehabilitation services. General employer information (e.g, size of company, employer's experience working with persons with disabilities) and job specific information (e.g., required speed, required academic skills, work schedule) are obtained. Additionally, a supported employment job analysis includes an examination of necessary social survival skills and job-related skills such as personal money management and grooming (Rusch, Schutz, & Agran, 1982). Additionally, detailed task analyses of job duties are developed.

These pieces of information are obtained through systematic observation of co-workers performing the job, or a highly similar job, and a validating interview with the prospective employer or supervisor (Rusch, Rusch, Menchetti, & Schutz, 1980). The individuality of each job and its setting is highlighted in the supported employment approach to job analysis. The skills identified through the job analysis form the basic content of the individual assessment and, ultimately, the training program (Hanley-Maxwell, 1986).

Assessment of the individual provides information regarding essential survival skills performance. This assessment is used to determine programmatic needs, not readiness or eligibility (Szymanski et al., 1987). Individual assessment determines the specific vocational skill training needs of the individual, as well as social and other job-related skills. Additionally, the individual assessment should include an examination of the individual's support systems to identify potential facilitating or inhibiting variables that may affect the successful job maintenance of the individual. Finally, individual assessment includes gathering information about the individual's interests and long-term goals.

Using the information obtained from the job analysis and the individual assessment, the congruence between the person and the job can be determined. Incompatibilities should not be used to rule out jobs. Job modifications, restructuring, assistive devices, or individualized interventions can be developed to accommodate or overcome discrepancies between the two.

Assessment in supported employment does not reflect activities that begin and end in a closed time set. Instead, assessment is a continuous, evolving, data-based process used to facilitate placement, evaluate the success of services, and problem solve when necessary. The content and process of assessment for the supported employee should be planned according to the individual needs of the consumer and the work environment. Additionally, the long-range perspective of employment histories and the job changes that naturally occur should be kept in mind. To be most valuable in meeting the short-term and long-term informational needs, assessment must be based on different activities, in multiple environments, and conducted over time. In addition, skills must be assessed for generalization across different settings, materials, and people.

PLACEMENT

Job placement for supported employment is slightly different than job placement for competitive employment. Both the service provider and the consumer must be accepted by the employer before the placement can be completed. Additionally, when facilitating the placement of several individuals into an enclave situation, many other variables (e.g., space, benefits, job sharing, wage sharing) that go beyond the scope of those considered with individual placements need to be evaluated (Szymanski et al., 1987).

When considering the individual consumer in the placement process, supported employment approaches examine data from many sources to ensure the optimal job-consumer match. The job analysis and consumer assessments described above are used to ensure the match between all aspects of the job and worker abilities, needs, and interests, as well as potential support systems. The use of such detailed matching appears to be highly correlated with successful placements (Martin, 1986).

Another variable critical to the success of supported employees is coordinated planning (Hanley-Maxwell & Bordieri, 1989). In addition to careful matching, planning requires the (a) coordination of all services across the consumer's ecosystem (e.g., residence, job placement); (b) development of consumer objectives based on assessed performance of skills critical to survival in the target environment; (c) identification of required environmental modifications; (d) identification and allocation of resources, especially those related to environmental modification; (e) identification of least intrusive methods of intervention; (f) re-examination of objectives and methods to ensure enhancement of independence and choice; and (g) identification of employer information needs. Finally, planning begins and ends with one primary question: Do all participants (i.e., service providers, employers, consumer, parents) agree on the total service plan?

TRAINING

Job-site training for supported employment is concerned with skill acquisition and the maintenance and generalization of those skills. Training must anticipate short- and long-term skill needs of consumers, both in terms of skill content and training methodology utilized. Content is usually covered by the use of thorough, individualized curricula that are developed through job analyses and assessment (Hanley-Maxwell, 1986). The training methodology used is behaviorally based. Skills are taught using preplanned, systematic methods that include (but are not limited to) the use of behavioral objectives, individualized reinforcement, graduated levels of assistance, error correction, and maintenance and generalization procedures (Mcloughlin, Garner, & Callahan, 1987; Szymanski et al., 1987).

Adaptation is also a critical aspect of training because (a) not all deficit skills can be trained, (b) training may be less efficient when adaptation is not considered first, and (c) adaptation or assistance may be needed to enhance the independence of the individual supported employee. Adaptation in supported employment, as in any other service delivery model, includes the development and implementation of assistive devices and technology, from the simplest to the most complex. These adaptations include: color highlighting of critical aspects of a task, use of picture lists to assist in task sequencing, computer-assisted communication, robotics, and other simple to complex adaptations. Adaptations are individual and job specific, and are developed to enhance the worker's perception of competence by fellow workers, as well as performance on the job. As such, all adaptations should be as discreet as possible, and acceptable to the supported employee and the persons in the working environment.

Adaptation also refers to adapting the skills of other persons involved with the supported employee. In this way, training does not always focus exclusively on the consumer. It may target others in the environment, including co-workers, employers, other service providers, and parents.

The length of training is dependent on on-going consumer and site assessment data, not agency or financial factors. As the employee adjusts to the job site through skill acquisition or site modification, assistance is gradually and systematically faded to a point where consumer performance is stabilized and maintained while staff involvement is minimized.

FOLLOW-UP

Follow-up is referred to in the *Federal Register* (May 12, 1988) as on-going support. It must be emphasized that follow-up services are not provided only to the consumer. They are also provided to those persons in the environments of the consumer (e.g., caretakers, employers, co-workers). Specifically, follow-up is usually concerned with the long-term maintenance of acquired skills. There are six purposes of a formal follow-up program. These include: identifying problems early, establishing follow-up schedules, providing on-the-job intervention, seeking validation of significant others, planning interventions by others, withdrawing follow-up, and evaluating adjustment (Rusch, 1986).

The follow-up service schedule is determined by individual worker needs. It should be designed to maximize consumer input and consumer control of the long-term support service. In so doing, it will enhance consumer flexibility when confronted with new or novel job demands. A follow-up process that improves consumer control and flexibility will reflect the unique disability-related needs of the individual, not just one model of on-going support (e.g., job coaching), and will target all persons involved with the supported employee (Hanley-Maxwell & Bordieri, 1989).

Summary

Supported employment is a relatively new service delivery system in vocational rehabilitation. To qualify as supported employment, the service must provide competitive work in integrated work settings to the employee with severe disabilities. On-going support must be provided for the duration of employment. The most frequently observed model of supported employment uses a job coach in both individual and group placements. Because individualization of service is a cornerstone of supported employment, variations of these models exist.

Regardless of the model of supported employment used, five processes must occur: (a) job development, (b) assessment, (c) job placement, (d) job-site training, and (e) on-going assessment and follow-along. Human service workers are encouraged to explore the supported employment opportunities available in their communities.

References

Bellamy, G. T., Rhodes, L. E., & Albin, J. M. (1986). Supported employment. In W. E. Kiernan & J. A. Stark (Eds.), *Pathways to employment for adults with developmental disabilities* (pp. 129-138). Baltimore: Paul H. Brookes.

Bellamy, G. T., Rhodes, L. E., Mank, D. M., & Albin, J. M. (1988). *Supported employment: A community integration guide.* Baltimore: Paul H. Brookes.

Federal Register. (1987, August 14). Rehabilitation Act Amendments of 1986: The State Supported Employment Services Program; Final Regulations (34 CFR Part 363). *52*(157), 30546-30552. Washington, DC: U. S. Government Printing Office.

Federal Register. (1988, May 12). Rehabilitation Act Amendments of 1986: The State Vocational Rehabilitation Services Program; Final Regulations. *53*(92), 16982-16983. Washington, DC: U. S. Government Printing Office.

Hanley-Maxwell, C. (1986). Curriculum development. In F. R. Rusch (Ed.), *Competitive employment: Issues and strategies* (pp. 187-198). Baltimore: Paul H. Brookes.

Hanley-Maxwell, C., & Bordieri, J. E. (1989). Purchasing supported employment: Evaluating the service. *Journal of Applied Rehabilitation Counseling, 20*(3), 4-11.

Hanley-Maxwell, C., Griffin, S., Szymanski, E. M., & Godley, S. H. (1990). Supported and time-limited transitional employment services for persons with blindness or visual impairment: An overview. *Journal of Visual Impairment and Blindness, 84*(4), 160-165.

Lagomarcino, T. R., & Rusch, F. R. (1989). A descriptive analysis of reasons why supported employees separate from their jobs. In C. Hanley-Maxwell & D. Harley (Eds.), *Special report: An examination of the impact of supported employment on our nation's citizens with severe disabilities* (pp. 45-49). Washington, DC: President's Committee on Employment of People with Disabilities.

Mank, D. M., Rhodes, L. E., & Bellamy, G. T. (1986). Four supported employment alternatives. In W. E. Kiernan & J. A. Stark (Eds.), *Pathways to employment for adults with developmental disabilities* (pp. 139-154). Baltimore: Paul H. Brookes.

Martin, J. E. (1986). Identifying potential jobs. In F. R. Rusch (Ed.), *Competitive employment: Issues and strategies* (pp. 165-186). Baltimore: Paul H. Brookes.

Mcloughlin, C. S., Garner, J. B., & Callahan, M. (1987). *Getting employed, staying employed.* Baltimore: Paul H. Brookes.

Moon, M. S., & Griffin, S. (1988). Supported employment service delivery models. In P. Wehman & M. S. Moon (Eds.), *Vocational rehabilitation and supported employment* (pp. 17-30). Baltimore: Paul H. Brookes.

Nisbet, J., & Hagner, D. (1988). Natural supports in the workplace: A reexamination of supported employment. *Journal of the Association for Persons with Severe Handicaps, 13*, 260-267.

Parker, R., Szymanski, E. M., & Hanley-Maxwell, C. (1989). Ecological assessment in supported employment. *Journal of Applied Rehabilitation Counseling, 20*(3), 26-33.

Perske, R. (1972). The dignity of risk. In W. Wolfensberger, *Normalization: The principle of normalization in human services* (pp. 202-205). Toronto: National Institute on Mental Retardation.

President's Committee on Employment of People with Disabilities. (1987). *Fact sheet on supported employment.* Washington, DC: Author.

Rehabilitation Act Amendments of 1986, 29 U.S.C. 701.

Rhodes, L. E., & Valenta, L. (1985). Industry-based supported employment: An enclave approach. *Journal of the Association for Persons with Severe Handicaps, 10*(1), 12-20.

Rusch, F. R. (Ed.). (1986). *Competitive employment: Issues and strategies.* Baltimore: Paul H. Brookes.

Rusch, F. R., Chadsey-Rusch, J., & Johnson, J. (1991). Supported employment: Emerging opportunities for employment integration. In L. Meyer, C. Peck, & L. Brown (Eds.), *Critical issues in the lives of people with severe disabilities* (pp. 145-170). Baltimore: Paul H. Brookes.

Rusch, F. R., & Hughes, C. (1989). Overview of supported employment. *Journal of Applied Behavior Analysis, 22*, 351-363.

Rusch, F. R., Rusch, J. C., Menchetti, B. M., & Schutz, R. P. (1980). *Survey-train-place: Developing a school-aged vocational curriculum for the severely handicapped student*. Unpublished manuscript, University of Illinois, Department of Special Education, Urbana.

Rusch, F. R., Schutz, R. P., & Agran, M. (1982). Validating entry-level survival skills for service occupations: Implications for curriculum development. *Journal of the Association for the Severely Handicapped, 7*, 32-41.

Shafer, M., & Nisbet, J. (1988). Integration and empowerment in the workplace. In M. Barcus, S. Griffin, D. Mank, L. Rhodes, & S. Moon (Eds.), *Supported employment implementation issues* (pp. 45-72). Richmond: Rehabilitation Research Training Center, Virginia Commonwealth University.

Szymanski, E. M., Hanley-Maxwell, C., & Parker, R. (1987). *Supported employment and time-limited transitional employment service delivery: An introductory guide for rehabilitation counselors*. Austin: University of Texas, Department of Special Education.

Szymanski, E. M., & Parker, R. M. (1988). Supported employment and time-limited transitional employment training: Options for rehabilitation counselors. *Journal of Applied Rehabilitation Counseling, 19*(2), 11-15.

U. S. Department of Education. (1988). Supported employment. *Rehabilitation Brief, 10*(1). Washington, DC: National Institute on Disability and Rehabilitation Research, Office of Special Education and Rehabilitative Services, Department of Education.

Wehman, P. (1988). Supported employment: Toward zero exclusion of persons with severe disabilities. In P. Wehman & M. S. Moon (Eds.), *Vocational rehabilitation and supported employment* (pp. 3-16). Baltimore: Paul H. Brookes.

Whitehead, C. (1989). Job opportunities today and tomorrow: Ensuring career choices, mobility, and employment (Reinforcing supported employment systems and programs). In C. Hanley-Maxwell & D. Harley (Eds.), *Special report: An examination of the impact of supported employment on our nation's citizens with severe disabilities* (pp. 51-62). Washington, DC: President's Committee on Employment of People with Disabilities.

Wolfensberger, W. (1972). *Normalization: The principle of normalization in human services*. Toronto: National Institute on Mental Retardation.

VI. Legal Services and Advocacy

Legal Aid and Public Interest Advocacy

Jill E. Adams, J.D.

Helping a client of limited means obtain legal services can be a frustrating experience. Resources are limited and restrictions on the allocation of these resources may impair the ability to find legal representation for the client who needs legal assistance.[1] Not all legal problems faced by a client with limited financial resources will require the client to seek assistance outside of the private bar. Some claims may arise under statutes which have fee-shifting provisions, which allow a prevailing plaintiff to recover attorneys' fees from the defendant. Most notable among these are statutes protecting civil rights.[2] Where a fee-shifting statute exists, a member of the private bar may take the case on a contingent fee basis. Under such an agreement, the client will pay no attorneys' fees unless suit is successful. Nevertheless, the client may be liable for litigation costs, even if the suit is unsuccessful. It is also common for personal injury actions to be handled on a contingent fee basis.

If a client has legal needs which cannot be handled by the private bar because the legal matter is not the kind of matter that can be handled on a contingent fee basis and the client does not have the resources to pay for legal services, then the client may seek help from a provider of legal aid.[3] These providers are basically of two types: providers who provide traditional legal services to poor people and public interest groups which will undertake impact litigation. Nationally, Legal Services Corporation is the primary funding source for providers of the first type; the American Civil Liberties Union (ACLU) is representative of the second type of provider.

Legal Aid

HISTORY

Until the early 1960s, legal aid for the poor in the United States was a matter of private charity. The legal aid movement began in New York with the establishment, by the German Society in 1876, of a legal aid society to protect recently arrived immigrants.[4] It was ten years later before a second legal aid society was founded.[5] The movement grew gradually until the publication, in 1919, of *Justice and the Poor* by Reginald Heber Smith. At the time of its publication, 41 cities had some kind of legal aid program.[6] Largely in response to Smith's book, the American Bar Association (ABA) formed a committee on Legal Aid in 1920[7] and there was rapid growth in the movement. In the ten years following the formation of the ABA committee, 30 new legal aid offices opened, and the total national expenditure on legal aid doubled.[8] The unorganized, local aid societies which preceded Smith's book found a voice in 1923 with the establishment of the National Association of Legal Aid Organizations (which later came to be known as the National Legal Aid and Defender Association).[9] In the Depression, however, legal aid declined as resources were insufficient to meet the demand, and frustrated clients stopped seeking assistance.[10] Following the Depression, the legal aid movement continued with private funding from religious and ethnic groups, bar associations, charitable funds (e.g., the Community Fund) and the donation of time by volunteer attorneys.[11] In 1962, just three years before federal funding for legal aid was first introduced, only $4 million was expended by all of the legal aid societies in the country.[12] Legal aid was able to provide only a ratio of one lawyer to every 120,000 income-eligible clients. The ratio of attorneys to the population able to afford legal counsel, was one attorney to 560 persons.[13]

The issue of whether there should be government funding of legal services of the poor was hotly debated, and is still debated today.[14] Federal funding was initiated during the 1960s *War on Poverty*. As part of that war, the Office of Economic Opportunity (OEO) was founded in 1964.[15] Although there was no specific congressional directive for OEO to undertake a legal service program, in 1965 the OEO began such a program.[16] Within 18 months of operation, the program increased the total expenditure on legal assistance to the poor eightfold, funding 800 new law offices and 2,000 new lawyers.[17] Subsequently, however, as expenditures on the Vietnam war increased, funding for the legal services program stagnated and efforts went into maintaining existing programs, rather than establishing new ones.[18]

The philosophy of the OEO Legal Services Program diverged, to some extent, from that of the historical legal aid movement which had focussed on providing the indigent equal access to the courts. Faced with inadequate resources to meet all of the legal needs of the poor, in 1967 the Legal Services Program announced that law reform was to be its primary objective.[19] As the director of the program who announced this policy put it, "[l]aw reform can provide the most bang for the buck."[20] Nevertheless, the great bulk of cases handled by grantees of the Legal Services Program were matters of individual client concern in such areas as welfare, housing, consumer matters, and so on.[21]

The law reform policy drew much criticism. Howard Phillips, who was director of OEO under President Nixon, set out to destroy the Legal Services Program.[22] Critics of the program also claimed that members of Congress interfered with the activities of the program on behalf of constituents who had been troubled by litigation brought by program grantees.[23] Among the most demoralizing attacks was one led by then Governor Reagan against California Rural Legal Assistance (CRLA), a program grantee.[24] CRLA had successfully challenged in the courts California's cutbacks in the Medi-Cal program. The result was that Governor Reagan was not able to meet his campaign promise of balancing the state budget. When CRLA received a $1.8 million grant from the Legal Services Program for 1971, Reagan vetoed the funding and filed a report, known as the Uhler Report, with the OEO charging CRLA with misconduct, including "a disposition to use their clients as ammunition in their efforts to wage ideological warfare...."[25] Although OEO had the power to override the veto, the charges required investigation. CRLA survived on interim funding while an OEO commission investigated. The OEO did not release the 400-page study produced by the investigatory commission until CRLA brought suit to force its release. The report, when released, provided,

> [T]he complaints contained in the Uhler Report and the evidence adduced thereon do not...furnish any justification whatsoever for any finding of improper activities by CRLA...The Commission expressly finds that in many instances [the Uhler Report] has taken evidence out of context and misrepresented the facts...[The Uhler Report] has unfairly and irresponsibly subjected many able, energetic, idealistic, and dedicated CRLA attorneys to totally unjustified attacks upon their professional integrity and competence....[26]

Despite the findings of the Commission, the OEO did not override the veto, but reached a compromise which provided some funding to CRLA and some funding to the state to develop an alternative program. The battle over CRLA diverted scarce resources and revealed the vulnerability of the Legal Services Program to political attack.

In 1973, President Nixon, by executive order, abolished OEO. The only program which survived was the Legal Services Program.[27] Although the program remained, funding stagnated and morale was low.[28] Critics complained of the law reform objectives of the program, and supporters feared political manipulation of the program since it was housed in the executive branch of government. The Nixon administration, the American Bar Association, and the National Legal Aid and Defender Association all came to support a private, nonprofit, federally funded corporation as the means of federally supporting legal services for the poor. Differences continued to exist on the structure of such a corporation and limitations which might be imposed on the activities of such a corporation.[29] A compromise bill enacted in 1974[30] created the Legal Services Corporation.

One of the major goals of placing control of legal services for poor people in a private corporation was to depoliticize the provision of legal services. Nevertheless, the board of the corporation is appointed by the president and funding must be authorized by Congress and approved by the president. The continued role of politics in funding for legal services for the poor is evident in the legislation creating the corporation itself. By statute, recipients of funding from the corporation may not provide legal assistance to persons seeking assistance with respect to proceedings or litigation to procure a nontherapeutic abortion.[31] Another provision prevents representation regarding the desegregation of elementary or secondary schools.[32] There are also limitations on conducting class action litigation.[33] The board of directors of the corporation attempted to impose regulations prohibiting recipients from engaging in representation relating to redistricting.[34] These regulations, however, did not withstand legal challenge.[35] In addition, the board has passed nonbinding resolutions discouraging recipients from handling cases brought by migrant farm workers, abortion-rights proponents, and persons summarily evicted from public housing for drug use.[36]

Further evidence of the continued politicization of the corporation is seen in the funding battles the corporation has faced. President Reagan proposed no funding of the corporation in seven of the eight budgets he presented to Congress.[37] Although Congress did fund the Legal Services Corporation during those years, funding for fiscal year 1982 was reduced by $80 million from the previous year, a cut of nearly 25%.[38] Current funding, when adjusted for inflation, is 27% less than in 1979.[39] Political battles are also fought over the appointment of directors of the corporation.[40] The existence and scope of the services funded by the Legal Services Corporation remains a hotly debated political issue.

PURPOSE/INTENT

The Legal Services Corporation is not a direct provider of legal services, but is a funding source for local providers. In the statement of purpose enacted by Congress as part of the Legal Services Corporation Act, the corporation is charged with "providing financial support for legal assistance in noncriminal proceedings or matters to persons unable to afford legal assistance."[41] It fulfills this purpose primarily by distributing congressionally appropriated funds to 284 independent field offices which provide direct legal assistance to clients.[42] These field offices are located in all 50 states, Puerto Rico, the Virgin Islands, Micronesia, and Guam.[43]

An 11-member board of directors governs the corporation.[44] Members of the board are presidential appointees who are confirmed by the Senate.[45] The majority of the directors must be attorneys, but the board must also include eligible clients.[46] No more than six of the board members may be from the same political party.[47] The officers and employees of the corporation are not considered federal employees, and the corporation itself is not deemed an agency of the federal government.[48] The role of the corporation is to make funding grants to local organizations which provide direct legal services to the poor and to ensure that the funded organizations comply with the provisions of the Legal Services Corporation Act.[49]

While independent, the local programs funded by the corporation must comply with its regulations. The corporation requires that 60% of the members of the board of directors of any recipient be attorneys licensed in the state in which the recipient is to provide legal services. In addition, one-third of the members must be eligible to be clients.[50]

Recipients may receive funding from sources other than the Legal Services Corporation, but restrictions on the expenditure of these funds are imposed on the recipients as a condition to receiving funding from the corporation.[51] Reliance on nonfederal funding has increased in recent years as federal funding for the corporation has been cut back. In 1979, recipients relied on the corporation for 87% of their funding.[52] By 1985, 22% of recipient funding was from sources other than the corporation.[53] These sources include other federal funding (7%); state and local government funding (5.3%); attorney fee awards (1.5%); Interest on Lawyer Trust Accounts (.6%); and other private sources, including bar associations, foundations, United Way, and other private donation (6.6%).[54] Although noncorporation funding has increased in the past decade, total funding is often well below funding in 1980. For example, Land of Lincoln Legal Assistance Foundation, Inc., which serves 60% of the geographic area of Illinois and 25% of the poor in Illinois, had its funding reduced by 50% from 1980 levels when the figures are adjusted for inflation.[55]

In addition to recipients, the legal services structure calls for state advisory councils.[56] These councils are composed of nine members appointed by the governor of the state, and are charged with notifying the corporation of violation of pertinent statutes or regulations by the recipients.[57]

Utilization Criteria

There are both income and subject-matter restrictions on eligibility for legal assistance from recipients of Legal Services Corporation grants. In addition, there are prohibitions on the representation of aliens who are not legally admitted to the United States.[58] The Legal Services Corporation Act provides that the corporation, in consultation with the director of the Office of Management and Budget and the governors of the states, shall establish maximum income levels for individuals eligible for legal assistance by recipients of corporation funding.[59] By regulation, the corporation has provided that, unless specially authorized, recipients are to establish income eligibility levels which shall not exceed 125% of the Federal Poverty Income Guidelines.[60] As of March 1991, this figure was $8,275 for a single individual, and $16,750 for a family of four.[61] A higher figure applies in Alaska and Hawaii.[62] A recipient may provide services to an individual whose income exceeds these amounts by no more than 150% if the individual seeks representation in obtaining benefits from a governmental program for the poor,[63] or if other factors (e.g., seasonal variations in income), debts, employment-related expenses (e.g., child care, transportation), or other significant factors make the individual unable to afford legal assistance.[64] Individuals whose income exceeds 150% of the national eligibility level (125% of the poverty level) may receive services if the person's income is primarily committed to medical or nursing home expenses.[65] Although a recipient is authorized to provide services to persons with incomes up to 125% of the federal poverty level, they are not required to set their financial eligibility criteria that high.[66]

Statutory restrictions exist with respect to representation regarding abortion and school desegregation.[67] Although there have been attempts to further restrict the subject matter of representation by regulation, these restrictions have been invalidated by the courts.[68] Nevertheless, recipients are required to develop priorities for the allocation of resources.[69] As a practical matter, this results in a subject-matter limitation on representation. There are insufficient resources for meeting the legal needs of all eligible clients in all permissible matters. While priorities are established by individual recipient agencies, representation is most common in matters of family law, housing, income maintenance (securing and maintaining governmental benefits [e.g., Aid to Families with Dependent Children, food stamps, social security, supplemental security income]), and consumer matters.[70] Other representation includes matters relating to education, juveniles, health (primarily Medicaid), employment, individual rights,[71] and utilities.[72]

Even within the categories where representation is common, resource allocation restrictions occur. For example, within the family law area, one recipient lists its highest priorities as representation of victims of domestic violence, representation of parents who have historically had physical custody of a child where child snatching is likely or has occurred, or where a proceeding is brought to change custody. The recipient lists representation of the noncustodial parent as a high priority only in defense of adoption proceedings.[73] Excluded from coverage are custodial modifications for any person not having custody historically, most adoption proceedings, enforcement of child support obligations, name changes, and so on.[74] While these priorities are only representative, they illustrate the limitation on the provision of legal services.[75]

Studies have indicated that one of the serious problems in providing legal services to the poor is that social service workers often do not have current information on representation priorities of the local Legal Services Corporation grant recipient.[76] In addition to lack of familiarity with established priorities, there are often assumptions made by providers of social services that the rejection of representation of one client means that another client with a similar problem will be rejected. Priority criteria, however, can be very case specific.[77] Factors which led to the rejection of one client may not lead to rejection of another. There are anecdotal reports of social service providers believing that no intake was being done by the local Legal Services Corporation grant recipient where, in fact, there had been suspension of intake a year earlier for only a week.[78] Better coordination of information between recipients and social service providers is fundamental to providing legal services to the poor.

OTHER PROVIDERS OF TRADITIONAL LEGAL AID

Although Legal Services Corporation recipients comprise a large portion of the providers of traditional legal aid, they are not the only providers of legal services to the poor. A recent study, for example, found 17 staffed, non-Legal Services Corporation-funded programs providing legal aid in one state, in addition to 12 private attorney programs.[79] These programs do not have the uniform characteristics of Legal Services Corporation programs, but are an important part of the network providing legal aid. Of the 17 staffed programs, six are law school clinics which provide training to law students under the supervision of law school faculty or staff attorneys while providing legal services.[80]

Funding for these additional programs come from a variety of sources. One important funding source is title III of the Older Americans Act.[81] Title III provides grants to states to establish services, including legal assistance services[82] to individuals 60 years old or older.[83] There are no income eligibility requirements for receiving services from a recipient of title III funding.[84] Thus, a recipient of title III funds may provide services to an individual who meets the age requirements for eligibility regardless of that individual's income.[85] Other staffed programs are diverse. Some are established to serve residents of a specific geographic area; others may serve specific populations.[86]

The final source of traditional legal aid is private attorney programs. Many of these programs are sponsored by local bar associations and provide volunteer attorneys who do not seek compensation or who seek a reduced fee for representation. Since 1985, recipients of Legal Services Corporation funds must devote 12.5% of their grant proceeds to developing Private Attorney Involvement (PAI).[87] Many private attorney programs receive funding from the PAI allocations of corporation-funded programs.

Public Interest Advocacy

In addition to traditional legal aid, which defines its mission as providing services to clients who would not otherwise be able to afford legal services, public interest advocacy groups may be a source of legal assistance. These groups are usually privately funded and give priority to issues that have precedential value or broad impact. For the public interest advocacy group, the potential for a broad impact is usually the most prominent criterion for case selection, rather than individual need.[88] The groups falling within the public interest category represent the broad array of the political spectrum. The Foundation for Public Affairs, a nonprofit research group which serves as a clearinghouse for information on public interest and public policy groups, reports that, in 1988, it monitored approximately 2,500 such groups, the majority of which were national organizations.[89] While not all of these groups list litigation as a method of pursuing their goals, many do. The Alliance for Justice, which surveys public interest groups that focus primarily on litigation, has estimated that there are now about 150 public interest law groups.[90]

The early forerunners of the public interest law groups were the American Civil Liberties Union (ACLU) and the NAACP Legal Defense Fund (NAACP/ LDF). The ACLU was founded in 1920 by Roger Nash Baldwin.[91] It was an outgrowth of several organizations founded during World War I to protect the free speech rights of pacifists.[92] Its mission is still defined as defending and preserving "individual rights and liberties guaranteed by the U. S. Constitution, the Bill of Rights, and federal statutes designed to implement those rights and liberties."[93] NAACP/LDF was established as a separate entity from the NAACP, in 1939, to combat segregation.[94] It was the NAACP/ LDF which litigated *Brown v. Board of Education*,[95] the case in which the Supreme Court, in 1954, declared segregation in the public schools illegal.

In the 1970s, public interest law groups proliferated. In 1969, there were only 23 such groups staffed by a total of 50 full-time attorneys. By 1984, there were 158 groups, with a total of 906 staff attorneys.[96] These organizations are modeled on the structure adopted by the ACLU and the NAACP/ LDF. Under this model, there are several dominant characteristics: (a) a full-time salaried staff of qualified lawyers is employed; (b) cases are selected on an impact, rather than a service basis; (c) litigation is used as a tool to initiate change—the posture is not reactive but reform oriented; (d) financial support is derived from a diverse nationwide membership; (e) the organization, through its legal work, attempts to create a political climate favorable to broad public policy changes; and (f) a network of volunteer attorneys takes cases to see that the broad theoretical changes achieved by the organization are given practical effect.[97]

The Internal Revenue Service has recognized that public interest law groups may qualify as charities and, therefore, contributions to qualifying groups are tax deductible. To maintain tax-exempt status, the group must accept no fees from clients, must account to the IRS as to how the work furthers the public interest, and must be directed by a citizen board independent of private interest.[98] In addition, as with any charitable organization, it may not participate in substantial lobbying activity.[99]

Funding for public interest law groups comes from membership dues, individual contributions, foundation grants, and court-awarded attorneys' fees.[100] Some groups obtain some funding from federal or state and local governments and other sources, including sales of publications and other materials.[101]

While public interest law groups maintain full-time staff attorneys, they also rely on cooperating attorneys who handle some litigation for the group, often on a volunteer basis.[102] In addition to attorneys, public interest law groups often rely on the work of legal interns, law students working over the summer or on a part-time basis while in school. This work may be paid or the student may receive academic credit for the work.[103] Nonlegal professionals may be employed as fund raisers, managers, editors of publications, and so on.[104]

Utilization criteria vary with the organization. A social service worker attempting to find legal assistance for a client may have to research the issue of whether there is an available public interest law group which addresses the kind of problem faced by the client.

Finding Legal Resources

Knowing that legal aid and public interest advocacy is sometimes available is not enough. One must know how to put one's client in touch with an appropriate provider of legal assistance. Because legal aid providers are either local organizations funded by Legal Services Corporation, or independent legal aid groups, there is no umbrella name by which to look up all groups. Yellow page listings are generally made only under the category of "attorneys."

A number of directories are published which provide listings of legal aid or public advocacy attorneys. The National Legal Aid and Defender Association (NLADA) publishes a directory of legal aid and defender offices. Directories may be found in law school libraries, some public libraries, at public defender offices, or may be purchased from NLADA. The Alliance for Justice publishes a Directory of Public Interest Law Centers. A directory of public interest groups, compiled by the Foundation for Public Affairs and entitled *Public Interest Profiles*, is published by Congressional Quarterly, Inc. Finally, the American Bar Association Private Bar Involvement Project publishes an annual directory of organizations which utilize volunteer private attorneys.

NLADA Directory
1625 K Street, NW
8th Floor
Washington, DC 20006

Alliance for Justice
600 New Jersey Ave., NW
Washington, DC 20001

Congressional Quarterly, Inc.
1414 22nd St., NW
Washington, DC 20037

American Bar Association
PBI Project
750 North Lake Shore Drive
Chicago, IL 60611

Endnotes

1. For example, one recent study found that in the state of Illinois, only 20% of the civil legal needs of low-income people are met. The Spangenberg Group, *Illinois Legal Needs Study* at 2 (1989). This chapter addresses only the issue of obtaining counsel for civil matters. The indigent criminal defendant can obtain

representation through a public defender or through court appointment of counsel where the defendant faces imprisonment if found guilty. *Gideon v. Wainwright*, 372 U.S. 335 (1963); *Argersinger v. Hamlin*, 407 U.S. 25 (1972).

2. Among the fee-shifting statutes are 42 U.S.C. § 1988 (1988) (providing for recovery of attorneys' fees by a prevailing plaintiff who brings an action under 42 U.S.C. §§ 1981, 1982, 1983, 1985, 1986 [1988] or title VI of the Civil Rights Act of 1964 which prohibits discrimination on the basis of race, color, or national origin in programs receiving federal financial assistance); 42 U.S.C. § 2000a-3b (1988) (providing for recovery of attorneys' fees in actions brought under title II of the Civil Rights Act of 1964 which prohibits discrimination at public accommodations on the basis of race, religion, color, or national origin); 42 U.S.C. § 2000e-5k (1988) (providing for recovery of attorneys' fees in actions brought under title VII of the Civil Rights Act of 1964 which prohibits discrimination on the basis of race, color, religion, sex, or national origin in employment); 42 U.S.C. §§ 1973(e) (1988) (providing for recovery of attorneys' fees for actions brought under the Voting Rights Act); 20 U.S.C.S. § 1415(e)(4)(B) (Law. Co-op Supp. 1991) (providing for attorneys' fees in actions to enforce the provisions of the Education of the Handicapped Act); 29 U.S.C. § 794a(b) (1988) (providing for attorneys' fees for actions brought to enforce provisions of the Rehabilitation Act of 1973); 42 U.S.C.A. § 12205 (1991) (providing for attorneys' fees for actions brought to enforce the provisions of the Americans with Disabilities Act of 1990). State provisions regarding civil rights also frequently provide for a prevailing plaintiff to recover attorneys' fees. *See*, e.g., *Ill. Rev. Stat.* ch. 68, ¶ 8A-104(G) (1989).

3. Members of the private bar may take some legal matters on a pro bono basis. The Model Rules of Professional Conduct adopted by the American Bar Association provide:

> A lawyer should render public interest legal service. A lawyer may discharge this responsibility by providing professional services at no fee or a reduced fee to persons of limited means or to public service or charitable groups or organizations, by service in activities for improving the law, the legal system, or the legal profession, and by financial support for organizations that provide legal services to persons of limited means.

A.B.A. Model Rule 6.1. There is increasing debate urging that the duty to provide pro bono service become mandatory rather than precatory. *See ABA/BNA Lawyers Manual on Professional Conduct*, 91:6001-6010 (1991).

4. C. Wolfram, *Modern Legal Ethics* § 16.7.2 (1986).

5. *Id.* This second society was founded in Chicago by the Protective Agency for Women and Children.

6. *Id.* (citing R. Smith, *Justice and the Poor* 135-36 [1919]).

7. Huber, Thou Shalt Not Ration Justice: A History and Bibliography of Legal Aid in America, 44 *Geo. Wash. L. Rev.* 754, 755-56 (1976).

8. E. Johnson, *Justice and Reform: The Formative Years of the OEO Legal Services Program*, 8 (1974).

9. *Id.* at 7.

10. C. Wolfram, *supra* note 4, at § 16.7.2.

11. *Id.*

12. E. Johnson, *supra* note 8, at 9 (citing 1962 Summary of Conference Proceedings, NLADA, at 13).

13. E. Johnson, *supra* note 8, at 9.

14. In 1951, Robert Storey, who was to become the president of the American Bar Association in 1952, wrote: "What are the trends toward regimentation of our profession? To me, the greatest threat, aside from the undermining influences of Communist infiltration, is the propaganda and campaign for a federal subsidy to finance a nationwide plan for legal aid and low-cost legal service." Storey, The Legal Profession versus Regimentation: A Program to Counter Socialization, *37, A.B.A. J.*, 100, 101 (1951). Throughout his presidency, Reagan tried to abolish the legal services program. D. Besharov, Introduction, *Legal Services for the Poor*, xiii (D. Besharov, ed. [1990]); *see also* Cramton, Crisis in Legal Services for the Poor, *26, Vill. L. Rev.*, 521 (1981) (noting that President Reagan's 1982 budget proposal contained no appropriation for the Legal Services Corporation).

15. Huber, *supra* note 7, at 757.

16. *Id.*

17. E. Johnson, *supra* note 8, at 71.

18. *Id.* at 99.

19. *Id.* at 126-34.

20. *Id.* at 133.

21. Huber, *supra* note 7, at 761 and n. 41. *See also* Cramton, *supra* note 14, at 535.

22. Huber, *supra* note 7, at 770-71 and n. 91. Phillips subsequently became head of the National Defeat Legal Services Committee of the Conservative Caucus. Cramton, *supra* note 14, at 532.

23. C. Wolfram, *supra* note 4, at § 16.7.3.

24. This discussion of the CRLA is based on the discussion in George, Development of the Legal Services Corporation, *61, Cornell L. Rev.*, 681, 683-87 (1976).

25. George, *supra* note 24, at 686 (quoting California Office of Economic Opportunity, *A Study and Evaluation of California Rural Legal Assistance, Inc.*, 191 [1971]).

26. George, *supra* note 24, at 686 (quoting OEO, *Report of the Office of Economic Opportunity Commission on California Rural Legal Assistance, Inc.*, 83-84 [1971]).

27. C. Wolfram, *supra* note 4, at § 16.7.3.

28. George, *supra* note 24, at 687.

29. For a thorough discussion of the political debate and compromise which led to the Legal Services Corporation Act, see George, *supra* note 24, at 690-99.

30. Pub. L. No. 93-355, 88 Stat. 378 (codified as amended at 42 U.S.C. §§ 2996 to 2996k [1988]).

31. 42 U.S.C. § 2996f(b)(8) (1988). Subsequent appropriation bills have broadened this restriction. For example, in the appropriation for fiscal year 1991, Congress provided, "...none of the funds appropriated under this Act to the Legal Services Corporation may be used by the Corporation or any recipient to participate in any litigation with respect to abortion." Departments of Commerce, Justice, and State, the Judiciary and Related Agencies Appropriations Act, 1991, Pub. L. No. 101-515, § 607, 104 Stat. 2101, 2152 (1991).

32. 42 U.S.C. § 2996f(b)(9) (1988).

33. 42 U.S.C. § 2996e(d)(5) (1988).

34. 45 C.F.R. § 1632.3 (1990).

35. *Texas Rural Legal Aid, Inc. v. Legal Services Corp.*, 740 F. Supp., 880 (D.D.C. 1990).

36. *76, A.B.A. J.*, 24 (1990).

37. Turmoil Continues at Legal Aid Agency, *Chicago Daily Law Bulletin*, Dec. 31, 1990, at 1, col. 5; Cramton, *supra* note 14, at 521 (citing Barbash, White House Wants to Cut Off Federal Aid for the Poor, *Washington Post*, Mar. 6, 1981, § A, at 1, col. 5; Taylor, Administration Seeks to Terminate U. S. Plan That Finances Legal Aid, *New York Times*, Mar. 6, 1981, § A, at 1, col. 2).

38. Besharov & Tramontozzi, Background Information on the Legal Services Corporation, *Legal Services for the Poor*, 211 (D. Besharov, ed. [1990]).

39. *Id.* This comparison reflects funding through fiscal year 1987.

40. *See*, e.g., Turmoil Continues at Legal Aid Agency, *supra* note 37.

41. 42 U.S.C. § 2996b(a) (1988).

42. Besharov & Tramontozzi, *supra* note 38, at 209 (citing Legal Services Corporation, *Budget Request for Fiscal Year 1989*).

43. Besharov & Tramontozzi, *supra* note 38, at 209.

44. 42 U.S.C. § 2996c (1988).

45. *Id.*

46. *Id.*

47. *Id.*

48. 42 U.S.C. § 2996d(e) (1988). The employees of the corporation are treated as federal employees for certain narrow purposes such as obtaining health insurance and pension benefits.

49. 42 U.S.C. § 2996e (1988).

50. 45 C.F.R. § 1607.3 (1990).

51. 42 U.S.C. § 2996i(c) (1988) provides:

> ...any funds [received from non-federal sources by a recipient] ... for the provision of legal assistance shall not be expended by recipients for any purpose prohibited by this subchapter, except that this provision shall not be construed to prevent recipients from receiving other public funds or tribal funds ... and expending them in accordance with the purposes for which they are provided, or to prevent contracting or making other arrangements with private attorneys, private law firms, or other State or local entities of attorneys, or with legal aid societies having separate public defender

programs, for the provision of legal assistance to eligible clients under this subchapter.

Section 1610.2 of the Code of Federal Regulations prohibits recipients from expending nonfederal funds in any manner prohibited by corporation regulations.

52. Besharov & Tramontozzi, *supra* note 38, at 212.

53. *Id.*

54. *Id.* at 213. "Interest on Lawyer Trust Accounts" (IOLTA) refers to funds generated from the interest earned on trust accounts maintained by attorneys of clients' funds where the funds held on behalf of the client would be too small or held too short of a time to draw interest in excess of service charges if segregated into separate accounts. Most states have IOLTA programs, and many states have mandatory programs.

55. The Spangenberg Group, *supra* note 1, at 63.

56. 42 U.S.C. § 2996c(f) (1988).

57. *Id.*

58. 45 C.F.R. part 1626 (1990). Although the regulations promulgated by the Corporation provide at § 1626.4(a)(1) that there may be no representation of "...an alien who has adjusted his status to that of temporary resident alien under the provisions of ... 8 U.S.C. § 1255a ...," this provision has been invalidated by the courts. *California Rural Legal Assistance, Inc. v. Legal Services Corp.*, 917 F.2d, 1171 (9th Cir. 1990).

59. 42 U.S.C. § 2996f(a)(2) (1988).

60. 45 C.F.R. § 1611.3(b) (1990).

61. 56 Fed. Reg. 9634 (1991) (to be codified as a revision to 45 C.F.R. part 1611, Appendix A).

62. *Id.*

63. 45 C.F.R. § 1611.4(a)(2) (1990).

64. 45 C.F.R. § 1611.5(b)(1) (1990).

65. 45 C.F.R. § 1611.5(b)(1)(B) (1990).

66. *See*, e.g., Land of Lincoln Legal Assistance Foundation, Inc., *Policy and Procedure Manual*, Tab 108, at 1 (March 1990) (establishing income eligibility at 100% of the federal poverty level).

67. 42 U.S.C. § 2996f(b) (1988); *see* note 31 *supra*.

68. *See*, e.g., *Texas Rural Legal Aid, Inc. v. Legal Services Corp.*, 740 F. Supp., 880 (D.D.C. 1990). In addition, the statute funding Legal Services Corporation for fiscal year 1991 provides, "...none of the funds appropriated in this Act for the Corporation shall be used, directly or indirectly, by the Corporation to promulgate new regulations or to enforce, implement, or operate in accordance with regulations effective after April 27, 1984, unless the Appropriations Committees of both Houses of Congress have been notified fifteen days prior to such use of funds...." Departments of Commerce, Justice, and State, the Judiciary and Related Agencies Appropriating Act (1991), § 607, *supra* note 31, 104 Stat. at 2152.

69. 42 U.S.C. § 2996f(a)(2)(C) (1988); 45 C.F.R. part 1620 (1990).

70. In 1984, the listed matters comprised 78% of the case load of Legal Services Corporation grant recipients. Besharov & Tramontozzi, *supra* note 38, at 219-20.

71. *Id.* at 220-21.

72. *See* Land of Lincoln Legal Assistance Foundation Inc., *Annual Report 1990 Priorities Review.*

73. *Id.*

74. *Id.*

75. For a thorough discussion of the resource limitations in one state, Illinois, see The Spangenberg Group, *Illinois Legal Needs Study* (1989).

76. *Id.* at 78.

77. *See id.* at 79.

78. *Id.* at 78.

79. *Id.* at 49-58.

80. *Id.*

81. 42 U.S.C. §§ 3021 to 3030p (1988).

82. 42 U.S.C. § 3027(a)(15) (1988).

83. 42 U.S.C. § 3022(9) (1988).

84. 42 U.S.C. § 3027(a)(15) (1988); 45 C.F.R. § 1321.71(d) (1990) ("A legal assistance provider may not require an older person to disclose information about income or resources as a condition for providing legal assistance under this part.")

85. Nonincome limitations on eligibility, such as subject matter limitations, apply to title III programs as well as to Legal Services Corporation programs. 42 U.S.C. § 3027(a)(15)(A) (1988).

86. For example, one such program, Chicago Legal Aid to Incarcerated Mothers, provides representation to women prisoners in Illinois, primarily on family law matters. Another, Travelers and Immigrants Aid of Chicago, provides representation to immigrants. The Spangenberg Group, *supra* note 1, at 52.

87. 50 Fed. Reg. 48591 (1985), published, as amended, at 45 C.F.R. § 1614.1 (1990).

88. *See* The Spangenberg Group, *supra* note 1, at 58.

89. Foundation for Public Affairs, *Public Interest Profiles 1988-89*, xix (1988).

90. *Id.* at 16.

91. C. Markmann, *The Noblest Cry*, 1 (1965).

92. *Id.* at 15-40; N. Aron, *Liberty and Justice for All: Public Interest Law in the 1980s and Beyond*, 8 (1989).

93. Foundation for Public Affairs, *supra* note 89, at 122.

94. N. Aron, *supra* note 92, at 9.

95. 347 U. S. 483 (1954).

96. N. Aron, *supra* note 92, at 27.

97. *Id.* at 9-10.

98. *See* Rev. Proc. 71-39, 1971-2 C.B. 575; Rev. Rul. 75-74, 1975-1 C.B. 152; Rev. Rul. 75-75, 1975-1 C.B. 154.

99. I.R.C. §§ 501(c)(3); 501(h) (1988).

100. N. Aron, *supra* note 92, at 41.

101. *Id.* at 50-62.

102. *Id. at 33.*

103. *Id.* at 36.

104. *Id.*

Civil Rights and Equal Employment/
Americans with Disabilities Act

Wendy York

Many human-service clients with physical or mental disabilities face discrimination. Sometimes the legal system can provide them with the help that they need. They may be able to regain a job from which they were wrongfully terminated or insist that a doctor's office remove physical barriers so they can freely enter and exit. The law regarding the rights of individuals with physical and mental disabilities is complex and ever changing. The purpose of this chapter is to give human-service workers an overview of the various statutes that can help persons with disabilities. It will assist the human-service professional in determining whether the client should contact a lawyer or the agency charged with enforcing the applicable statute.

History/Legislation

Although the first Civil Rights Act was enacted in 1871, it was not until the Civil Rights Act of 1964 that a broad-based statute was enacted prohibiting discrimination on the basis of race, color, religion, national origin, or sex. The Act barred discrimination in public accommodations, federally assisted programs, employment, and a wide range of businesses engaged in interstate commerce. The Act created the Equal Employment Opportunity Commission (EEOC) to enforce the rights provided for under the Act. The Act also permitted individuals to bring their own private lawsuits. Even though the Civil Rights Act of 1964 was very broad, it did not address discrimination against persons with physical or mental disabilities.

Legislation to assist individuals with disabilities was first enacted by Congress to aid returning World War II veterans with disabilities. The thrust of the assistance was vocational training. Slowly Congress realized, however, that vocational training was insufficient to meet the tremendous problems faced by all Americans with disabilities.[1]

In quick succession, Congress enacted a variety of bills that went beyond providing vocational training. Congress first enacted the State and Local Assistance Act of 1972, as amended, which prohibited discrimination against those with handicaps by state and local governments receiving federal revenue-sharing moneys. One year later, Congress enacted the Rehabilitation Act of 1973. It prohibited discrimination against people with disabilities by certain federal contractors and programs receiving federal assistance. In 1974, a third act was enacted to assist Americans with disabilities: The Vietnam Era Veteran's Readjustment Assistance Act. Its purpose was to prevent discrimination against, and establish employment preference for, returning Vietnam veterans with disabilities. Finally, Congress enacted The Developmentally Disabled Assistance and Bill of Rights Act of 1975 whose purpose was to assist individuals with disabilities. The act provided federal grants to states to eliminate architectural barriers for those with disabilities. In return, the states agreed to take affirmative action in hiring individuals with disabilities.

Fifteen years after the 1973 Rehabilitation Act, Congress evaluated existing legislation for people with disabilities. Despite some gains through prior legislation, millions of the disabled remained unemployed, isolated, and segregated. Congress took action once again, and by using much of the same language contained in the Rehabilitation Act of 1973, Congress enacted the Americans with Disabilities Act (ADA). The ADA goes far beyond the 1973 Rehabilitation Act because it prohibits discrimination against people with disabilities by all employers of 15 or more employees, not just federal contractors. Called by its chief sponsor the "Emancipation Proclamation for those with disabilities,"[2] it gives "civil rights protections to individuals that are like those provided to individuals on the basis of race, sex, national origin, and religion."[3] President Bush signed the ADA on July 26, 1990.

Purpose/Intent

Despite prior legislation, as of 1990 people with disabilities remained, in Congress' words, "a discrete and insular minority"[4] subjected to unequal treatment and "political powerlessness in our society"[5] arising from "stereotypic assumptions not truly indicative" of their individual ability.[6] As a result of its findings, the Americans with Disabilities Act of 1990 (ADA) was enacted as a national mandate for elimination of discrimination against people with disabilities.

The purposes of the ADA as set forth in the act are:

1. To provide a clear and comprehensive national mandate for the elimination of discrimination against individuals with disabilities
2. To provide clear, strong, consistent, enforceable standards addressing discrimination against individuals with disabilities
3. To ensure that the federal government plays a central role in enforcing standards established in this Act on behalf of individuals with disabilities
4. To invoke the sweep of congressional authority, including the power to enforce the fourteenth amendment and to regulate commerce in order to address the major areas of discrimination faced daily by people with disabilities.[4]

Since the ADA is so new, it is difficult to know exactly how its provisions will be interpreted. Detailed regulations are currently being developed to explain what employers, owners of public accommodations, and others who are bound by the ADA must do to comply with the act. Those who are bound by the ADA are termed *covered entities*. The focus of this chapter is the Americans with Disabilities Act since it is the broadest of all acts affecting the disabled. However, if a client has a potential claim under the ADA, he or she may have a claim under the Rehabilitation Act of 1973 if the employer is a federal contractor. Likewise, Vietnam Era veterans may have claims under the Vietnam Era Readjustment Act. Given the broad language of the ADA, a disabled client's most powerful weapon is probably the ADA.

HOW TO DETERMINE IF THE AMERICANS WITH DISABILITIES ACT MAY APPLY TO A CLIENT

During an interview, the human-service worker may learn that a client with physical or mental disabilities has been fired from a job, denied access to a store or hotel or, perhaps, prevented from using a public bus because of his or her disability. The human-service worker should determine whether the client may be able to avail himself or herself of congressional legislation, most notably the ADA. The following questions should assist the professional in making that determination.[5]

Is the client considered disabled under the act?
The ADA applies to persons (a) with any physical or mental impairment that substantially limits one or more of the person's major life activities; (b) with a record of such an impairment; or (c) regarded as having such an impairment. It may, therefore, include clients who do not have a particular impairment but were misdiagnosed and have "a record of the impairment." It may also include clients who have HIV or AIDS-related complex, even if it does not substantially limit their major life activities since they may be "regarded as having an impairment."[6]

Impairment has been defined by the EEOC under the Rehabilitation Act of 1973[7] as including any physiological disorder or condition, cosmetic disfigurement, or anatomical loss affecting one or more of the major body systems, or any mental or psychological disorder, such as mental illness, retardation, or even specific learning disabilities. Since the ADA uses the term *impairment*, it is likely that it will be interpreted in the same way as the Rehabilitation act of 1973.

The ADA specifically excludes from the disability definition homosexuals, bisexuals, sexual behavior disorders, compulsive gamblers, kleptomaniacs, pyromaniacs, and certain disorders arising out of current drug use. Additionally, illegal drug users and alcoholics who cannot perform their job duties or whose employment presents a threat to property and safety are excluded from the protection of the ADA, and no longer have protection under the Rehabilitation Act.

If the client may be considered disabled, what does the ADA prohibit generally?

The ADA prohibits discrimination against qualified individuals with disabilities in four different areas: employment, public services with a focus on transportation, public accommodations, and telecommunications. Once the human-service worker determines that the client would be considered disabled under the ADA and has, perhaps, been subjected to discrimination as a result of the disability, the professional must consider the area of discrimination. Was the client discriminated against by an employer or potential employer, a bus company, a public accommodation (e.g., a hotel), or was a hearing-impaired client denied meaningful access to the phone system?

How does the ADA apply in employment areas?

The ADA prohibits discrimination against individuals with disabilities who can perform the essential functions of the job without reasonable accommodation, in other words, without any modification to the facilities or job structure by the employer. However, the ADA goes further because individuals with disabilities who can perform the job with reasonable accommodation cannot be discriminated against by an employer. For example, if a person could do the job if the employer installed an inexpensive mechanism on a piece of equipment, then the employer is required to make that *reasonable accommodation* and cannot refuse to hire or promote an individual solely because of his or her disability.

The discrimination can occur through an employer's failure to hire, promote, or train a qualified individual with a disability. If an employer fails to hire a qualified applicant because he or she does not want to make existing facilities accessible to that applicant, the applicant may have a claim under the ADA. Discrimination can also occur by segregating employees in such a way as to adversely affect career opportunities. For example, if an individual with a disability is placed in an isolated area to the detriment of his or her career, the ADA may prohibit such isolation.

What is the reasonable accommodation *that an employer must make to an individual with a disability?*

To determine what is *reasonable accommodation*, the agencies and courts will look at the financial resources of the employer and examine the impact of providing the accommodation on the employer's financial resources. Employers may be required to do such things as modify work schedules, provide readers, or modify equipment. An employer is not required to make the accommodation if it means undue hardship. An undue hardship may occur when the *accommodation* is unduly costly, extensive, substantial, disruptive, or will fundamentally alter the nature of the program. In making that determination, it is important to look at the size of the business, the type of operation the employer runs, and the nature and cost of the accommodation.

Must the employer shoulder the entire cost of the reasonable accommodation?
Employers may be eligible for funds from their state rehabilitation agencies. They may also be eligible for substantial tax savings under the *Targeted Jobs Tax Credit.* "Undue hardship" is determined by examining the cost to the employer, not the total cost of the accommodation if the employer receives governmental assistance.

Is the client's employer covered under the act?
The ADA applies to most employers of 15 or more workers. However, although the employment section becomes effective on July 26, 1992 for employers of 25 or more, it does not become effective for employers of 15 to 24 until July 26, 1994.

Covered employers include private employers, the states, employment agencies, and labor organizations. Indian tribes, bona fide tax-exempt private clubs, the federal government, and government-owned corporations are not covered under the ADA. Government-owned corporations, however, are probably covered under the Rehabilitation Act of 1973.

May the employer discriminate against a person with a contagious disease?
This is a highly controversial issue which resulted in a compromise. The Secretary of Health and Human Labor has drafted a list of infectious and communicable diseases which may be communicable through food. If a client has one of these diseases and the danger of its transmission through food cannot be eliminated by reasonable accommodation, an employer may refuse to have this individual handling food.

Does the employer have any defenses to a charge of discrimination?
The employer can assert that the alleged discrimination is job-related, consistent with business necessity, and that the individual cannot perform the job even with reasonable accommodation. The employer can also claim that any accommodation to the employee would present an undue hardship to the employer.

Does a client who was fired for alcohol or illegal drug use have an ADA claim?
Any employee who is using illegal drugs during his or her employ is not considered a "qualified individual with a disability." However, if the client is participating in drug rehabilitation and is no longer using drugs, the employer cannot fire or refuse to hire her or him simply because of prior drug use. Similarly, a recovering alcoholic cannot be discriminated against simply because of her or his status as an alcoholic.

The employer may prohibit the use of alcohol and illegal drugs in the workplace and fire those who do not comply. Additionally, the employer may hold alcoholics and users of illegal drugs to the same standards as other employees. In other words, there is no duty to reasonably accommodate alcoholics and illegal drug users.

May an employer conduct a pre-employment physical to determine whether a client is an individual with a disability or the nature and extent of a disability?

The employer may not conduct pre-employment physicals to determine whether an individual is disabled. The employer is limited to asking questions regarding the applicant's ability to perform job-related functions.

May the employer conduct employment examinations?

Once a person is hired, the employer may require an examination if all new employees are subjected to the examination and if access to the information is restricted. Supervisors may be informed of necessary accommodations, medical personnel may be informed if emergency treatment may be necessary, and government officials may be informed to determine whether the employer is complying with the act.

How does the ADA apply to public transportation?

The ADA bars discrimination by any state or local government provider of public transportation against any qualified individual with a disability from participating in, or receiving benefits from, the services, programs, or activities they provide. A qualified individual with a disability under this section is one who, with or without reasonable modification of policies or architectural, communication, or transportation barriers, or the provisions of auxiliary aids, meets the essential eligibility requirements of the system. The focus of these provisions is the public bus systems, public rail systems, and privately operated bus and van companies.

What is a public bus system's obligations under the ADA?

A public bus system has three major obligations under the ADA. First, all new vehicles, other than new buses, purchased after August 26, 1990 must be accessible to individuals with disabilities. *Accessibility* means accessible to individuals with physical disabilities including individuals in wheelchairs. The public entity can, however, purchase inaccessible used vehicles, but only if it can first demonstrate a good faith effort to purchase an accessible used vehicle.

Secondly, the public entity must provide a paratransit system to those individuals with disabilities who cannot use the fixed route system unless it would present an undue burden. For example, if a client cannot reach a fixed bus stop, the public entity must provide comparable public transportation service through, for example, an accessible van. However, this paratransit system is not required if it would unduly burden the public entity.

The third, and final, obligation of a public bus system, is that new bus stations and alterations to existing stations must be made accessible to persons with disabilities. Alterations must be accessible "to the maximum extent feasible."[8]

What are a public rail system's obligations under the ADA?

A public rail system has two major obligations under the act. The first obligation is that all new rail vehicles purchased after August 26, 1990 must be accessible to persons with disabilities. Obligations regarding purchase of used rail vehicles are the same for rail companies and bus companies. However, by July 26, 1995 all existing rail systems must have one accessible car per train.

The second obligation of a public rail system is that new rail stations and alterations to existing stations must be accessible. Existing key stations must be made accessible by July 26, 1993 unless an extension is granted. Extensions may, in certain circumstances, be granted up to thirty years. Finally, existing intercity rail stations or Amtrak® stations, must be made accessible to people with disabilities by July 26, 2010.

What are the obligations of privately operated bus and van companies?

Privately operated buses and vans and privately operated terminals are considered public accommodations. Therefore, the public accommodations requirements of the ADA apply. However, the public services section of the ADA does require that absent an extension, new buses purchased after July 26, 1996 must be accessible. The deadline is July 26, 1997 for small companies. The ADA requires that new vehicles, other than new buses, which were purchased after August 26, 1990 must be accessible to people with disabilities.

How does the ADA apply to public accommodations?

The ADA prohibits discrimination that would interfere with the "full and equal enjoyment" of the goods and services provided by a public accommodation. A public accommodation is not complying with the ADA by providing unequal or separate participation.

Who is covered under the public accommodation provisions?

Public accommodations include privately run hotels, restaurants, bars, movie theaters, lecture halls, retail stores, shopping centers, libraries, museums, galleries, parks, zoos, professional offices, laundromats, day-care centers, schools, gymnasiums, health spas, homeless shelters, and bowling alleys. Almost any private business in this country with 15 or more employees cannot prevent persons with handicaps from full and equal enjoyment of the goods and services that business provides. The Act does not apply to private clubs and religious organizations.

When is the effective date of these provisions?

The effective date for employers with 25 or more employees is July 26, 1992. For those with 15-24 employees, the effective date is July 26, 1994. If a public accommodation runs a transportation service, vehicles it purchases after August 26, 1990 must be accessible. This section of the ADA does not apply to employers of less than 15.

What must a covered provider of a public accommodation do or not do to comply with the act?

Regulations from the Attorney General fully explain what a covered entity must do to comply with the ADA. The ADA says that a provider of a public accommodation must not generally impose eligibility criteria that would screen out or tend to screen out those persons with disabilities from fully enjoying their goods and services. It would be discriminatory to refuse to serve a deaf person or forbid blind people from entering a store.[9]

The covered public accommodation must make reasonable modifications in its procedures to provide goods and services to people with disabilities unless the modification would fundamentally alter goods. For example, a drug rehabilitation clinic could not refuse to treat drug addicts simply because they tested positive for HIV.[10]

The covered public accommodation must take necessary steps to ensure that individuals with handicaps are not treated differently because of the absence of auxiliary aids, unless providing the auxiliary aid would fundamentally alter the goods or services or present an undue burden on the provider. An auxiliary aid need not be provided if the business has another method to provide meaningful access. For example, a restaurant need not provide braille menus if a server is available to read the menu aloud.[11]

The covered public accommodation must remove architectural barriers and transportation barriers in existing vehicles used to transport the public unless the removal is not readily achievable. Removal is readily achievable if it can be done without too much difficulty or expense.

Finally, all new public accommodations and alterations must be readily accessible. This applies to all public accommodations built after January, 1993. Accessibility is not mandated if it is structurally impracticable.

How does the ADA apply to telecommunications?

Effective July 26, 1993, all common carriers engaged in the business of communication by wire or radio must ensure meaningful access to hearing- and speech-impaired individuals. Meaningful access is provided through keyboards called a *Telecommunication Devices for the Deaf* (TDD). The Act requires the phone carrier to provide operators who know how to use the TDD. The hearing-impaired person contacts that operator and relays who they want to call and what they want to say. The operator then calls the person and reads to them what appears on the operator's terminal. The person gives the operator his or her response and the operator types the response into the keyboard to transmit to the hearing-impaired individual.

What steps should a client take if he or she has a potential ADA claim?

The steps a client should take depend on whether the claim is related to employment, transportation, public accommodations, or telecommunications.

Employment claims. The ADA employment provisions are administered in the same way as title VII of the Civil Rights Act of 1964. The primary enforcement agency is the Equal Employment Opportunity Commission (EEOC), although suits may be brought through the Attorney General or privately. If the client alleges discrimination against a state or local government employer, the Attorney General is responsible for investigating and prosecuting the claim.

The EEOC is a five-member organization, only three of whom may be of the same political party. The members serve five-year terms. Although the main office is in Washington, DC, the commission has over 40 field offices throughout the country.

If a client has a potential employment discrimination claim under the ADA, she or he should immediately contact the nearest EEOC and file a written charge which contains a general description of the parties and the alleged discrimination. If the state in which the client resides has a state or local law which might apply and an organization for enforcement, the state is given the first opportunity to try to resolve the dispute. In that case, the EEOC must transfer the charge to the state or the client must first file a charge with the state enforcement agency. The state has 60 days to act on the complaint. If the state fails to act, the client has 300 days from the date of the discrimination or 30 days from the date of receiving the notice that the state has terminated its involvement to file a charge with the EEOC. If no state or local law applies, the client must file a charge with the EEOC within 180 days after the alleged discrimination.

Once a charge is filed with EEOC, the commission notifies the person against whom the complaint is made within 10 days. The EEOC then proceeds to investigate the charge, determining whether reasonable cause exists to believe that the discrimination occurred. This determination should be made 120 days from the filing of the charge.

If the EEOC determines that no reasonable cause exists, the EEOC still provides the client with a right-to-sue letter. The client is given the right-to-sue letter because the EEOC was utilized as required under the statute. If the client does not receive a right-to-sue letter, one may be requested. Once he receives the letter, a complaint must be filed in the U. S. District Court within 90 days.

If the EEOC determines that reasonable cause exists, it will attempt to informally resolve the dispute. It does this by meeting with the parties individually and in confidence. If the dispute is not resolved through this conciliation process, the EEOC may file a suit on behalf of the client in the U. S. District Court. Alternatively, the EEOC may issue a right-to-sue letter and the client can file suit on his or her own behalf. If the EEOC agrees to pursue the case on behalf of the client, the client still retains the right to bring his or her own action if, for example, she or he is dissatisfied with the EEOC representation.

If the employer is a state or local government, the Attorney General is charged with enforcement. The Attorney General will investigate complaints and undertake compliance reviews.

Transportation claims. Enforcement procedures in section 505 of the Rehabilitation Act of 1973 apply to enforcement of the ADA transportation regulations. The client may file a complaint with the U. S. Department of Transportation or file a private lawsuit.

Public Accommodations claims. The aggrieved client can file a complaint with the Attorney General or can file a private lawsuit.

Telecommunication claims. Enforcement of these provisions is through the Federal Communication Commission (FCC). A client must file a complaint with the FCC, with the FCC handing down a final order within 180 days. If a state has been certified by the FCC to implement state relay services, the state will be in charge of enforcement. If, however, the state does not respond to the complaint within 180 days, the FCC may enforce the regulations.

What remedies are available to the client?

Employment claims. The remedies for employment discrimination are designed to try to make the client whole. Therefore the remedies include hiring or reinstatement of the disabled person with or without back pay, attorneys' fees, and costs.

Transportation claims. Remedies under section 505 of the Rehabilitation Act of 1973 are available for violations under this section of the ADA. These include requiring the entity to comply through an injunction, as well as awarding attorneys' fees.

Public Accommodation claims. The remedies available for discrimination by public accommodations include ordering accessible alterations, ordering that auxiliary aids be provided, monetary damages, and civil penalties up to $50,000 for a first violation and $100,000 for a second violation.

Telecommunication claims. If the common carrier has not complied with the ADA, the FCC may revoke its license to do business as a common carrier for telephone services.

Conclusion

The ADA is a powerful tool to all individuals with disabilities. It is too early to tell exactly what will be required of covered entities. Detailed regulations and court battles will be required before it will be known if this legislation is truly the "Emancipation Proclamation" for the disabled. Until then, the human-service professional who knows generally about the ADA and the other legislation available to aid the disabled, can be of great assistance to his or her clients. If, from the questions above, it appears that a client is a qualified individual with a disability who has been discriminated against, the client should be referred to the appropriate agency or a private attorney.

Endnotes

1. Civil Rights and the Disabled: A Comparison of the Rehabilitation Act of 1973 and the Americans with Disabilities Act of 1990 in the Employment Setting, Vol. 54 *Albany Lase Review*, 123 (1989).
2. G. Elsasser, "Senate OK's Rights Bill for Disabled," *Chicago Tribune*, Sep. 8, 1989, Sec 1, at 1.
3. Fact Sheet: National Organization on Disability, The Americans with Disabilities Act of 1990.
4. The Americans with Disabilities Act of 1990, Section 2(a)(7)(1990).
5. *Id.*
6. The Americans with Disabilities Act of 1990, Section 2(b)(1-4)(1990).
7. The Americans with Disabilities Act of 1990, Section 3(2)(a-c)(1990).
8. Cubra and Jackson, The Americans with Disabilities Act of 1990, Vol. 18. *The New Mexico Trial Lawyer Journal*, p. 1, no. 10 (November/December 1990).
9. 29 U.S.C. 791 et seq.
10. Turley and Beck (Eds.). Americans with Disabilities Act of 1990, Section 227 (1990).
11. The Americans with Disabilities Act of 1990, Section 227 (1990).
12. Turley and Beck at 99.
13. *Id.* at 101.
14. *Id.*

Guardianship and Advocacy

Richard Kern

Guardianship

HISTORY/LEGISLATION

Guardianship appeared in ancient Rome. The practice of guardianship was codified in 13th century England, and guardianships, modeled on Roman practices, were in use throughout Europe by the end of the Middle Ages. In France and Germany, relatives of a proposed ward have strong rights in deciding who is appointed guardian, and public agencies administer guardianships in most European countries. However, the courts are the principle administrator of guardianships in the United States.

Standards to ensure quality guardianship programs were proposed by the Select Committee on Aging (Chairman of the Subcommittee on Housing and Consumer Interests of the Select Committee on Aging of the U. S. House of Representatives [Select Committee on Aging], 1989). The committee called for the development of alternative services, expanded oversight of guardians, increased funding for guardianship programs, improved training of service professionals and guardians, and further research on how guardianship services are imposed and provided.

Guardianship is a court's appointment of a guardian to make decisions for, and handle the affairs of, another individual, called a ward, whom the court has found to be incompetent (Center for Social Gerontology, 1986). Other terms used to describe different types of guardians include *guardian of the person*, *guardian of the estate*, *conservator of the person*, and *conservator of the estate*. Guardianship often allows guardians to decide such issues for their wards as where they live, how they spend their money, and which prescriptions they receive. Under some guardianships, a ward is reduced to the legal status of a child.

Some forms of guardianship allow the ward to maintain more independence than others. The most restrictive form, and the one most often used by the courts, is plenary guardianship, which grants guardians power over their wards' persons and estates (Center for Social Gerontology, 1986). A conservatorship is a guardianship with power over a ward's financial affairs only. In a limited guardianship, a court allows a guardian control over one or more areas of a ward's life (e.g., paying bills, making decisions about medical care). Currently, courts tend to use limited guardianships more than in the past. In some cases, a guardian may be appointed to oversee a single transaction (e.g., the sale of a home). Temporary or emergency guardianship may be imposed for a few months if a guardian dies suddenly or cannot perform his or her duties due to an emergency.

An individual is termed *legally incompetent* when he or she is found to come within a jurisdiction's definition of incompetence (Center for Social Gerontology, 1986). Traditionally, a condition affecting mental capacity (e.g., mental or physical disability, mental illness) and a resulting disability must be proven to find an individual incompetent.

Generally, statutes allow any capable and willing individual to be a guardian. There are usually no qualifications beyond competency and stability, though some categories of people (e.g., providers of residential services, convicted felons) may be barred. Most guardians are relatives or friends of the ward, and many state laws grant relatives, especially spouses and children, preference as guardians.

Sometimes, a ward has no one willing to act as a guardian and no funds to pay for one. In such situations, some jurisdictions provide guardianship services through a public guardian, either an agency or an individual. These publicly funded offices are often composed of one or more state or county employees. One example is the agency operating in Illinois, where more than 6,000 people are under state guardianship. The agency not only is *guardian of last resort* for those wards, but is also a support system for families that are guardians.

In addition to public guardians, private, not-for-profit organizations (funded through contracts with public agencies), and volunteer programs also offer guardianship services (Center for Social Gerontology, 1986).

Little statistical information is available concerning the number of guardianships. However, demographic and federal policy trends suggest the number of guardians and payees is increasing. These trends include (a) an increase in the number of elderly, (b) a movement toward mainstreaming, (c) a proliferation in the number of elder abuse reporting laws, and (d) an increasing reliance on guardianship by health care institutions (Select Committee on Aging, 1989).

The need for good guardians will increase as the number of older adults increases. During the 1970s, the population aged 65 and over grew by 28%, and the number of people aged 85 and over increased by 59%. In 1989, nearly 30 million persons were aged 65 and over (Select Committee on Aging, 1989). This growth has likely been accompanied by an increase in the number of people outliving their support networks, savings, and ability to care for themselves.

The movement toward mainstreaming the chronically mentally ill has also probably increased reliance on guardianship services. Between 1955 and 1975, the number of patients within state hospitals fell by 75% (Select Committee on Aging, 1989). Some of those who have been released cannot handle all their own affairs, and alternative living settings and service systems have not been adequate to meet their needs for assistance, support, and care.

Elder abuse reporting laws also seem to be a factor in an increase in the amount of public attention paid to older individuals and reliance on guardianship (Select Committee on Aging, 1989). More than 40 states have enacted laws requiring professionals to report suspected abuse and neglect to public agencies. Typically, people who resist an investigation of these reports and refuse to accept services face the possibility of becoming an unwilling recipient of guardianship services. Many states lack funds to pay for services that allow the elderly to live independently and so resort to pursuing guardianship.

Hospitals and nursing homes also seem to be asking for guardianship services more often now than they did in the past (Select Committee on Aging, 1989). A fear of lawsuits and matters of finance or convenience seem to be fostering this trend. Some nursing homes, finding it easier and more financially secure to deal with a guardian than an elderly person, require an individual to be a ward before admitting him or her. In some jurisdictions, nursing homes have filed guardianship petitions against many of their residents.

PURPOSE/INTENT

State-imposed guardianship, when responsibly exercised, helps physically and mentally disabled adults make and carry out decisions. Guardianship also is designed to protect vulnerable individuals from people who want to take advantage of them. For many wards, the system works well (Center for Social Gerontology, 1986; Select Committee on Aging, 1989).

The procedural safeguards surrounding most guardianship proceedings are traditionally lax (Center for Social Gerontology, 1986). Guardianship hearings are customarily informal and nonadversarial. Rules of evidence are relaxed, and there is often no legal counsel to represent the proposed ward.

Because of differing statutes, the process of establishing guardianship varies from state to state and between jurisdictions within a state (Center for Social Gerontology, 1986). In addition, case law and the differing practices of judges influence guardianship proceedings. Some states also differentiate between potential wards—whether adults, minors, or persons with developmental disabilities.

The proposed ward or one of his or her relatives or friends usually files a petition for guardianship with a court. A change in the proposed ward's behavior or ability to function or communicate usually leads the petitioner to take action. All petitions allege the incompetence of a potential ward to care for himself or herself or to manage his or her estate.

In nearly all jurisdictions, the proposed ward must be notified of the guardianship hearing, and most jurisdictions require an interested third party, usually a relative, also to receive a notice. This notice is designed to protect the ward from his or her own confusion and from the petitioner.

The amount of time that must pass between the notice and the hearing is not often specified in the statutes. Notices often fail to convey what is at stake, the possible defenses open to the proposed ward, or his or her rights. Therefore, wards often lack representation at their hearings, and, in a few jurisdictions, he or she has no right to such representation (Center for Social Gerontology, 1986).

The potential ward is presumed competent until the petitioner proves otherwise. In establishing the ward's incompetence, courts traditionally have sought proof of two factors: a condition affecting mental capacity (e.g., mental or physical disability, mental illness) and a resulting disability. However, there is often little concrete evidence of the disabilities, so the courts rely on a medical diagnosis of the condition alone (Center for Social Gerontology, 1986). Often, a medical diagnosis is also used to establish the link between the condition and the disability.

Judges usually decide whether to impose a guardianship after a hearing lasting only a few minutes. Most jurisdictions do not provide for a jury trial or allow them only on request.

The letter appointing a guardian usually specifies his or her duties and powers. Generally, guardians must have enough contact with a ward to be aware of his or her status and needs. A guardian may see to a ward's comfort, living situation, medical treatment, financial arrangements, and other lifestyle matters. However, the guardian's duties are not always clearly set out in state statutes or in letters of appointment.

Courts implement supervisory mechanisms to ensure that guardians carry out their duties. These mechanisms may include requiring a guardian to post bond and to report on his or her handling of the ward's estate. However, many courts fail to enforce these requirements or examine the reports (Center for Social Gerontology, 1986).

Guardianships are not often removed. The guardian usually lacks an incentive to do so, and the ward is often unable to handle the legal intricacies of the removal process. Most statutes require the ward to prove that he or she is no longer incompetent.

In addition, it is difficult to reverse a judgement of incompetence. Many statutes barely address the process of restoring a ward to the legal status of competence. There are fewer procedural safeguards surrounding that process than there are around guardianship hearings (Center for Social Gerontology, 1986).

Due process protections in guardianship hearings have been improved as states recognize how guardianship strips wards of their constitutional freedoms and stigmatizes them with a declaration of incompetence (Center for Social Gerontology, 1986). These improvements include meaningful notices of guardianship hearings, mandatory attendance of potential wards at hearings, and their representation by adequate counsel there.

Many states have taken steps to protect potential wards from inappropriate guardianship by increasing the importance of their functional abilities and emphasizing their thought and communication processes (Center for Social Gerontology, 1986). In some jurisdictions, guardianship cannot be imposed without showing a functional disability. Courts also are tending to examine the effect of an impairment on a potential ward's ability to make responsible decisions.

In addition, court visitors are sometimes appointed to investigate the circumstances surrounding the petition for guardianship and make a recommendation about it to the court. This procedure is designed to improve the reliability of the proceedings (Center for Social Gerontology, 1986). Courts also appoint guardians ad litem, who help protect the rights of potential wards and guard against unneeded guardianships.

Despite these safeguards, the guardianship system sometimes unnecessarily strips individuals of their civil rights (e.g., right to marry, right to vote) (Select Committee on Aging, 1989). All wards are stigmatized with a ruling of incompetence. In addition, some guardians abuse their power and neglect wards, endangering their financial, physical, and emotional welfare.

CLIENT SERVICES

The increasing need for guardianship services has led to the creation of three types of programs (Select Committee on Aging, 1989). Some states and communities have established a public guardian's office to provide services. Second, private, nonprofit programs, supported by contracts with state and local agencies, have been created. Volunteer programs—run by churches, social service agencies, and courts—are a third source of guardianship services.

Each type of guardianship program has advantages. In some states, the public guardianship system assures an oversight of wards' care. Contracts for guardianship services from nonprofit organizations are sometimes beneficial and cost saving. Well-trained volunteers can be a very positive influence and resource.

Courts are increasingly resorting to less restrictive alternatives—such as protective services, money management, and durable powers of attorney (Select Committee on Aging, 1989). Protective services involve the use of home health care, house repair, and other options that allow independent living. Money management includes automatic banking, which allows the payment of routine bills, and direct deposit of regular sources of income. Durable powers of attorney allow an individual, while competent, to choose who will be his or her decision maker should they become incompetent.

Advocacy

HISTORY/LEGISLATION

During the last 30 years, there has been an increasing recognition of the rights of the handicapped, the mentally retarded, the elderly, and the mentally ill. Rights protection services have been developed to ensure that these rights are honored and to improve them (Freddolino, 1983).

Changes in the guardianship system have occurred through advocacy by government agencies, citizen groups, parents and families, attorneys, and consumers. State, county, and local agencies have prepared bills, funded advocacy programs, and developed advocacy positions within service delivery systems. The advocacy movement seems to have reached its apex in the late 1970s, when many advocacy programs were created (Freddolino, 1983). Advocacy groups have continued to operate in the 1990s.

Advocacy involves speaking on the part of a person or issue (Freddolino, 1983). An advocate helps persons who are handicapped secure the same rights and services other citizens enjoy by representing their interests. People in the human services profession have widely adopted advocacy (Roeher, 1984). They speak out to safeguard the rights of individual clients and to force changes for whole classes of people. Advocacy can take many different forms—protege/advocate type programs like Parent-to-Parent, human and civil right agencies, legal aid programs, ombudsman offices, crisis intervention groups, and consumer networks (Roeher, 1984).

All advocacy involves conflict over the distribution of power, authority, and resources (Freddolino, 1983). Therefore, advocates struggle against those who hold power to secure the rights of populations, including those who are wards. Advocacy helps humanize bureaucracy and enables special groups to be heard in the political arena (Roeher, 1984).

Guardianship can be one form of advocacy, in which a person or group represents the interests of a ward and takes responsibility for his or her property (Rogers, 1984). Advocates work on the behalf of wards who need services but cannot seek them out. Advocacy can also help the court specify the things that a limited guardian can do, allowing the ward more independence and personal development.

Advocacy programs almost always focus their efforts on a particular disability group. Their work may or may not include advocacy within the guardianship system for clients in the group or the group as a whole. For example, state agencies for the protection and advocacy of the developmentally disabled provide, among other services, advocacy for clients who are wards. The state of Illinois has an advocacy program within an agency providing guardianship services.

Most funds for advocacy programs come from government sources (Freddolino, 1983). Programs providing legal services and public advocacy programs operate with support from state and federal agencies, and state and local government departments. Consumer-organized groups, such as those operated by former psychiatric patients and the parents and families of those with disabilities, received money largely from donations, dues, charities, and foundations.

Staffing patterns for advocacy programs vary widely (Freddolino, 1983). Typically, advocacy programs are small; most of them are staffed by two to five people. Programs offering legal services and public advocacy programs are often staffed by attorneys, paralegals, and social workers. Members of consumer-oriented groups perform much of the work done by their groups on a volunteer basis. Advocacy associations are usually staffed by administrative personnel supported by volunteers.

PURPOSE/INTENT

Advocacy programs offer services to individuals and attempt to bring about changes in legal or service delivery systems (Freddolino, 1983). Help given to individuals may include notifying them of their rights, providing legal services, investigating complaints, offering support groups, training in self-advocacy, and offering clients information about services and public benefits. In addition, many programs engage in lobbying, public speaking, and other activities tending to improve the position of the disability groups in the community and within the legal system.

Rights issues are also commonly addressed by advocacy groups (Freddolino, 1983). Issues addressed include the right to mental health services, the right to confidentiality, and the right to a humane environment. Rights problems concerned with freedom from stigma and guardianship are often addressed. Consumer-organized and operated programs have reported addressing a larger number of rights problems than do other types of advocacy programs.

Advocacy groups use varied methods to affect change. One method is legal action (e.g., lawsuits on behalf of institutionalized people) to force resources from the institutions toward smaller, community-based facilities. Besides taking an adversarial stance, advocacy groups also affect change by bargaining, negotiating, and pleading with governmental agencies (Larsen, 1984).

CLIENT SERVICES

Advocacy on behalf of persons involved in the guardianship process is provided through five types of programs: legal organizations, associations, consumer groups, parent and family groups, and internal advocacy programs (Freddolino, 1983). Legal organizations include providers such as legal aid offices, public defenders, and public interest law firms. Consumer groups are largely composed of members of a disability group such as former psychiatric patients or the developmentally disabled. Advocacy can also be done by associations—most of which are private, nonprofit, volunteer groups—or by groups made up of the parents and families of people within a disability group. In an internal advocacy program, an advocacy program is provided within an organization that offers broader services (e.g., department of mental health), an agency to provide protection and advocacy for the developmentally disabled, or a private program for care of the mentally retarded.

Examples of internal advocacy programs expressly for those involved in the guardianship process exist in Illinois and California. In Illinois, a legal advocacy service exists in the same office as the state guardian. This program is mandated to help a client find private counsel before providing him or her services through an attorney employed by the program (Guardianship & Advocacy Commission, 1990). In California, court investigators attempt to catch abuses of guardianship arrangements. Their duties include checking on proposed wards who will not appear in court, checking on wards, and investigating allegations of fraud and abuse (Castaneda, 1987).

Some parent-based associations are also involved in guardianship services and advocacy. The Foundation for the Handicapped, a Washington State-based corporate guardianship program for children with handicaps, has challenged governmental agencies by administrative means and in court (Larsen, 1984). Court cases involving foundation clients are concerned with rights advocacy. In addition, The Guardianship, Advocacy, and Protective Services Program of Oregon (GAPS), part of the Association for Retarded Citizens of Oregon, offers nonlegal advocacy, temporary or limited guardianship, and long-term or plenary guardianship services (Soenneker, 1984).

References

Castaneda, L. (1987, September 29). Investigators: Backbone of conservatorships. *The Los Angeles Daily Journal*, pp. 1, 12.

Center for Social Gerontology. (1986). *Guardianship and alternative legal interventions: A compendium for training and practice.* Ann Arbor, MI: Author.

Chairman of the Subcommittee on Housing and Consumer Interests of the Select Committee on Aging of the U. S. House of Representatives. (1989). *Model standards to ensure quality guardianship and representative payeeship services.* (Committee Publication No. 101-729). Washington, DC: U. S. Government Printing Office.

Freddolino, P. P. (1983). Findings from the national mental health advocacy survey. *Mental Disability Law Reporter, 7*(5), 416-421, 435.

Guardianship and Advocacy Commission. (1990). *The Guardianship and Advocacy Act and other statutes pertaining to the Guardianship and Advocacy Commission.* (Publication No. JB9101-700). Springfield: State of Illinois.

Larsen, E. J. (1984). The foundation for the handicapped. In T. Apolloni & T. P. Cooke (Eds.), *A new look at guardianship* (pp. 223-261). Baltimore: Paul H. Brookes.

Roeher, G. A. (1984). The changing context of the human services movement: Implications for the disability field and the need for more adequate backup systems. In T. Apolloni & T. P. Cooke (Eds.), *A new look at guardianship* (pp. 13-33). Baltimore: Paul H. Brookes.

Rogers, P. R. (1984). Understanding the legal concept of guardianship. In T. Apolloni & T. P. Cooke (Eds.), *A new look at guardianship* (pp. 35-48). Baltimore: Paul H. Brookes.

Soenneker, A. J. (1984). Guardianship, advocacy, and protective services (GAPS) Program. In T. Apolloni & T. P. Cooke (Eds.), *A new look at guardianship* (pp. 265-284). Baltimore: Paul H. Brookes.

Client Assistance Programs

Nancy Schade

History/Legislation

THE 1973 AMENDMENTS (P. L. 93-112): THE CREATION OF THE DISCRETIONARY CLIENT ASSISTANCE PROGRAM (CAP)

The original stimulus for establishing CAP in 1972 came from citizens with disabilities who addressed a long-held belief that a bureaucratic maze often prevented persons with handicaps from understanding, receiving, or using appropriate vocational rehabilitation (VR) services. In response, Congress established a pilot project closely related to the state VR agency in an effort to avoid adversarial relationships between clients and VR agencies. The Act authorized a minimum of seven projects and a maximum of 20. The projects, which were not requested to be statewide, were to be initiated by state VR agencies through a competitive grant application. Legislative limitations against an adversarial advocacy system were balanced by the assurance that project staff have direct communication with top state administrators and could not have dual allegiance to other VR duties.

Initial funding for CAP began at $500,000, with 11 projects being funded by May, 1974. When the funding was increased to $1,000,000 in 1975, the number of projects rose to 18. Although the funding remained level for the next three years, the number of projects increased to 20. In 1978, Congress lifted the 20 program limitation and provided $3.5 million in funding. Thirty-six CAP programs existed in 1979, and 42 in 1980. As a result of budget cuts, the mandated minimum level was modified in the 1981 Reconciliation Act and the number of CAPs dropped back to 36, with $2.8 million in funding being provided. As part of the new administration's efforts to contain the federal deficit, the appropriation for CAP was decreased to $942,000 in fiscal year 1982 with no funds budgeted initially in fiscal year 1983. During this period of decreased funding, the number of CAPs was reduced to 17 by the end of fiscal year 1983. Many of these projects survived on carry-over funds or state appropriations, with a few being entirely state funded. Congress restored funding to previous levels the following year.

The majority of the CAPs were operated by the state VR agencies themselves, either using existing personnel or staff hired expressly to provide CAP services. CAPs were established in state VR agencies for the blind, as well as general VR agencies. In some states (e.g., Virginia), a CAP was established in each. A few CAPs were designated to the state VR agency with CAP services being contracted to external agencies, including the Protection and Advocacy (P & A) systems for people with developmental disabilities and other private agencies or not-for-profit organizations (e.g., United Cerebral Palsy, Easter Seals Society, Legal Services). Many of the CAP directors were people with disabilities, as were many of the staff members they hired.

Although the administration recommended no funding for CAP in 1984, hoping that the states would assume the burden of funding any further CAPs, the 1984 reauthorization of the Act resulted in the discretionary CAP being converted into a mandatory formula grant program.

Section 112(a) of the Rehabilitation Act of 1973, as amended, establishes CAP and outlines the areas where CAP may provide assistance. It mandates that states be given grants to establish and carry out CAPs to provide assistance in informing and advising all applicants and clients of all available benefits under the Act, and, upon request of such applicants and clients, to assist such applicants and clients in their relationships with projects, programs, and facilities providing services to them under this Act. CAPs are required to have the ability to pursue legal, administrative, or other appropriate remedies to ensure the protection of the rights of such individuals under the Act. The 1986 amendments expanded CAP's mandate to include providing information on the services and benefits available under the Act to any individual with a disability in the state.

THE 1984 AMENDMENTS (P. L. 98-221): CAP AS A MANDATORY PROGRAM

During the 1984 reauthorization of the Act, the Senate version of the proposed amendments contained language that would change the fundamental character of CAP by mandating that each state and territory operate a CAP as a condition for receiving payments from its allotment under section 110 of the Act (i.e., the Basic Vocational Rehabilitation Program).

The Senate's proposed changes to the Act met with great resistance in the House of Representatives. A compromise, which was reached in the conference committee, resulted in the following provisions being incorporated into the 1984 amendments and being addressed in the governing regulations.

Governor's Designation: The governor in each state and territory was given the responsibility of designating a public or private agency to conduct the state's CAP. The Governor could only designate one agency within the state to operate the CAP. No state could receive payments from its section 110 (Basic Vocational Rehabilitation Program) allotment under the Act in any fiscal year unless the state had a CAP in effect before October 1, 1984.

Independence Requirement: The governor must designate an agency which is independent of any agency which provides treatment, services, or rehabilitation to individuals under the Act. However, a grandfather clause provided that the governor could designate an agency which provided treatment, services, or rehabilitation to individuals with handicaps under the Act if there was an agency in the state that both (a) served as a CAP under section 112 of the Act by directly carrying out a CAP; and (b) was, at the same time, a grantee under section 112 or any other provision of the Act.

Conflict of Interest Prohibition: With the exception of the CAPs that were designated to service providing agencies based on the "grandfather clause" referenced above, no employee of the designated agency can, while so employed, serve as a staff member of, or consultant to, any rehabilitation program, project, or facility in the state which receives assistance under the Rehabilitation Act of 1973, as amended.

Consultation Requirement: In designating an agency to conduct the CAP, the governor must consult with the director of the state VR agency (or, in states with both a general agency and an agency for the blind, the directors of both agencies), the head of the developmental disabilities protection and advocacy agency, and representatives of professional and consumer organizations serving individuals with handicaps in the state.

Authority of the Designated Agency: The agency designated by the governor to operate the CAP must have the authority to pursue legal, administrative, and other appropriate remedies to ensure the protection of the rights of individuals with handicaps who are seeking or receiving treatment, services, or rehabilitation under the Act within the state. This authority must include the authority to pursue those remedies against the state VR agency(ies) and other appropriate state agencies.

Prohibition Against Class Actions: CAPs are prohibited from bringing any class action lawsuits in carrying out their responsibilities.

Identifying and Addressing Systemic Issues: The director of the designated CAP must be afforded reasonable access to policy-making and administrative personnel in the state and local rehabilitation programs, projects, and facilities. The CAP program is authorized to advise state and other agencies of identified problem areas in the delivery of rehabilitation services to individuals with handicaps and suggesting methods and means of improving agency performance. CAP is not authorized to act as a general advocacy agency for individuals with disabilities. Therefore, systemic issues which are identified and addressed by CAP must directly relate to programs, projects, and facilities funded under the Act.

THE 1986 AMENDMENTS (P. L. 99-506): THE CAP MANDATE IS EXPANDED

Three changes were made in the CAP program when the Act was reauthorized in 1986. First, the CAP mandate was expanded to include providing information on the available services and benefits under the Act to any individuals with handicaps in the state. Second, a governor's authority to move the designation from one agency to another was limited; a governor was required to demonstrate "good cause" before redesignating the CAP, and then only after providing public notice of the intention to make such redesignation and providing an opportunity for public comment on the proposed redesignation. The requirements applying to the original designations made in 1984 also had to be met for the newly designated agency. Third, after the initial designation process, any change in the designation of a CAP required that it be placed in an agency independent of any program providing services funded under the Act.

Purpose/Intent

CAP ASSURANCES—OMB NO. 1820-0520

To receive funds, each state, through its governor, must submit written assurances to the Rehabilitation Service Administration (RSA) that it will operate an appropriately compliant Client Assistance Program. The following assurances are signed by the Governor and submitted to the Rehabilitation Service Administration:

Assurance 1: In designating the CAP, the governor consulted with the director of the state VR agency (or, in states with both a general agency and an agency for the blind, the directors of both agencies), the head of the developmental disability protection and advocacy agency, and with representatives of professional and consumer organizations serving individuals with handicaps in the state.

Assurance 2: The governor will not redesignate the agency designated without good cause and only after notice and an opportunity for public comment has been given of the intention to make such redesignation.

Assurance 3: The designated agency is independent of any agency which provides treatment, services, or rehabilitation to individuals under the Rehabilitation Act; or the state is excepted from such independence requirement.

Assurance 4: The designated agency has the authority to pursue legal, administrative, and other appropriate remedies to ensure the protection of the rights of individuals with handicaps who are receiving treatment, services, or rehabilitation under the Act within the state.

Assurance 5: The authority to pursue remedies described in item 4 includes the authority to pursue those remedies against the state VR agency and other appropriate state agencies. The designated agency meets this requirement if it has the authority to pursue these remedies either on its own behalf, or by obtaining necessary services (e.g., legal representation) from outside sources.

Assurance 6: No program employee will, while so employed, serve as a staff member of, or consultant to, any rehabilitation project, program, or facility receiving assistance under the Rehabilitation Act in the state.

Assurance 7: The program director will be afforded reasonable access to policy-making and administrative personnel in the state and local rehabilitation programs, projects, or facilities.

Assurance 8: The state will advise all clients and client applicants of the existence of the Client Assistance Program, the services provided by the program, and how to contact the program.

Assurance 9: The designated agency will implement procedures designed to ensure that, to the maximum extent possible, mediation procedures are used prior to resorting to administrative or legal remedies. The regulations define mediation to include good faith negotiations, but does not require the use of a third party before resorting to administrative or legal remedies.

Assurance 10: The designated agency will not bring any class action on carrying out its responsibilities under the CAP.

Assurance 11: The designated agency will submit to the secretary an annual report on the operation of the agency's program during the previous year, including a summary of the work done and the uniform statistical tabulation of all cases handled by the program.

Assurance 12: The designated agency will provide the Secretary of Education with the information needed to conduct evaluations and studies of the program.

Assurance 13: In carrying out the program, the Governor will consult with the director of the state VR agency (or, in states with both a general agency and an agency for the blind, the director of both agencies), the head of the developmental disability protection and advocacy agency, and with representatives of professional and consumer organizations serving individuals with handicaps in the state.

Assurance 14:
   a. The state legally may carry out each provision of its request for assistance.
   b. The agency specified in the request for assistance has authority under state law to receive, hold, and disburse federal funds made available under the program.
   c. The state's request for assistance is the basis for state operation and administration of the program.

Assurance 15: The designated agency will obligate funds received under this program by the end of the fiscal year for which they are made available.

Client Services

FEDERAL REGULATIONS

The federal regulations promulgated to supplement section 112 of the Act set forth below describe the kinds of activities in which CAPs may engage, the manner in which the Program Director may be afforded access to policy-making and administrative personnel, and a clarification of what mediation entails. Sections which merely reiterate the Act are not included in the following discussion.

AUTHORIZED ACTIVITIES

CAP's role and responsibilities are consistent throughout the VR process. Funds are available under section 112 of the Act for the following authorized activities:
- *Helping* applicants/clients to understand rehabilitation services programs available under the Act;
- *Advising* applicants/clients of all benefits available to them through rehabilitation programs authorized under the Act, and of related federal and state assistance programs, as well as of their rights and responsibilities in connection with such programs and benefits;
- Otherwise, *assisting* applicants/clients in their relationships with programs, projects, and facilities providing rehabilitation services under the Act;
- *Helping* applicants/clients by pursuing, or assisting them in pursuing, legal, administration, and other available remedies when necessary to ensure the protection of their rights under the Act;
- *Advising* state and other agencies of identified problem areas in the delivery of rehabilitation services to individuals with handicaps and suggesting methods and means of improving agency performance;
- *Providing information* to the public concerning the CAP; and
- *Providing information* on the available services under the Act to any individuals with handicaps in the state.

REHABILITATION SERVICE ADMINISTRATION (RSA) ISSUANCES

The following section outlines some of the key RSA issuances concerning the governor's designation of an agency to operate the CAP, the nature and scope of CAP services, and the state's responsibility to notify applicants/clients about the availability of CAP, and so on.

Recipient of CAP Allotment

CAP grants can be paid directly to the designated agency if state law permitted it or did not prohibit it. Although the grant was technically being awarded to the state, the designated agency was also held responsible for the expenditure of funds.

Designation

RSA confirmed that such agencies could include private, for-profit organizations. RSA also made it clear that a governor could not appoint more than one state VR agency to administer the CAP and reaffirmed that no CAP employee can serve as an employee of the VR agency. RSA also clarified that once an agency has been designated to administer the CAP, it may contract with another organization to provide CAP assistance, but only if the independence requirement set forth in the Act is not violated.

Target Population

RSA reiterated that those individuals seeking or receiving services under the Act are deemed eligible for services provided by CAP. Consequently, individuals served by CAP are *not* limited to applicants/clients of the state VR agency or persons participating in independent living activities.

Outreach and Recruiting

RSA clarified that CAP outreach should be directed to current applicants and clients of programs, projects, and facilities funded under the Act. Outreach activities are not intended for generating enrollment of clients into VR programs and projects. Providing information to the public is an additional function of the CAP outreach policy. Public contact services may be used as a means of generating inquiries about, and applications for, CAP services.

Nature and Scope of CAP Services

CAP services are authorized only for applicants/clients of rehabilitation services and benefits funded under the Act. This target population is further defined as, "an individual receiving or seeking services under the Act." Hence, individuals seeking or receiving services under any project, program, or facility funded under the Act would be included.

Generally, the appropriateness of providing a CAP service can be judged based on whether the applicant/client's problem or concern is related to a service or benefit available under the Act. Hence, the pursuit of remedies is directly related to an individual's rights in connection with services and benefits available under the Act. CAP does not have the authority to pursue remedies for the protection of rights in relationship to issues which do not involve services funded under the Act. Consequently, a CAP may assist an applicant/client in pursuing, for example, a discrimination issue against a service provider funded under the Act, but not against an outside entity (e.g., a private employer, a government program) which is not funded under the Act.

Although CAPs were created primarily to handle individual cases and, hence, were not given the authority to pursue "general advocacy" regarding the overall needs of persons with disabilities through class action litigation, CAPs are mandated to pursue system's advocacy activities with respect to applicants and clients of programs, projects, and facilities funded under the Act and, in general, with respect to services provided under the Act.

Specifically, CAPs are authorized to advise state VR and other state agencies of identified problem areas in the delivery of rehabilitation services and to suggest methods of improving the performance of agencies which provide services under the Act. Furthermore, the regulations require that CAP directors be afforded reasonable access to policy-making and administrative personnel in state and local rehabilitation programs. The purpose of this requirement is interpreted for use not only in resolving individual cases, but also in identifying problems in the rehabilitation services delivery systems and in suggesting ways of making needed improvements.

CAPs are also authorized to provide information to the public concerning services and benefits under the Act and the availability of CAP services. CAPs may advise applicants/clients of benefits available to them through federal and state assistance programs, and their right in relation to these programs; however, they are not authorized to assist in relationships with or pursue remedies with regard to these programs. Nevertheless, CAPs are not precluded from "helping" with outside programs when such help is limited to assistance in completing forms, organization of information and facts, or referral to legal aid or enforcement agencies. Any efforts regarding other programs should be limited and based upon individual circumstances.

CAP's Authority to Pursue or Pay Costs for Pursuit of Legal Remedies

A designated CAP agency must have the authority to pursue legal remedies on behalf of an applicant or client. This authority must include the ability to pursue administrative and legal remedies against the state VR agency(ies) and other appropriate state agencies. The designated agency meets this requirement if it has the authority to pursue those remedies either on its own behalf or by obtaining necessary services (e.g., legal representation) from outside sources.

The pursuit of legal remedies by a CAP agency is allowable only in connection with the provision of services to ensure the protection of applicant and client rights under the Act. Therefore, CAP may not furnish or purchase legal assistance for an applicant or client in the pursuit of a claim against an individual. In addition, CAP does not have the authority to litigate on an applicant's or client's behalf for monetary damages, since money is not a benefit or service under the Act.

CAP Services to Individuals with Handicaps in Rehabilitation Facilities

An individual in a rehabilitation facility must be an applicant for, or a recipient of, services provided by funds or grants from RSA or the National Institute on

Disability and Rehabilitation Research (NIDRR), which include client services as an approved activity, to be eligible for CAP services. However, information on available services may be given to any individual with a handicap within the state.

CAP's Discretion to Determine Services to be Provided

CAP is not obligated to assist an applicant or client when the CAP has determined that the client's dispute lacks merit. Although CAP has the discretion to determine when it is appropriate to provide services to an individual, CAP is expected to meet its basic purpose of assisting applicants and clients in resolving differences and finding alternative solutions whenever possible.

Informing Clients and Applicants of CAP

The state will advise all clients and client applicants of the existence of the client assistance program, the services provided by the program, and how to contact the program. RSA further clarified that this responsibility applies to all programs, projects, and facilities which provide services under the Act.

The Role of CAP in the Rehabilitation System

The role CAP plays in the rehabilitation system has significantly changed since its inception in 1973. Originally established as a discretionary program, its primary purpose was to serve as an ombudsman program and to improve communication between applicants and clients and VR counselors, and between other rehabilitation staff and the clients referred to them by counselors. CAPs were initially created to help clients understand the rehabilitation process and the benefits available to them under the Act. Congress envisioned CAP providing "assistance" to applicants and clients to ensure that the rehabilitation system worked well for them.

Some of the provisions included in the 1984 amendments to the Act changed the nature of CAP, causing it to become a more integral part of the rehabilitation service delivery system. The provisions which were instrumental in causing this change are:

- Each state and territory had to establish and operate a CAP in order to receive its state allotment under section 110 of the Act.
- The agencies designated to operate the CAP had to have the ability to pursue legal, administrative, and other appropriate remedies to ensure the protection of the rights of individuals seeking or receiving services under the Act.
- CAP had to be afforded reasonable access to policy-making and administrative personnel in state and local rehabilitation programs, projects, and facilities.

As a result of these provisions, CAP's role has expanded and CAP has become an integral part of the rehabilitation service delivery system. CAP now serves as a vital link between the programs, projects, and facilities funded under the Act and the community, enabling persons with disabilities to meaningfully access the rehabilitation system. CAP also advises the state VR agency of identified problem areas in the delivery of rehabilitation services, providing important input into policy development and implementation.

Finally, as a result of the changes described above, CAP is increasingly viewed as an advocacy program for persons with disabilities who are seeking or receiving rehabilitation services under the Act. Since 1984, CAPs have been required to use mediation as a primary method of resolving the concerns of applicants and clients. CAP does *not*, however, function in the role of a traditional mediator, that is, always acting as a neutral third party between the client and the state VR agency. This fact is recognized in the federal regulation where mediation is defined as including good faith negotiations, and the use of a third party is not required before resorting to administrative or legal remedies. The regulations indicate an understanding that CAP often has to act as an advocate for its clients; otherwise, there would be no requirement that CAP negotiate with the state VR agency in good faith. When the 1984 amendments required CAPs to have the capacity to pursue administrative, legal, and other available remedies, CAP's role was broadened to include individual advocacy. However, CAP's approach to advocacy differs from many approaches to advocacy in that CAP can only address issues and problems that are related to services and benefits available under the Act.

Summary

CAP was created to facilitate consumer use of rehabilitation services. CAP provides a forum for applicants and clients to air grievances. CAP can assist applicants and clients in understanding and utilizing the appeals process. When deemed necessary, CAP has recourse to legal remedies. In its role as a system's advocate, CAP provides a check and balance system which can assist rehabilitation programs in identifying and remedying systemic problems and policy concerns. Hence, CAP can assist in facilitating the expansion and improvement of rehabilitation services. CAP can also assist in removing program barriers (e.g., inappropriate policies and procedures attitudinal problem) which function to inhibit equal access to rehabilitation services funded under the Act.

Note: Adapted from *Client Assistance Orientation Manual*, Sallie R. Rhodes, M. S., National Association of Protective and Advocacy Systems, 900 2nd St. N.E., Suite 211, Washington, DC 20006, under a grant from Rehabilitation Services Administration.

VII. Education

Vocational Education

Clora Mae Baker, Ph.D.
John S. Washburn, Ed.D.

The vocational education program is one of the most complex and misunderstood aspects of American education. It is distinguished from other educational programs in that it includes participation by students of all ages—elementary through adult. Vocational education is sometimes defined as a *process* of vocational development which prepares youth and adults for employment in occupations requiring less than a baccalaureate degree. Or, it may be defined as a *program* (e.g., agriculture, home economics, trades and industries, health, business/office occupations).

This chapter is intended to define and describe the vocational education program and clarify its role in preparing youth and adults for work for both educators and counselors alike. A summary will define changes anticipated in the future which will result from new federal legislative initiatives.

Purpose/Intent

Vocational education is one of several major systems in the U. S. which prepares people for work. The military, Job Training Partnership Act (JTPA), business and industry, apprenticeship, public school vocational education, and private vocational schools primarily emphasize preparation of individuals (at less than the baccalaureate level) for work (National Council on Employment Policy, 1982). Universities are the primary source of training for professions requiring advanced degrees. There are substantial student transfers among the various employment and training systems (e.g., JTPA funds may be used to purchase training from the vocational education system, the military may buy training from public education).

Vocational education has two broad purposes—preparation of youth and adults for work, or for further education to prepare for work. Most vocational education programs occur in high school, technical institute, and community college settings.

Vocational education programs can only be distinguished by the nature and level of preparation students receive for work, not by the age of the student. Students enrolled in vocational education courses in the public school have markedly different expectations. Many of the students will have repeated contact as adults with institutions that offer job training experience. Some students may enroll in one or two courses (e.g., keyboarding), while other students will concentrate on a sequence of courses to master job entry level skills (e.g., dental assistant, welding). There are vocational programs designed to prepare students for a particular occupation (e.g., nursing) or for a cluster of occupations (e.g., building trades). Other programs prepare students for job specific programs (e.g., clerk typist). Yet other programs are designed to prepare students for a particular job for a specific employer.

Generally, high school and adult-age students have the opportunity to participate in coursework in one of several clusters in agriculture, health, business, home economics, and the industrial areas. In those clusters, agricultural production (farming), general merchandising, nursing, child care, accounting, secretarial, electronics, auto mechanics, and drafting enroll the largest number of students.

Approximately two-fifths of the students who enroll in vocational education in the high schools are in courses which are not designed for particular jobs or occupations. These are courses designed to orient students to work (e.g., general business). Most of the students enrolled in vocational programs in community colleges are preparing for a particular job or occupation. Therefore, a vocational program may be very general in nature (e.g., general business), or very specific (e.g., training word processing operators).

Of all high school seniors who graduated in 1982, more than 90% took at least one vocational education course. However, after a series of educational reform reports, many states approved new requirements for high school graduation and enrollments in vocational education courses and other elective subjects such as music and art have declined.

The American Vocational Association (1990a) notes that across the United States there are approximately 26,000 institutions that teach vocational education to more than 16 million students at any one time. The vocational education system in the country graduates more than 2 million students each year.

History/Legislation

During the decades immediately after 1900, there was a major impetus for vocational education, with strong support from the business community. Industrialists focused on the need for highly skilled labor and alleged that the factory system had made the apprenticeship system obsolete. It had become difficult and economically inefficient to allow informal, on-the-job learning in modern factories.

Business leaders argued that better trained workers would be more satisfied with their jobs because of increased understanding and appreciation of their role in an industrial economy; that industrial accidents, absenteeism, and labor turnover would decrease; and that increased productivity would be the result of a satisfied, more stable work force. The political influence of the business community and the impact of its arguments was evidenced by the establishment of numerous study committees and advocacy groups. Ultimately, a report from the Commission on National Aid to Vocational Education led to the passage of the Smith-Hughes Act, which provided the first federal aid for vocational education (Barlow, 1967).

The Smith-Hughes Act of 1917 initiated the first program of federal grants-in-aid to promote vocational education below the collegiate level. Money was made available for teachers of agriculture, trade, home economics, and industrial subjects. Subsequent legislation added provisions for funding for health, business, and office occupations.

A major shift in the nature of vocational education legislation occurred in 1963. The Vocational Education Act of 1963 and subsequent legislation focused on service to students in contrast to prior legislation which provided for training personnel in a few selected occupational categories. The intent of Congress was to provide vocational education for all people and all occupations, except those which were identified as professional occupations requiring a baccalaureate or higher degree. Recently, the Congress passed new legislation for vocational education.

The Carl D. Perkins Vocational and Applied Technology Education Act of 1990 continues the focus on services to students, however, its purpose has been expanded. Resources are allocated to integrate more fully academic and occupational skills provided for students. Also, the Congress intends an economic development focus for new federal vocational education legislation. Vocational education is seen as a program to prepare America's work force in a more competitive, global economy (American Vocational Association [AVA], 1990b).

The 1990 Act continues to focus on the special needs of singles parents, displaced homemakers, single pregnant women, criminal offenders, disadvantaged, handicapped, and limited English proficient youth and adults. There are special programs for community-based organizations, consumer and homemaking education, career guidance and counseling, and business/labor/education partnerships, among others.

ADMINISTRATIVE STRUCTURE

In all 50 states, there is one state agency responsible for the administration of vocational education. The state agency might be the agency responsible for elementary and secondary education, the agency responsible for higher education, a separate board of vocational education, or some other entity. However, each state must have a sole state agency to distribute federal funds for vocational education available through the Carl D. Perkins Vocational and Applied Technology Education Act.

Vocational programs are financed largely by local funds with small amounts of federal funding. Some states also allocate funds for vocational programs. Federal and state funds available for vocational education are intended to pay for the excess costs of offering vocational education programs beyond those costs associated with a regular program (e.g., English, mathematics).

Vocational Education Programs

In the United States, Bottoms and Copa (1983) identified various types of institutions which offer vocational education programs. *High schools* will typically offer programs in home economics, business education, agriculture, industrial arts/technology education, or health occupations. Academic and vocational subjects are offered in the comprehensive high school.

Some school districts support *vocational high schools*. These are usually specialized schools where a majority of students are enrolled in vocational education subjects. Students in these schools will often receive academic coursework in the vocational high school.

The National Center for Research in Vocational Education (Mitchell & Russel, 1990) noted several of the vocational high schools which have received national attention. For example, the Chicago High School for Agricultural Sciences is a magnet school offering agricultural subjects not common in an urban environment. The Murry Bergtraum High School for Business Careers in New York City is recognized for networking with the business community and serves 2,500 students from New York City's five boroughs. The minority population constitutes 80% of the 2,400 student body at the John H. Francis Polytechnic High School in Sun Valley, California. This school serves students throughout the Los Angeles Unified School District.

In the 1960s, many states supported the development of *area vocational centers*. Some area vocational centers are designed to serve high school age youth. Other area vocational centers are designed to serve post-secondary age youth. Most secondary area vocational centers are shared-time facilities which provide vocational education to students from a number of high schools in a region. These students will normally receive their academic coursework in the regular high school and travel to the area vocational center two or three hours a day for vocational training. Similarly, post-secondary area vocational schools often provide instruction only for vocational education programs, not academic coursework.

Many states have *community colleges* which are two-year, degree granting institutions. Most of the community colleges provide general and vocational education programs. Many of the community colleges' associate degree programs will be designed so that students can transfer to colleges or universities. Other programs will be designed for students who wish to receive an associate of applied science or certificate in an occupational area.

Some states have *technical institutes* which are degree granting institutions offering (primarily) vocational education programs. Technical institutes normally focus on training to provide immediate job placement.

Some *four-year institutions* across the United States offer two-year programs. For example, Southern Illinois University at Carbondale offers extensive associate degree programs in the College of Technical Careers in a number of vocational education program areas (e.g., dental hygiene, electronics, office systems).

Finally, some states support *skill centers* which are somewhat different than other institutions described earlier. These are usually very specialized institutions that provide vocational education to economically disadvantaged students.

TYPES OF COURSE SEQUENCES

Each vocational education program offers a series of courses, designed in a logical learning sequence, for job entry or further education. Ideally, the school modifies course sequences based on community and student interest, labor market information, and the availability of resources. A program at the secondary level for a general office clerk occupation might include a course sequence as follows:

> *Ninth Grade—Orientation*
>> Orientation to General Business–one semester
>> Keyboarding I–one semester
> *Tenth Grade—Orientation*
>> Keyboarding II–one semester
>> Computers in Business–one semester
> *Eleventh Grade—Skill Preparation*
>> Accounting I–one semester
>> Office Equipment Applications or Word Processing–one semester
>> (or)
>> Machine Transcription–one semester
> *Twelfth Grade—Skill Preparation*
>> Office Procedures and/or Model Office–one year *or*
>> Cooperative Office Occupations–one year

It is important to note there are several patterns of participation for students enrolled in high school vocational education courses. While some students may enroll in a complete sequence of courses designed to prepare them for a career, other students may only take one or two courses in a vocational sequence. In high school, some youth are ready to take courses that will help them achieve well-defined career goals; others are not. Students completing a sequence of courses in a vocational area may choose to enter employment upon graduation from high school. Other students will continue their education at a post-secondary institution.

For example, at a local community college the student, or returning adult, may choose to pursue an associate degree in banking and finance. In addition to general education coursework, a typical banking and finance program might include the following occupational courses:

> *First Year—Fall Semester*
>   Accounting I
>   Business Mathematics
>   Principles of Banking
>   Business Seminar
>   Introduction to Business
> *First Year—Spring Semester*
>   Accounting II
>   Principles of Management
>   Money and Banking
> *Second Year—Fall Semester*
>   Economics
>   Bank Accounting
>   Data Base Management
>   Basic Programming
> *Second Year—Spring Semester*
>   Business Correspondence
>   Business Electives
>   Bank Marketing

Students enrolled in post-secondary banking and finance program might also be working part-time in a financial institution. It is not unusual for a graduate to enter a full-time position for a few years, then decide to continue his or her education at a university level. However, baccalaureate degree programs at the university level do not receive vocational education funding.

Ideally, programs are articulated from one educational level to the next. However, there is some unnecessary duplication of effort among vocational education providers. Students may not necessarily be guaranteed that all of their vocational training at one level will be considered at they progress to the next. A new federal legislative initiative titled *Tech-Prep* is addressing this problem by funding programs which link occupational preparation in grades 11-14. New Tech-Prep initiatives require the collaboration of secondary and post-secondary institutions.

COURSE DELIVERY

Vocational education courses are provided in a number of different ways. Many agencies share instructional responsibilities with other public and private agencies in the surrounding area. Sometimes, the school will provide experiences in cooperation with business, industry, or government. Listed below are examples of the different strategies which schools use to provide vocational education:

- *In-school vocational instruction*: classroom and laboratory experiences conducted within the school's existing facilities.

- *Cooperative agreements*: instructional responsibilities for a course(s) within a particular vocational program shared by schools of the same type. The area vocational center described previously is an example of this type of arrangement.
- *Contractual arrangements*: instructional responsibilities for contractual ventures shared by schools of different types. For example, a private cosmetology school might provide instruction for high school students.
- *Extended classroom*: community facilities utilized as extensions of specific programs. For example, a nursing home might be used as a site to provide instruction for nurse assistants.
- *Cooperative vocational education*: paid work experiences where students alternate study in school with on-the-job training.
- *Apprenticeship training*: vocational education programs which are offered for apprentices who are employed to learn skill trades (e.g., carpenters, plumbers).
- *Supervised occupational experience*: a cooperative effort on the part of the school and students' parents or guardians wherein vocational experiences are provided at home, school, or another suitable location under the supervision of an instructor. For example, an agriculture student might have a special summer project on the family farm.

ISSUES FOR THE FUTURE

Certainly, the vocational education program will change in the future. The new definition of vocational education in the Carl D. Perkins Vocational and Applied Technology Education Act notes that vocational education programs should focus on competency-based applied learning which contributes to an individual's academic knowledge, higher order reasoning and problem solving skills, work attitudes, general employability skills, as well as the occupational skills necessary for economic independence (American Vocational Association, 1990b).

The continued success of the vocational education program will require new curriculum, teacher retraining, outlays for new equipment, and expanded partnerships with the private sector. Continued student participation in traditional vocational offerings will have dilatory consequences on students' futures— unless they have access to the content of new technologies such areas as fiber optics, information processing, bio-technology, and electronics.

Changes in skill requirements for jobs must also be viewed in the context of significant demographic shifts in the work force. The Hudson Institute's (Johnston & Packer, 1987) *Workforce 2000* report notes that:

> The work force will grow slowly, becoming older, more female, and more disadvantaged. Only 15% of the new entrants to the labor force over the next 13 years will be native white males, compared to 47% in that category today. (p. xiii)

The vocational education program of the future must be sensitive to changes in work force patterns and characteristics of the work force such as age, ethnicity, and gender patterns among workers. Programs for adults needing training or retraining and for special populations should grow in number. Also, vocational education programs must continue to be sensitive to the intensive investment in new technology by U. S. business and industry. Many believe that the U. S. cannot be competitive in the global economy with large numbers of job/skill mismatches. Partnerships between the schools that offer vocational education and business, industry, and government will likely expand.

The vocational education program is only one of several major systems which prepare people for work. However, it is likely it will continue to serve as the prime system in the educational arena which assists youth and adults to prepare for work or further education in preparation for later employment.

References

American Vocational Association. (1990a). *Fact sheet: Vocational education today*. Arlington, VA: Author.

American Vocational Association. (1990b). *The AVA guide to the Carl D. Perkins Vocational Applied Technology Education Act of 1990*. Arlington, VA: Author.

Barlow, M. L. (1967). *History of industrial education in the United States*. Peoria, IL: Bennett.

Bottoms, G. L., & Copa, P. (1983, January). A perspective on vocational education today. *Phi Delta Kappan*, 348-354.

Johnston, W., & Packer, A. (1987). *Workforce 2000*. Indianapolis, IN: Hudson Institute.

Mitchell, V., & Russel, E. (1990). *Exemplary urban career-oriented secondary school programs*. Berkeley, CA: National Center for Research in Vocational Education.

National Council on Employment Policy. (1982). *A vocational education policy for the 1980's*. Washington, DC: National Council on Employment Policy.

Adult Education

Henry D. Wong, Rh.D.

Adult education in America is a complex, multifaceted phenomenon character-ized by divergent definitions, philosophies, settings, and providers. For the purpose of this chapter, adult education may broadly be defined as any systematic and purposeful effort by adults to elicit changes in knowledge, skills, attitudes, and/or values (Darkenwald & Merriam, 1982). More specifically, it has been defined as:

> ...instruction or services below the college level for adults [any person 16 years old or above] who do not have (1) the basic skills to enable them to function effectively in society; or (2) a certificate of graduation from a school providing secondary education (and who have not achieved an equivalent level of education). (Adult Education Act, 1984, p. 2366)

History/Legislation

HISTORY

Historically, adult education has its roots in the colonial period whereby young women and men could participate in boarding schools, dancing schools, grammar and evening schools, churches, apprenticeships, and home activities (Long, 1975). A wide range of potential topics were offered depending upon the provider. For example, boarding schools for young women provided reading, writing, arithmetic, embroidery, dancing, and music. Grammar and evening schools not only focused on the "three r's," but also on bookkeeping, architecture, and navigation (Long, 1975). Girls and boys could be apprenticed in such trades as bakers, barbers, tailors, seamstresses, blacksmiths, gunsmiths, painters, and many others. Of prime importance during the mid-1600s, was the home. Parents were expected to educate their children in some craft/trade, caring for the home, and/or to be literate and well-mannered. Parents neglecting this responsibility were threatened with the possibility of having their children removed from the home by *selectmen* whose tasks were overseeing parental instruction and examination of children (Jernigan, 1965).

Early evidence of the federal government's commitment to adult education was indicated when federal funds were expended in 1777 to instruct soldiers of the Continental Army in basic math, and again in 1867 with the establishment of the National Department of Education (now the U. S. Department of Education) (Taylor, 1983).

LEGISLATION/AUTHORITY

President Lyndon B. Johnson signed the Economic Opportunity Act of 1964 heralding a national commitment to adult basic education (Ellis, 1984). Its mandate provided literacy training to adults (age 18 and above) having difficulty reading and/or writing the English language posing substantial barriers to their ability to maintain or obtain employment, thereby inhibiting their participation as citizens.

Two years later, the passage of the Adult Education Act of 1966 transferred the adult basic education program from under to the Commissioner of Education. This bill expanded educational programs for adults who had not graduated from a secondary school. It also created the National Advisory Committee on Adult Basic Education whose purpose was to advise the Commissioner on adult educational policy, services, and funding (Ellis, 1984).

Since that time, there have been thirteen amendments to the Adult Education Act of 1966 representing incremental services and funds to the program (National Advisory Council on Adult Education Annual Report FY 1987). Only a few select highlights of this legislative history will be presented.

According to Ellis (1984) the Adult Education Act Amendments of 1970 redefined adults (age 16 and above) and provided additional secondary-level educational programs for those who had not completed high school. American Indians were targeted specifically under the amendments to the Adult Education Act of 1972 to receive basic literacy training (i.e., reading, writing, and arithmetic) for the purpose of improving their employment. With the passage of the 1974 Amendments signed by President Ford, adults who were institutionalized, elderly, and/or limited in their English-speaking ability were included to receive education. Additionally, agencies providing educational, recreational, and cultural services were eligible to receive federal funding under this legislation and a National Clearinghouse was established to collect and disseminate adult education information.

The 1978 Amendments to the Adult Education Act extended programs to immigrants, especially Indochinese, for the purpose of enhancing their English language. Adult educational programs could now be provided by "business, labor, libraries, colleges, and community organizations" (Ellis, 1984, p. 9).

Currently, the 1984 Amendments to the Adult Education Act encourage the private sector and volunteers to provide literacy skills rather than increasing federal funds. Private, for-profit agencies/institutions are allowed to deliver adult education. The definition of adult was broadened to include those beyond the "age of compulsory school attendance under state law" (Ellis, 1984, p. 10). Women, American Indians, and immigrants were specifically targeted to receive services. Additionally, under title VII of the Act, the establishment of bilingual, educational programs were mandated to facilitate equal educational opportunities for students with limited English proficiency at the preschool, elementary, secondary, and adult program levels. Primary emphasis was given to students who were not born in the United States, or who were American Indian or Alaskan, coming from environments where another language (other than English) had a substantial impact on their English proficiency (i.e., reading, writing, speaking, and/or comprehension).

Finally, with the enactment of the Stewart B. McKinney Homeless Assistance Act in July of 1987, the Adult Education Act was amended to extend literacy and basic skills remediation to homeless adults and homeless children.

FUNDING

Federal funding levels under the Economic Opportunity Act of 1964 totaled over $18 million and served 37,991 people (Taylor, 1983). There have been steady and moderate increases since that time, with less federal involvement under the Reagan administration. For example, in 1981, federal expenditures were $100 million serving over 2 million adults. In 1988 and 1989, funding totaled just over $105 and $115 million respectively, with services to over 3 million people (National Advisory Council on Adult Education Annual Report FY 1987). Currently, the federal/state funding match ratio is 9:1 (National Advisory Council on Adult Education Annual Report FY 1987).

PERSONNEL

The diversity of adult educational needs manifests itself in a myriad of providers and settings. Settings in which adult education may occur include "private industry, professional associations, trade unions, government service, federal manpower programs, military services, agricultural extension, city recreation departments, community organizations, churches and synagogues, free universities, and parks and forests" (Long, 1987, p. 13). Additionally, the home is another setting in which self-directed learning occurs (Swicegood, 1980). Correctional institutions (federal and state) provide other avenues for adult learning (Goldin & Thomas, 1984).

Teachers, mentors, facilitators, and counselors are just a few of the descriptions ascribed to personnel in this field (Darkenwald & Merriam, 1982). Although the majority of teachers of adults are volunteers, others hold such occupational titles as social worker, recreational specialist, clergy, vocational education teacher, public relations specialist, kindergarten and elementary school teacher, librarian, secondary school teacher, administrator (U. S. Dept. of Labor, 1990), as well as various specialists in government, industry, and business (Darkenwald & Merriam, 1982).

TRAINING

Due to the diverse nature of educational settings, providers, and adult needs, no clear distinct training requirements can be identified as characteristic of a teacher of adults. Rather, a majority of teachers of adults receive little formal education, with few possessing teaching licenses. They are primarily employed by noneducational agencies and are selected based upon their subject matter expertise (Darkenwald & Merriam, 1982).

Generally, training requirements vary by subject matter and by state (U. S. Department of Labor, 1990). These requirements may include (a) work experience; (b) certificates and/or licenses; (c) bachelor's, master's, or doctoral degrees; (d) completion of continuing education programs; (e) in-service training; and/or (f) subject matter expertise without credentials (Darkenwald & Merriam, 1982; U. S. Department of Labor, 1990).

Purpose/Intent

RATIONALE

Brookfield (1985) suggests that the purpose of adult education is to empower adults to control their lives and interpersonal relationships within society, as well as enhance self-worth and self-actualization. Long (1987) indicates five broad purposes of adult education include:

Americanization: cultural assimilation and citizen development
Application: enhancement of occupational skills and/or employability
Personal enlightenment
Social improvement: health, personality, arts, and literature
Literacy

The aims and objectives of this field therefore reflect national socioeconomic and political goals among diverse groups. Consequently, adult education's mission is to provide social/educational equal opportunity, an adequate supply and competent human resources for work, the development of citizenship, and national defense needs (Long, 1987).

Many philosophical orientations characterize adult education contingent upon the provider and setting. Such philosophies have included, but are not limited to:

Perennialism: past knowledge over the centuries is important focusing on activities disciplining the mind (e.g., memorization, reading, writing);
Essentialism: preservation and socialization of culture for future generations emphasizing historical and contemporary knowledge (e.g., history, the classics, math, natural sciences);
Progressivism: all things are relative emphasizing the value of human experience and problem solving;
Reconstructionism: focuses on the relativity of truths/consequences and value of the scientific method;

Existentialism: individual self-fulfillment and value of autonomy through education (Long, 1987).

Darkenwald and Merriam (1982) suggest six philosophies prevalent in America today influencing adult education (i.e., liberal, progressivism, humanistic, behaviorism, radicalism, and philosophical analysis). Liberalism emphasizes broad-based knowledge/theory, content of learning, and impact upon logical reasoning and rational behavior. Humanism focuses on self-directed learning, freedom, and independence. Behaviorism emphasizes behavioral objectives and controlled learning activity, whereas radicalism centers on the use of knowledge for power and socio/political/economic change. Philosophical analysis addresses procedures of inquiry about terms, concepts, and values (Long, 1987).

Lastly, the corporate or certification philosophy is newly emerging with utility as an underlying principle. This philosophy values certificates, activities, and skills useful in employment. It is quite popular among business, industry, government, and professional associations for the purpose of meeting policy and human resource needs (Long, 1987).

UTILIZATION CRITERIA

The specific criteria used in the determination of which adults receive education varies considerably based upon public policy, setting, providers, and individualized needs of adults. Numerous factors exist influencing adult educational participation. A survey of 1,893 adults conducted by the National Center for Education Statistics indicated that over one-half of all adults state the primary reason for their participation in educational pursuits is work related (Darkenwald & Merriam, 1982). The remaining sample cited other reasons as personal/family interests, gaining general information, and social/recreational interests. Valentine and Darkenwald (1990) suggest five deterrents to participation include those deterred by personal reasons (e.g., child care, health, disability, location), those deterred by lack of confidence, costs, those disinterested in organized education, and those disinterested in course offerings.

Another explanation is based on the Psychosocial Interaction Model (Darkenwald & Merriam, 1982). According to this model, variables influencing participation can be divided into pre-adulthood and adulthood. Pre-adulthood variables include intelligence, socioeconomic status, values, and family characteristics. Adulthood variables include socioeconomic status, social participation in community activities, occupation, and lifestyle preferences. Generally, the probability of adult participation is lowest for those persons at the lower levels of socioeconomic status and highest for those at the upper levels.

SPECIAL CASE MANAGEMENT NEEDS

Andragogy, the art and science of empowering adults to learn, is a popular concept in adult education. The assumptions of this concept are that adults (a) become more self-directed and less dependent as their self-concept matures, (b) draw upon their experiences for learning, (c) readiness to learn is tied to their social roles, and (d) wish to apply knowledge in a practical, immediate way with a focus on solving problems (Long, 1987, p. 174).

Consequently, the learning environment must be conducive to conditions fostering comfort, trusting and respectful relationships, free expression, and opportunities whereby learners perceive the goals of learning as their own through participating actively (Knowles, 1970).

Additionally, schools, colleges, universities, and other programs receiving federal funds are sensitive to the needs of personnel and the adult learner through the Rehabilitation Act of 1973 Sections 502-504. For persons with disabilities, Section 502 mandates the accessibility of programs and buildings, whereas Section 503 prohibits discrimination and advocates affirmative action in the employment setting. Section 504 mandates equal opportunities for such persons to participate in programs/activities receiving federal funds which has a major impact on educational settings.

Under the Adult Education Act of 1984 specially targeted groups (e.g., women, American Indians, Alaskans, elderly, immigrants, other adults with literacy deficits) could obtain educational services to assist them in retaining or acquiring work and/or meet adult responsibilities of citizenship.

Generally, participants of adult education in contrast to nonparticipants are young, Caucasian, better educated, of higher socioeconomic status, employed full-time in human services, living in the suburbs and western states, and receiving veterans' benefits (Darkenwald & Merriam, 1982). Additionally, of those 26 million participating in adult education based upon the 1980 Census, 72% were Caucasian, 14% were Black, 11% were Hispanic, 1% were Asian, and 1% were Native American. Analyzing this sample by age reveals that 51% were 60 years old and above, 23% were between the ages of 45-59, 18% were between the ages of 25-44, and 8% were 16-24 years old (National Advisory Council, 1987). Between the years 1985-1986, 1.6 million women and 1.4 million men received one or more formal adult education courses. Other estimates of participation range from 21-50 million people depending on the definitions one uses for adult education and the settings in which it occurs (Long, 1987).

Client Services

DESCRIPTION OF SERVICES

The hallmark of adult education is its connection to living and learning for self-actualization. Its emphasis is on practical application to daily tasks. According to Darkenwald & Merriam (1982) five general categories comprise the field in descending order: (a) work related, (b) general and academic, (c) social life/recreation, (d) personal/family life, and (e) community life.

Long (1987) indicates that over 37 million adult education courses were provided in 1981. Almost one-half of these courses involved business (23%), health care/education (14%), and engineering (10%). Business courses were most popular for men and women; a majority of men prefer engineering, whereas women prefer health-related courses. The remaining courses reveal more participation by women with exceptions in agriculture and social science. Men participate primarily for reasons of certification/licensure, whereas women cite their interests are meeting new people, learning about culture, and spiritual improvement. Overall, 60% of adult education courses were taken for work-related purposes and the rest for personal/social reasons.

Of growing interest and participation are adults who are elderly (age 55 and above) (Long, 1987). Those aged 60-64 primarily took vocational and safety related courses. Civic, public service, and courses in religion were taken by adults age 70 and above.

Adults with disabilities who are homebound or hospitalized are finding greater opportunities to learn through the use of special telephone/video equipment transmitting course information on job skills, survival skills, basic literacy, and the arts (Shworles & Wang, 1980). McCollum (1980) indicates that adults in correctional settings are now able to access courses for postsecondary education, social skills, physical education, the arts, and recreational activities in contrast to earlier times when only basic literacy and General Educational Degree courses were available.

TYPICAL REFERRAL QUESTIONS

Professionals and other providers of human services are often instrumental in providing adult educational opportunities facilitating self-actualization, employability, literacy, and citizenship. Considerations of empowerment and the mandates under public policy may suggest the following referral questions:

What professionals and diagnostic tools are available in the community for the purpose of identifying strengths of the adult and her or his deficits (e.g., medical, psychological, vocational, educational, transportation) impacting upon access to adult education?

Human-service providers should be cognizant of the community resources available to assist adults in their quest for self-actualization. First, some understanding of various diagnostic evaluations/tools can facilitate the provider's understanding of the adult's needs across a wide range of areas previously mentioned. Second, depending on one's role, organizational mission and goals, and available resources, service providers may be able to refer, coordinate services, or cover the costs, equipment needs, and transportation needs related to access of educational programs. Third, identifying, establishing, and maintaining relationships with educational settings within the community and other teachers of adults should enhance the human-service provider's ability to keep the pulse of local conditions.

How can I identify adults who might pursue additional education?

Human-service providers may consider a marketing strategy that outreaches to adults in the community, encouraging their referral and involvement in available educational settings. Secondly, such a strategy could include the collaboration and involvement of those settings and teachers of adults to consider methods of promotion, presentation of services, determining accessible places, especially for adults with transportation barriers, and identification of costs (if any) for adults to receive services.

References

Adult Education Act of 1984. (1984). Public Law 98-511, 98 Stat. 2366. Washington, DC: U. S. Congress.

Brookfield, S. (1985). A critical definition of adult education. *Adult Education Quarterly, 36*(1), 44-49.

Darkenwald, G., & Merriam, S. B. (1982). *Adult education: Foundations of practice.* New York: Harper & Row.

Ellis, J. (1984). *A history and analysis of the Adult Education Act, 1964-1984.* (CE No. 040 193). Washington, DC: U. S. Department of Education. (ERIC Document Reproduction Service No. ED 252 658)

Goldin, C., & Thomas, J. (1984). Adult education in correctional settings: Symbol or substance. *Adult Education Quarterly, 34*(3), 123-134.

Jernigan, M. W. (1965). *Laboring and dependent classes in colonial America, 1607-1783.* New York: Frederick Unger.

Knowles, M. (1970). *The modern practice of adult education: Andragogy versus pedagogy.* New York: Association Press.

Long, H. B. (1975). The education of girls and women in colonial America. *Journal of Research and Development in Education, 8*(4), 66-82.

Long, H. B. (1987). *New perspectives on the education of adults in the United States.* New York: Nichols.

McCollum, S. G. (1980). Adult education in corrections. In E. J. Boone, R. W. Shearon, & E. E. White and Associates (Eds.), *Serving personal and community needs through adult education* (pp. 250-258). San Francisco: Jossey-Bass.

National Advisory Council on Adult Education Annual Report FY 1987. (CE No. 050 188). Washington, DC: Author. (ERIC Document Reproduction Service No. ED 295 004).

Rehabilitation Act of 1973, Public Law 93-112, 87 Stat. 335. Washington, DC: U. S. Congress.

Shworles, T. R., & Wang, P. H. (1980). Education for handicapped adults. In E. J. Boone, R. W. Shearon, & E. E. White and Associates (Eds.), *Serving personal and community needs through adult education* (pp. 155-159). San Francisco: Jossey-Bass.

Stewart B. McKinney Homeless Assistance Act of 1987. Public Law 100-77, 101 Stat. 482. Washington, DC: U. S. Congress.

Swicegood, M. L. (1980). Adult education for home and family life. In E. J. Boone, R. W. Shearon, & E. E. White and Associates (Eds.), *Serving personal and community needs through adult education* (pp. 250-258). San Francisco: Jossey-Bass.

Taylor, P. G. (1983). The Adult Education Act: Issues and perspectives on reauthorization. *Lifelong Learning, 7*(1), 10-11, 26-27.

U. S. Department of Labor. (1990). *Occupational outlook handbook* (1990-1991 ed.) Indianapolis: JIST Works.

Valentine, T., & Darkenwald, G. (1990). Deterrents to participation in adult education: Profiles of potential learners. *Adult Education Quarterly, 41*(1), 29-42.

Special Education

Norma J. Ewing, Ph.D.
Debra A. Harley, M.A., C.R.C.

The meaning and significance of *special education* is often unclear to persons who have not formally studied or been actively involved in the area for some reason (e.g., consumer, parent, advocate). Much of the ambiguity and confusion that exists is created by semantic and philosophical differentials surrounding a plethora of terminology used to communicate in the field. In addition to the perplexing nomenclature, constant change (e.g., labels, delivery systems, public policy, legislation) occurring in the discipline causes continuous confusion. The interaction of these potent factors works against development of an understanding of special education as a discipline or practice.

After many years of commitment and reflection in the field, many professionals experience *information anxiety*. This trepidation is caused by the struggle to stay abreast of emerging information and a conscious effort to integrate "sifted" information into the existing information bank. In the process, emotions often run rampant as professional exchange occurs in lecture halls, seminars, conferences, and academic outlets (e.g., professional journals). Receptivity to change, an open mind, and critical analysis of new information are the primary antidotes for reconciling continuous consternation over matters associated with the area.

The Meaning and Scope of Special Education

A functional understanding of the meaning and scope of special education can be achieved through assimilation of concepts related to key terminology. The integration of important concepts provides the basis for a theoretical, as well as practical, understanding of what can be a complex and puzzling education enigma. A cursory understanding is too often the end result.

The phrase *special education* is sometimes used to refer to an area of specialization in the education profession. Most frequently it is used to connote the existence of an activity or a specific program option within the broad spectrum

of the overall educational system. Meyen and Skrtic (1988) extend the meaning
by including functionality (i.e., who receives it and what it is they receive) in their
definition. They define special education as:

> ...a broad term covering programs and services for children who
> deviate physically, mentally, or emotionally from the normal to an
> extent that they require unique learning experiences, techniques,
> or materials in order to be maintained in the regular classroom,
> or specialized classes and programs if the problems are more
> severe. (p. 592-93)

Another definition frequently referenced in the literature is credited to the United
States Office of Education (USOE) (1977). That definition indicates special
education is:

> ...specially designed instruction, at no cost to the parent, to meet
> the unique needs of a handicapped child, including classroom
> instruction, instruction in physical education, home instruction,
> and instruction in hospitals and institutions. (p. 42478)

The USOE definition accentuates the breadth of the delivery system for special
instruction and indicates it is "free" to parents. Concepts inherent in any definition
of special education have reference to persons from birth through age 21, as
established by federal law. This concept translates into an educational practice in
which persons with a disability are referred to as "aged out," meaning at age 22
they are no longer eligible for special education services. Administrative and direct
service responsibilities are subsequently shifted to rehabilitation or other social
service agencies. Ideally, prior to the shift, the special education system and
rehabilitation agency have collaborated and cooperated in making the transition
smooth and successful.

The isolated definitions in the above text provide a rather perfunctory
understanding of special education. A clear, functional understanding of the
meaning of special education is hardly possible without integration of the meaning
of other key terms. Related terminology used today include "exceptional children,"
"handicapped," and "children or persons with disabilities." These terms provide
additional substance for understanding special education as a discipline, and
appends a utilitarian perspective to the profession. All three are common terms
that allude to a wide range of individuals who do not meet expectancy in term of
"normal" growth and development.

Increased human rights advocacy, political forces, elevated respect for dignity
of persons with a disability, and carefully considered language incorporated in
federal and state legislation repudiate use of the terms synonymously. Over the
past few decades, society has made a conscious effort to eliminate the use of terms
that promote prejudice, stereotyping, discrimination, and exclusion of persons who
require special provisions to develop or function at their maximum level. The
search for more acceptable language to classify or identify persons has meant
replacing commonly used terms with other words that communicate a more
positive message, and indicates advancement in the attitude of society. This
positive humanistic force has encouraged society to discontinue or de-emphasize

terminology that perpetuates negative connotations and promotes a disposition known as *handicappism*. Handicappism is manifested as a set of ideas, assumptions, and practices that promote different and unequal treatment of people because of visible or presumed physical, mental, and behavioral differences (Meyen & Skrtic, 1988). Both laypersons and professionals apply labels and stereotypes to persons with disabilities that negatively affect the way these persons are viewed and treated (Yoshida, Wasilewski, & Friedman, 1990).

Historically, the term *exceptional* has a long history of use in the field. The International Council for the Education of Exceptional Children (CEC), the major parent professional organization, was founded in 1922 and since its inception has maintained the term *exceptional* as an important component in the title. More than likely, the term was used because of the inclusive accuracy in meaning. The range of individual differences encompassed in the conceptual framework of the term included persons that represent both the upper and lower limits of the behavioral or intellectual continuum. The range included the gifted at upper limits and the mentally retarded at the lower limits. Even today, the term conveys more positive connotations than negative perceptions associated with the terms *handicapped* or *disabled*. However, use of *exceptional* does result in some confusion outside the field, as many persons tend to interpret the term as applicable only to the gifted.

The term *handicapped* is restrictive in meaning and conveys negative messages. It is difficult to communicate using the term without being pejorative. The word literally means "cap in hand" and originates from a time when the disabled begged in the streets in order to survive (Avoiding Handicappist Stereotypes, 1977). The word is used to refer to persons who are perceived as impaired or lacking in capability. Until recently, *handicapped* was the sanctioned term used by the federal government, as illustrated in the landmark legislation, Education for All Handicapped Children Act of 1975 (EHA) and Amendments of the Education of the Handicapped Act, 1986. However, in October 1990, EHA was renamed the Individual with Disabilities Education Act (IDEA). This change indicates a shift in language for the federal government. In IDEA the phrase "children with disabilities" was substituted for the phrase "handicapped children" (U. S. Congress, 1990). In both instances the phrases are used prior to the delineation of categorical labels and definitions that establish who is eligible for special education.

Although many persons still use the terms *handicapped* and *disabled* synonymously, an increasing number of persons have emphasized the past few years that *disability* is a matter of objective fact; whereas, the term handicapped embodies an attitudinal interpretation of the effect of an actual or perceived status, as viewed by self or others. In this way of thinking, a disability may become a handicap primarily as a function of how people think about it (Sage & Burrello, 1986) and subsequently, inadvertently becomes a "self-fulfilling prophecy" without conscious intent.

U. S. Office of Education, through regulations to implement EHA in 1977, set forth terms/labels and definitions for use in labeling children handicapped (now referred to as *children with disabilities*) and declaring them eligible for special education. Those terms/labels are: deaf, deaf-blind, hard of hearing, mentally retarded, multihandicapped, orthopedically impaired, other health impaired, specific learning disability, speech impaired, and visually impaired. Autism and traumatic brain injury were added as labels in the 1990 EHA amendments (National Association of State Directors of Special Education, 1990). Individuals from birth through age 21, who exhibit behaviors that resulted in being classified in any of the above categories are eligible for special education services.

LEGISLATION/AUTHORITY

Federal and state legislation has exerted tremendous influence on delivery of special education services. The history of legislation to provide services for persons with a handicap or disability dates back more than a century and a half. Prior to 1950, the laws were primarily aimed at providing institutional care or rehabilitative services. In the 1950s, the spotlight on legislation began to change with emphasis on research and training, vocational education, assessment, and special education services became a major focus (Ysseldyke & Algozzine, 1990). Then, in the mid-1970s, a major revolution occurred in the field, resulting in changes that promoted significant steps forward for a technological society. During this decade, many of the landmark legal cases on the right to education for the handicapped were considered in the courts and established precedent on which to base important state and federal legislation. The decade of 1990 is being referred to as the decade of full implementation.

In 1971, the Pennsylvania Association for Retarded Citizens (PARC) filed a class-action suit on behalf of retarded children who were excluded from public education on the basis of intellectual deficiency (*PARC v. Commonwealth of Pennsylvania*, 1971). The court ordered Pennsylvania schools to provide a free public education to all mentally retarded children, ages six to 21 commensurate with their individual learning needs.

In 1972, the case of *Mills v. District of Columbia* expanded the PARC decision to include all handicapped children. The District of Columbia schools were ordered by the court to provide a free and appropriate education to every school-age, handicapped child. The court also ordered alternate educational services be made available when regular public school assignments were not appropriate. These two court cases, PARC and Mills, established the right of handicapped children to an education, and served as major catalysts for several court cases and pieces of legislation that have continued to provide for improved services for children with a disability.

NATIONAL LAW MANDATES EDUCATION
OF CHILDREN WITH A DISABILITY

Current practices in special education are driven essentially by specific state and federal laws that mandate services for individuals with a disability. In November, 1975, the United States Congress passed the Education of All Handicapped Children Act. This piece of legislation capitalized on prior outcomes of court cases and state and federal legislation to generate a national law with broad reaching effect. The law was "passed in perpetuity" and by enormous margins (404 to 7 in the House; 87 to 7 in the Senate) and can be rescinded only by an act of Congress (Cartwright, Cartwright, & Ward, 1989). It mandates a free, appropriate public education for handicapped students between the ages of three and 21. Major components of the law are:

- Individualized education program (IEP);
- Nondiscriminatory and multidisciplinary assessment;
- Education in the least restrictive environment; and
- Rights of children with handicaps and their parents (due process).

The law was a blueprint for educational reform for students with a disability. Major provisions in the law targeted past educational practices that were blatantly unfair, discriminatory, and resulted in undue, lasting, harmful effects. Nondiscriminatory and multidisciplinary assessment distinctly related to determining eligibility or classifying children for special education. There was a need to reduce problems inherent in deciding who should receive special education. The indisputable, disproportionate representation of minorities in special education was a factor considered when including the assessment provisions. The least restrictive environment and individual education provisions were also aimed at elimination of practices that were unfair and discriminatory treatment. Students could no longer be labeled, "silently" barred from public school programs, or segregated in isolated classrooms apart from their peers without appropriate reason or justification.

AMENDMENTS TO THE EDUCATION OF THE HANDICAPPED ACT

The Education of the Handicapped Act Amendments of 1986 extended all rights and protection of P. L. 94-142 to preschoolers with handicaps. It mandated a free and appropriate education for all handicapped children ages three through five, and established a new early intervention program for infants and toddlers, birth through two years of age. Through the amendment, Congress also established a new state grant program for infants and toddlers with handicaps. This provision does not mandate states must provide services to all infants and toddlers who are developmentally delayed, but it does establish strong financial incentives for state participation. However, for years, a handful of states have mandated special education from birth. Others still delay service until school age, but most are somewhere in between ("Four States Respond," 1990).

One major difference between requirements of the original law and its amendments is that states are not required to report preschool children by handicap labels or categories. Students are not identified by such categorical labels as learning disabled, mentally retarded, and behavior disordered. They are referred to primarily as *at-risk* or *developmentally delayed* children.

INDIVIDUALS WITH DISABILITIES EDUCATION ACT

Recent reauthorization of the Education of the Handicapped Act (EHA), referred to as Education of the Handicapped Act Amendments of 1990, renamed EHA as Individuals With Disabilities Education Act (IDEA). There are several major changes in the Act resulting from amendments to EHA. One important message the federal government communicates is a change in the broad encompassing term used to refer to persons eligible for special education services. As reported in the *Federal Register*, (September 25, 1990) the secretary (Secretary of Education) has determined that it is more appropriate to use the term *children with disabilities* in place of *handicapped children*. The term *children with disabilities* has the same meaning as *handicapped children* which is defined in section 602 of the Education of the Handicapped Act (EHA).

Some other major changes in the reauthorization of the EHA are: (a) added two new categories of disabilities: autism and traumatic brain injury; (b) added rehabilitation counseling and social work services to the definition of related services; (c) strengthened transition services; (d) added a new program to serve severely emotionally disturbed children; (e) required the Secretary of Education to solicit public comments regarding the appropriate components of an operational definition for the term *attention deficit disorder* (ADD); and (f) directed new special education grants to historically black colleges and universities (HBCUs) to support an increase in the number of minority special education teachers. These zealous changes indicate a continued strong commitment and firm belief that persons with a disability are entitled to an appropriate education, not as a charity, but as fair treatment.

INCREASE IN POPULATION SERVED IN SPECIAL EDUCATION

It is widely known that the number of students receiving special education has continued to increase in recent years. The Twelfth Annual Report to Congress on the Implementation of the Education of the Handicapped Act (U. S. Department of Education, 1990) indicates that during the 1988-89 school year, 4,587,370 children from birth through age 21 were served under Part B of the Education of the Handicapped Act (EHA) and Chapter 1 of the Elementary and Secondary Education Act, State-Operated Programs (ESEA/SOP). This represents an increase of 2.1% over the number of handicapped children served in 1987-88, the largest increase since 1980-81.

According to the Twelfth Annual Report to Congress (U. S. Department of Education, 1990), the vast majority of the children served (87%) were between six and 17 years of age. Four types of handicaps account for the vast majority (94%) of children served in special education programs in 1988-89; learning disabled (48%), speech impaired (23%), mentally retarded (14%), and emotionally disturbed (9%). These proportions have changed over the past decade. The percentage of learning disabled served has increased, while speech impaired and mentally retarded have declined. Growth in the number of poor and culturally and linguistically different children in our schools, of which a disproportionate number are placed in special education, have likely had some direct impact on the overall increase in the number of students served in special education. Provisions in EHA mandating nondiscriminatory testing and multidisciplinary assessment coupled with an increase in awareness of the undisputable evidence of over representation of minorities classified as mentally retarded (Baca & Chinn, 1982; Mercer, 1973) are likely reasons for the decrease in the number of minorities labeled mentally retarded and speech impaired.

The epidemic of "drug babies" and children with Acquired Immune Deficiency Syndrome (AIDS) is expected to increase the number of students manifesting physical and mental impairments over the next generation. These two overwhelming social problems are ultimate challenges that many believe are certain to produce an onerous proportion of school children with impairments. Evidence of the significant responsibility educators, physicians, and other related service personnel will assume in serving these students is mounting and frustrating because so much is unknown about the effects of these conditions and what educators will be faced with in the classroom.

Nationally, about 10% of new babies have been exposed prenatally to maternal substance abuse. In certain inner-city hospitals, as many as 60% of babies are born to drug abusers ("Drug-exposed Babies," 1990). A growing number of educators are concerned about the explosion of drug-exposed babies, many of whom are certain to require special education services. According to Greer (1990), these "drug babies" will not only exhibit *post-drug impairment syndrome* (e.g., poor abstract reasoning and memory, poor judgment, inability to concentrate, inability to deal with stress, frequent tantrums, wide variety of behavior disorders, violent acting out) but other critical impairments as well. At birth, many crack addicted babies have strokes and seizures, and are born with small heads, missing bowels, and malformed genitals, as well as yet to be determined birth defects. These children are likely to experience the same dysphoria and thought and mood disorders as a recovering abuser (Greer, 1990). Educators, parents, and advocacy persons must begin to plan now on the most feasible way to deliver a "free, appropriate public education" for these children with complex behavioral manifestations that are not understood.

There is mounting evidence that children with AIDS will be entering the special education delivery system in an increasing number in the not-too-distant future. These students have also become a growing concern to educators, particularly with the inclusionary and due process provisions inherent in Public Law 94-142 and Public Law 99-457. Educators have moved beyond the issue of whether the children should be excluded from school, to concern for the effect of the disease on the neurological development of children and impact on learning. Due to the erratic course of neurological deterioration, these children will present a definite challenge for special education professionals (Byers, 1989). Given the numerous complex problems (e.g., increasing number, neurological impairments, lack of sufficient educational and medical research, negative attitudes) associated with these children, special education strategy awaits further research. Special educational services must be guided by careful inquiry that will provide direction for effective classroom instruction and practices.

Service Delivery System

Students with disabilities are educated in a variety of settings. One major provision of the Education for Handicapped Children Act requires children with a disability receive their education with "normal" peers, to the maximum extent possible. This practice is referred to as placing students with a disability in the *least restrictive environment* (LRE). LRE is a setting that is, as much as possible, like that of students in the "mainstream" or "normal" school environment. The placement should not have negative effect on learning and development of the student with a disability. To achieve this legal directive, school systems make available educational program options ranging from regular classroom placement with support services (e.g., consultant, itinerant teacher) to homebound and hospital programs. The range of educational program options are regular class placement, resource room placement, segregated class placement, separate special school placement (i.e., residential facility), and homebound or hospital instructional program. Depending on the severity of the disability, the most appropriate program option is provided for each student based on a multidisciplinary team decision aimed at making a placement determination that retains the student in the LRE. Inherent in this practice, is the premise that all children with a disability have the legal right to learn in an environment consistent with their intellectual, physical, and emotional needs.

Some interesting data are available regarding program options serving children with a disability. In 1987-88, 93% of students age three through 21 with a disability received services in regular school buildings (regular classes, resource rooms, or separate classes). About 30% were served in regular class placements, 38% were served in resource rooms, and 25% were served in separate classrooms (U. S. Department of Education, 1990). These data indicate that, indeed, a range of program options is being used to provide service for students with a disability.

When students with a disability remain in the regular classroom, regular teachers assume responsibility for educating the students. Many regular classroom teachers assume total responsibility for selecting materials or adapting instruction to meet the needs of the students. Some plan instruction or teach the students with the help of instructional consultants or itinerant teachers who provide assistance in the regular classroom. This delivery system option is commonly referred to as a *stay put* program option, in which students receive special education services without being removed from the regular classroom. Ysseldyke and Algozzine (1990) identify six basic types of stay put programs, they are:

- Using special educators in the regular classroom;
- Team teaching;
- Using staff support teams or intervention assistance teams;
- Using special educators as instructional consultants;
- Peer networks; and
- Using special education assistants.

When students with a disability require more assistance than can be provided in the regular classroom, they receive more intensified, specialized, direct instruction in a resource room. This option in the program delivery system removes students from the regular classroom and is referred to as *pull out* programs. Instruction in a resource room is under the direction of a certified special education teacher. The amount of time a student spends in a pull out setting varies according to student need. The time can range from a few minutes a day to several hours a day. The instruction can be supplemental, remedial, or compensatory. In a resource room, a student receives necessary assistance to assure achievement in classes with regular education peers.

Students who require more intensive instruction than that provided in a resource room are placed in self-contained classrooms. Such settings are within regular school buildings, but students are segregated from their normal peers for more than 50% of the school day. Such classrooms primarily serve students with moderate and severe disabilities. The students spend the majority of the school day receiving instruction in a separate class, but participate in regular classroom activities to the maximum extent possible. Provisions are made for the students to be mainstreamed or integrated with regular education peers for nonacademic subject areas (e.g., art, music, physical education) and some social functions (e.g., recess, lunch hour, athletic events).

Some students, because of the severity of their disability, are unable to attend a public school or school system program and must receive services through special day schools, residential schools, or home- or hospital-based program. In such settings, appropriate staff, facilities, and program opportunities are provided to meet the unique needs of the students.

Special Education and Rehabilitation

Because of the population the two disciplines target or serve, special education and rehabilitation are indisputably related. Conversely, the two disciplines are often viewed in a subliminal manner as separate or detached by many educators, rehabilitation practitioners, consumers, and advocates. The distinction has been sustained through definitions that refer to separate roles without pointing out similarity or compatibility. Rehabilitation has been defined in terms of *re-education* and special education in terms of *education* (Whitehouse, 1953). The distinction routinely conveyed is that rehabilitation implies "a readaptation process" and special education "a learning process" (Bitter, 1979). Viewing the two areas as separate, limits the potential scope and magnitude of service provisions to persons with a disability and impedes service and research advancement in both fields.

The two fields are connected through several linkages. The links are based on the common responsibility of providing services to persons with a disability. Persons with a disability are of primary interest to both fields. A major difference exists in terms of roles, responsibilities, and service provisions based primarily on the age of the target group. This difference is somewhat artificial at the upper age limits for special education and the lower age limits for rehabilitation. The transition state between special education and rehabilitation allows many persons with a disability to "fall between the cracks" and languish in a suspended state of despair because artificial barriers prohibit appropriate interagency collaboration and service provisions.

Special education and rehabilitation are also linked through a common goal of maximizing the abilities of persons with disabilities in the least restrictive environment. In order to facilitate maximum functioning in the least restrictive environment, three factors must be considered: (a) physical capacity, (b) intellectual functioning, and (c) acquired vocational, social, and economic levels and skill acquisition potential (Rubin & Roessler, 1983).

Also, a relationship between the two disciplines is evident in cooperative vocational training programs that have existed in the public schools since the 1950s (Bitter, 1979). The program commonly referred to at the high school level as "co-op program" was designed to integrate rehabilitation services with school programs for students with a disability while they were still enrolled in school. The intent of this joint effort was to provide students with relevant vocational materials within the secondary school curriculum and reduce the dropout rate of special education students. The transition of students with disabilities from high school to successful adult functioning is a national goal, and supported through the U. S. Department of Education. This focal point requires interagency agreement and collaboration of both fields, as well as other human service areas. Elrod (1987) pointed out that this alliance is a necessary ingredient for special needs students who need support to assist them in gaining access and successfully acquiring skills for competitive employment and independent living in the adult life cycle.

Special education and rehabilitation share the individualized approach to service delivery. A major provision in special education legislation is the Individual Education Plan (IEP) which is an educational plan tailored to an individual student's needs and is required by law. Rehabilitation requires an Individual Written Rehabilitation Program (IWRP) which is a detailed plan of objectives, goals, and services that will move the individual from dependency to employment. The IEP and IWRP require the consumer's goals and objectives be individualized to fit the student or client's needs, and that the goals and objectives be validated by appropriate assessment. Both individual plans move the consumer from a passive role to an active role in the service planning process. Through this mode, both special education and rehabilitation have become more consumer centered rather than teacher or counselor centered.

Lastly, the two disciplines are linked through major pieces of legislation with common goals. The Vocational Rehabilitation Act of 1973, section 504, was a precursor to the Education for All Handicapped Children Act of 1975. Section 504 clearly articulated the message that individuals with disabilities cannot be excluded from participation in, denied benefits of, or subjected to discrimination under, any program or activity receiving federal financial assistance. It simply prohibits discrimination against people who have a disability. Most of the provisions of section 504 were incorporated into and expanded The Education for Handicapped Children Act, but section 504 is broader and the provisions are not restricted to a specific age group or to education. These two pieces of revolutionary legislation are closely aligned in terms of their intent and purpose.

The Americans with Disabilities Act of 1990 (ADA), is another important piece of legislation that links special education and rehabilitation. This piece of legislation was approved by the Congress after long and thorough deliberation, and signed by President Bush on July 26, 1990. ADA gives civil rights protection to individuals with disabilities in private sector employment, all public services, public accommodations, transportation, and telecommunications. The Act is patterned after section 504 of the Rehabilitation Act of 1973. In as much as special educators serve students who will be seeking employment and independent lifestyles at some point in life, it is important that educators apprise individuals of their rights and protections under the ADA (Council for Exceptional Children, 1990).

Conclusion

This chapter has provided the framework for a functional understanding of the meaning and scope of special education, and the relationship between special education and rehabilitation. Because of the wide range of terminology used to communicate, semantic and philosophical differences, and constant changes in the field, it is difficult to develop a "comfort zone" with the topic. Because the field is relatively new in some instances (e.g., pedagogy for some categorical areas) many ideas, concepts, and facts are emerging more rapidly than the system and society are prepared to accept with blind confidence. Without question, the consumers, parents, and professionals look to the future in terms of continued advancement in the field.

Service and support for persons with a disability are both enriched and expanded by the interdisciplinary interaction between special education and rehabilitation services. Interagency collaboration can facilitate the expansion of program efforts aimed at enhancing employment opportunities and social integration for persons with disabilities. Through combined human and fiscal resources, research efforts, and training programs, the two disciplines can succeed at enabling and empowering persons with a disability.

References

Avoiding handicappist stereotypes. (1977). *Interracial Books for Children Bulletin, 8*(6,7), 1.

Baca, L., & Chinn, P. (1982). Coming to grips with cultural diversity. *Exceptional Children, 2*, 33-45.

Byers, J. (1989). AIDS in children: Effects on neurological development and implications for the future. *Journal of Special Education, 23*, 5-16.

Bitter, J. A. (1979). *Introduction to rehabilitation.* St. Louis: C. V. Mosby.

Cartwright, G., Cartwright, C., & Ward, M. (1989). *Educating special learners.* Belmont, CA: Wadsworth.

Council for Exceptional Children. (1990, October/November). American with Disabilities Act of 1990: What should you know? *Supplement to Exceptional Children, 57.*

Drug-exposed babies not a lost generation, experts say. (1990, November 7). *Education of the Handicapped*, p. 1. Alexandria, VA: Capitol.

Elrod, F. G. (1987). Academic and social skills pre-requisite to success in vocational training: Perceptions of vocational educators. *Journal for Vocational Special Needs, 10*(1), 17-21.

Federal Register. (1990, September 25). *55*(163), 39244.

Four states respond to infant, preschool programs. (1990, November 7). *Education of the Handicapped*, p. 1. Alexandria, VA: Capitol.

Greer, J. (1990). The drug babies. *Exceptional Children, 56*(6), 382-384.

Mercer, J. (1973). *Labeling the mentally retarded.* Berkeley, CA: University of California.

Meyen, E., & Skrtic, T. (1988). *Exceptional children and youth* (3rd ed.). Colorado: Love.

Mills v. Board of Education of District of Columbia. (1971). 1939-71 (D. D. C. 1971).

National Association of State Directors of Special Education. (1990). *Education of the Handicapped Act amendments of 1990 (P. L. 101-476): Summary of major changes in parts A through H of the act.* Washington, DC: Author.

Pennsylvania Association of Retarded Citizens v. Commonwealth of Pennsylvania. (1971). 343 F. Supp. 279, 297 (E. D. PA. 1971).

Rubin, S. E., & Roessler, R. T. (1983). *Foundations of the vocational rehabilitation process* (2nd ed.). Baltimore: University Park Press.

Sage, D., & Burrello, L. (1986). *Policy and management in special education.* New Jersey: Prentice Hall.

U. S. Office of Education. (1977, August 23). Implementation of part B of the Education of the Handicapped Act. *Federal Register, 42*, 42474-42518.

U. S. Department of Education. (1990). *Twelfth annual report to congress on the implementation of the Education of the Handicapped Act.* Washington, DC: U. S. Government Printing Office.

U. S. Congress. (1990, October). Proceedings and debates of the 101st Congress, second session. *Congressional Record.* Washington, DC: Government Printing Office.

Whitehouse, F. A. (1953). Habilitation: Concept and process. *Journal of Rehabilitation, 19*(2), 3-7.

Yoshida, R., Wasilewski, L., & Friedman, D. (1990). Recent newspaper coverage about persons with disabilities. *Exceptional Children, 56*(5), 418-423.

Ysseldyke, J., & Algozzine, J. (1990). *Introduction to special education.* Boston: Houghton Mifflin.

VIII. Human Services

Centers for Independent Living

Robert F. Kilbury, M.S.
Barbara J. Stotlar, M.E.

History/Legislation

According to Lachat (1988), "Independent living (IL) emerged as a concept in the 1960s with the creation of self-help networks among individuals with severe disabilities who were attempting to live in the community" (p. 1). Some say this movement began in Berkeley, California when the administration of the University of California tried to prohibit Ed Roberts from going to college because he was too severely disabled (Levy, 1988). Others point to the story of Judy Heumann, who, despite passing the oral and written portions of the licensure exam for teachers in New York City, was prohibited from teaching by the Board of Education because she could not pass the physical examination due to her disability (Levy, 1988).

In any case, it can be said indisputably that the IL movement was begun more than 20 years ago by a segment of citizens with severe physical disabilities. Persons with spinal cord injuries, multiple sclerosis, polio, and cerebral palsy were among the disability groups most widely represented (DeJong, 1979). These individuals were hindered by a world which was inaccessible to them and they began to fight to change that world. Roberts eventually attended UC-Berkeley, wrote a grant to start the Disabled Students' Program there, founded the prototype Center for Independent Living (CIL) within a community at large, became the director of the California Department of Rehabilitation in 1976, and is the co-founder of the World Institute on Disability (WID). Heumann won her lawsuit involving the Board of Education and worked as a teacher at her former elementary school prior to joining Roberts at the CIL in Berkeley in 1973. She later co-founded the WID.

Such social movements as civil rights, deinstitutionalization, demedicalization, consumerism, and self-help had profound influences on the Independent Living movement (DeJong, 1979). IL is both a reaction against, and an alternative to, the traditional vocational rehabilitation (VR) model which had not effectively served persons with severe disabilities. Independent living is both a social movement as well as a unique service delivery model. It is this innovative model of service delivery that this chapter shall attempt to describe.

While there are many definitions for independent living programs, Frieden (1983) describes them as "a community-based program with substantial consumer involvement that provides directly or coordinates indirectly, through referral, services severely disabled individuals need to increase their self-determination and to minimize their dependence on others" (p. 62). Many authors describe three types of IL programs: Centers for Independent Living (CILs), IL Residential Programs, and IL Transitional Programs (Frieden, 1983; Rubin & Roessler, 1987). While residential components are generally viewed as countermanding the intent of the movement due to their segregatory nature, transitional and residential programs have nevertheless proven their worth throughout the history of rehabilitation. For the sake of brevity and consistency, this chapter will focus on CIL programs.

CILs, then, are not-for profit, nonresidential, community-based programs run by Boards of Directors, 51% of whom must be persons with disabilities. CILs are mandated by the National Council on the Handicapped (now named the National Council on Disability) to provide the four core services of Information and Referral (I & R), Advocacy, Peer Counseling, and Independent Living Skills Training.

The first true CIL, with the help of Ed Roberts and, later, Judy Heumann, was established in 1972 in Berkeley, California (Levy, 1988; Rubin & Roessler, 1987). Shortly thereafter, CILs sprung up in Boston, Houston, Chicago, and New York. Today there are more than 200 nationwide.

LEGISLATION

The groundwork for federally funded CIL programs was laid by the passage of such legislation as the Architectural Barriers Act of 1968, the Urban Mass Transit Act Amendments of 1970, the historic Rehabilitation Act of 1973, and the Education of All Handicapped Children Act in 1975 (Goldman, 1985). Importantly, with its emphasis on civil rights, active client participation, and serving persons with severe disabilities, the Rehabilitation Act paved the way for consumerism and empowerment in rehabilitation. Section 504 of title V, patterned after the Civil Rights Act (Rubin & Roessler, 1987), significantly reinforced the notion that persons with disabilities had rights. It states that:

> No otherwise qualified handicapped individual in the United States...shall, solely by reason of his handicap, be excluded from participation in, be denied the benefits of, or be subjected to discrimination under any program or activity receiving federal financial assistance (Sherman & Zirkel, 1980, p. 331).

Widely described as the "Bill of Rights for persons with disabilities," section 504 took years to be implemented (Rubin & Roessler, 1987). In fact, it was only after nationwide demonstrations by individuals with varying disabilities that Joseph Califano, then Secretary of the Department of Health, Education, and Welfare, finally signed the federal regulations pursuant to the Act on April 28, 1977 (Levy, 1988). Through that effort, people with disabilities empowered themselves and discovered they had a potent voice. They also learned that in order to attain their rights, coordinated advocacy would be required. A continuation and expansion of this empowerment led to the overwhelming passage of the landmark Americans with Disabilities Act (ADA), signed by President George Bush on July 26, 1990.

FUNDING

While section 130 of the 1973 Rehabilitation Act provided for several demonstration grants for CILs, it was not until the passage of the Rehabilitation, Comprehensive Services, and Developmental Disability Amendments of 1978 that centers were legislatively legitimized by the appropriation of funding (Rubin & Roessler, 1987; Valera, 1983). Valera (1983) describes this legislation as "the single most far-reaching piece of legislation ever offered to the disabled community" (p. 45). The law mandated that citizens with disabilities be involved in the management, direction, and provision of services in these centers (Laurie, 1979).

Title VII of the 1978 amendments provided federal funding which enabled CILs to proliferate in the late seventies and eighties. Part A of title VII provided moneys for state rehabilitation agencies to develop IL programs. Part B moneys allowed agencies and other entities to start CILs. Part C funding, never authorized until 1986, was targeted to provide IL services to older, blind individuals (Rubin & Roessler, 1987). It is important to note the total of all three portions of this federal funding amounted to only $40 million in 1986, a tiny sliver of the total rehabilitation pie (approximately 3%). As with most federally funded services, these federal funds are matched by state funds.

PERSONNEL

All CILs are directed by a Board of Directors which is responsible for setting policy for the center as a service provider. As indicated, CIL boards are comprised of a majority of persons with disabilities who reflect the needs of the community through their policy-making powers. Some states go beyond this requirement by mandating that centers be membership organizations. For example, Illinois CILs are required to solicit involvement from consumers in the communities served (members), who are in turn responsible for electing the board.

Direct service and administrative staff are responsible for policy implementation and daily service provision. The backbone of all CILs are the direct service providers who provide a multitude of IL services as described below. Service providers, while usually either full- or part-time paid employees of the center, may be volunteers whose particular background or experience is more effective in dealing with a consumer's issue(s). Whether paid staff or volunteers, direct service providers are generally persons with disabilities.

Depending on the needs of their particular communities and their level of funding, many CILs hire individuals who serve as Independent Living Specialists, Deaf Services Coordinators, Blind Services Coordinators, Outreach Specialists, Advocacy Specialists, Housing Specialists, Transportation Specialists, Personal Assistant (PA) Coordinators, and so on. With the passage of the Americans with Disabilities Act, many CILs also have staff who are becoming experts in educating the public concerning the ADA Regulations.

Purpose/Intent

The rationale for CILs is that individuals with disabilities are often the best resources in facilitating the consumer's (never referred to as a "client" in IL) choice of options. All too often, the VR system has been perceived by the disability community as being too narrow in its definition of "rehabilitation." With VRs primary focus on "vocational closure," other aspects of daily living are easily overlooked. Independent living has a more holistic definition of rehabilitation and provides services which reflect this broader definition.

Independent living focuses on serving individuals with severe disabilities, regardless of vocational rehabilitation eligibility. Such services promote empowerment, self-help, consumerism, and changing the environment rather than the individual. This orientation provides an alternative paradigm to VR. Gerben DeJong (1983) has provided us with a conceptualization of how IL and VR differ. While in VR the focus is on changing the individual "client" or "patient" by professional intervention (VR Counselor, Physical Therapist, or Physician); in IL the focus is on removing barriers to full participation and integration, reducing dependence on "professionals," and facilitating the empowerment of the "consumer." In the VR model, the focus is on the individual with the disability; in the IL model the focus is on the "disabling environment." In the former paradigm, the professional is in control; in the latter, the consumer of services assumes control over these services. Finally, the desired outcomes of VR include employment, maximizing activities of daily living, and improved motivation; in IL the goals include self-direction, integration into the least restrictive environment, and social productivity.

CILs attempt, through both individualized and community-wide programs, to create a world which is more accessible for everyone. This might entail training an individual who is deaf to use a telecommunication device for the deaf (TDD) so that they can call the police, fire department, hospital, or (through a message relay center) the local pizza delivery person. It might involve referring PAs to consumers so that they can live in an apartment rather than in a nursing home. It could include assisting a consumer in finding an accessible apartment, or in filling out employment or housing applications, or in completing public aid or social security forms. Disability awareness presentations, which create a more accessible attitudinal environment, also epitomize this purpose.

UTILIZATION CRITERIA

Should the human service provider have a consumer with a disability who might benefit from peer counseling or IL skills training (whether this training is in the use of adaptive equipment, wheelchair maintenance, or the attainment of entitlements), referral to a CIL would be appropriate. If the provider knows of a situation where an individual might benefit from housing or PA referral, a CIL referral should be made. Additionally, CILs are equipped to deal with situations where a parent of a child with a disability would benefit from advocacy services. If there is a need to determine whether or not your facility is accessible to individuals with varying disabilities, you might call the local CIL for technical assistance. If you ever ask yourself concerning disability issues or policies: "I wonder what a person with a disability would say," call your local CIL.

SPECIAL CASE MANAGEMENT NEEDS

As all services are consumer directed, active consumer participation in goal development, as well as subsequent service delivery, is necessary for positive outcomes. While federal funding sources require proof of disability for services to individuals (exceptions being services to families, community services, and requests for I & R), most centers also receive state and/or local funding which is more discretionary in nature. Through such funding, consumers or their advocates are often deemed eligible for services.

Independent Living Services

With the exception of the four core services required by law, CILs pursue their mission though a variety of programs and services which are defined by the needs of individuals within their catchment area. For example, variables which may affect the services provided include whether the catchment area is urban or rural, the type and scope of existing resources within the area, the sources of CIL funding available, and the priorities given to identified service needs by the potential consumers of such services. While this diversity makes describing CIL service delivery from state to state, or even county to county, difficult, it is this flexibility to respond to the needs of the individual communities that make services from CILs both effective and unique.

Persons considering referral to a CIL should contact the center in their area for a listing of the services that center provides. The following sections are meant to encourage the reader to do so, as well as to acquaint the professional with common CIL services. This portion begins with the four core services federally mandated of all CILs and concludes with other services that CILs typically provide.

INFORMATION AND REFERRAL

Information and referral (I & R) is a service response to requests from individuals or community entities for practical information relating to disability issues or concerns. Such information is provided with the intent of "increasing public knowledge about the needs, issues, resources, services, and advancement of persons with disabilities and independent living" (Budde, Lachat, Lattimore, Jones, & Stolzman, 1987, p. 16). CILs can therefore be thought of as clearinghouses of information needed by consumers, their families, other service providers, communities at large, or anyone else interested in increasing options for persons with disabilities or removing architectural, attitudinal, or communicative barriers from society. Typically, the type of information requested ranges from situation specific (e.g., local options for transportation, housing, community resources and benefits, adaptive equipment, daily living techniques) to more general inquiries concerning accessibility, disability awareness, disability law, statistics, trends, and the like.

Persons requesting I & R from a CIL need not have a disability nor must they reside within the catchment area served by the CIL. Referring parties may expect to receive a listing of additional resources and/or a referral to another appropriate agency or person for additional details; if CILs themselves do not have the answers to your questions, they often can provide direction to someone who will.

ADVOCACY

The provision of advocacy by CILs takes two distinct tacks, both of which are required by law. *Consumer advocacy* includes an array of services which either train or support individual consumers or consumer groups in presenting their position or needs to others in order to "achieve, maintain, or improve their independent living goals" (Budde et al., 1987, p. 11). The gist of such services is to assist individuals in attaining their rights, entitlements, or access to activities which have been denied them on the basis of disability. Under some circumstances, and only upon consumer request, CIL staff may act (temporarily) on their behalf, at the same time providing whatever adjunct services are necessary to empower the individual to advocate for themselves in the future.

Community or *systemic advocacy* includes an array of services which articulate the position of the disability community at the local, state, or federal level. These services are provided to affect the removal of barriers and disincentives to integration and choice for persons with disabilities, the development of community options, or changes in policies which are "disabling" the populations served by the CIL (Budde et al., 1987).

PEER COUNSELING

Peer-counseling programs and services vary widely from center to center. However, peer support/assistance is usually provided by a nonprofessional who has made a successful transition into community living and has disability-related experiences, knowledge, and coping skills. These individuals provide information, a common experiential base, support, and direction to others who desire to make a similar transition (Schlatzlein, 1978). This orientation is the cornerstone of all service provision at CILs.

Depending on the center's funding and method of service delivery, peer counseling may be provided by either a staff person or by a peer volunteer (sometimes a former consumer of services), either in the center itself or in the field. Some CILs utilize an instructional approach wherein peer counselors are viewed as educators providing training in independent living skills (e.g., personal assistant management), thus deemphasizing the traditional therapeutic expectations associated with the role of "counselor." Other centers use an I & R approach in which peer counseling is conducted either by phone or by mail. Regardless of the process utilized, consumers will receive peer counseling from a service provider who views the consumer as an equal, who is capable of acting as a role model and a link to resources within the community, and who is willing to share personal experiences to facilitate the consumer's ability to assume control of and choice over life options.

IL SKILLS TRAINING

CILs assist consumers, either individually or in groups, in developing the skills they identify as needing to achieve their goals for independence and choice. Areas of training are varied, but typically include the management of personal assistants, the use of adaptive equipment, assertiveness or self-advocacy skill development, and activities of daily living.

SPECIALIZED SERVICES

Many centers respond to the needs of their communities and populations by creating new services or by adapting core services to better accommodate special needs or underserved groups. These specialized services include interpreter or reader referral, mobility training, TDD training, brailling services, and support groups to name a few. Some centers are bridging the gap between IL and VR, becoming involved in such traditionally controversial services as job coaching.

PERSONAL ASSISTANCE SERVICES

For many persons with severe physical disabilities, the difference between living in the community and institutionalization is the availability of and the consumer's ability to hire and manage qualified personal assistants (PAs). PAs are individuals who do not generally have formal medical training, are hired and managed by individual consumers, and are often paid by the local rehabilitation agency. These individuals provide a variety of services which are defined by the consumer according to their unique circumstances. Services provided by PAs include housekeeping, transportation, laundry, as well as more intimate personal care. The value of such services is easily measured by the observable effect they have on the consumer's quality of life and level of independence.

Given the importance of the availability of qualified PAs, many CILs provide a variety of services to facilitate the consumer's ability to hire and manage them. Typically, centers maintain an updated list of PAs which can be forwarded to consumers for review. The degree to which centers screen and match PAs to individual consumer needs is a function of the funding source(s), consumer circumstance, and how strictly the center interprets the IL philosophy of consumer control.

Additionally, basic skills training may be offered to persons interested in becoming PAs or who are currently working as PAs and wish to upgrade their skills. Such training packages are provided in a general manner that does not infringe upon the consumer's responsibility to instruct the PA in their specific needs. PA training programs may also be supplemented with in-service training, PA support groups, advocacy training, and so on.

COMMUNITY SERVICES

Through their commitment to the creation of a barrier-free environment, CILs provide services within their communities which promote this mission. *Community education* and *outreach projects* include public presentations, workshops, and in-service training designed to increase public awareness of the needs and rights of citizens with disabilities, as well as the dissemination of the IL philosophy. Centers generally have written materials, videotapes, and other media available which promote the empowerment of people with disabilities to strive for self-imposed independent living goals, both as individuals and as a minority group. *Technical assistance* is provided by most CILs and includes consultation with city planners, building contractors, and businesses concerning architectural and communicative accessibility, as well as community initiatives to increase the opportunities for equal participation in classrooms, worksites, recreational facilities, and other public settings.

TYPICAL REFERRAL QUESTIONS

The consumers of CIL services are typically either self-referred or referred from other agencies. By far, the most important question the consumer or referring agency should explore is "Does the consumer wish to increase independent functioning in one or more areas of their life?" Other potential referral questions include "What barriers to independence has the consumer identified?" and "Are they willing to take responsibility for change in their own lives?"

References

Budde, J. F., Lachat, M. A., Lattimore, J., Jones, M., & Stolzman, L. (1987). *Standards for independent living centers*. Lawrence, KS: RTC/IL.

DeJong, G. (1979). Independent living: From social movement to analytic paradigm. *Archives of Physical Medicine and Rehabilitation, 60*, 435-446.

DeJong, G. (1983). Defining and implementing the independent living concept. In N. M. Crewe & I. K. Zola (Eds.), *Independent living for physically disabled people* (pp. 4-27). San Francisco, CA: Jossey-Bass.

Frieden, L. (1983). Understanding alternative program models. In N. M. Crewe & I. K. Zola (Eds.), *Independent living for physically disabled people* (pp. 62-72). San Francisco, CA: Jossey-Bass.

Goldman, C. D. (1985). Disability rights: A perspective on advocacy. *Journal of Intergroup Relations, 13*(2), 34-40.

Lachat, M. A. (1988). *Independent living service model: Historical roots, core elements, and current practice*. Hampton, NH: Center for Research Management.

Laurie, G. (1979). Independent living programs. *Rehabilitation Gazette, 22*, 1.

Levy, C. W. (1988). *A people's history of the independent living movement*. Lawrence, KS: Research and Training Center on Independent Living.

Rubin, S. E., & Roessler, R. T. (1987). *Foundations of the vocational rehabilitation process* (3rd ed.). Austin, TX: Pro-Ed.

Schlatzlein, J. E. (1978). *Spinal cord injury and peer counseling/peer education*. Unpublished manuscript. Minneapolis, MN: University of Minnesota.

Sherman, M., & Zirkel, P. (1980). Student discrimination in higher education: A review of the law. *Journal of Law and Education, 9*(3), 301-341.

Valera, R. A. (1983). Changing societal attitudes and legislation regarding disability. In N. M. Crewe & I. K. Zola (Eds.), *Independent living for physically disabled people* (pp. 28-48). San Francisco, CA: Jossey-Bass.

Therapeutic Recreation

Joseph D. Teaff, Ed.D.

History/Legislation

HISTORY

Persons with disabilities and special needs have not had the opportunities to participate in recreation programs and activities as evidenced by early historical practices. However, these individuals are now being given these opportunities because of various legislative acts.

Recreation did not play a major role in the lives of individuals with disabilities until the twentieth century. In 1906, the Playground Association of America, later known as the Playground and Recreation Association, and ultimately as the National Recreation Association, was formed. As a service organization, it promoted the cause of community recreation for more than half a century. The organized recreation and park movement stated from the beginning that its services were for all people. During the 1920s and 1930s, public schools began offering after school recreation programs for individuals with disabilities. The National American Red Cross was active during World War II in providing recreation opportunities for military personnel. It was not until the late 1940s that the recreation programs began to appear on a wide scale in public hospitals. The Veterans' Administration was a pioneer in this effort, particularly in working with individuals who were emotionally disturbed. The first significant effort to provide therapeutic recreation services occurred in veterans' hospitals and state institutions serving persons with mental illness.

Summer camps for children and adolescents began in the United States in 1861, but it was not until the 1940s that camping became a popular service to meet the needs of persons with disabilities. During the 1940s, the concept of using the outdoor wilderness as a therapeutic milieu began to be developed. Therapeutic wilderness programs can be defined as outdoor activities taking place in a wilderness environment that are designed to improve the emotional and behavioral adjustments of the participants. Therapeutic wilderness programs may range from a half-day outing to a year around operation, and may include activities such as backpacking, mountaineering, rock climbing, canoeing, camping, and cross-country skiing.

LEGISLATION

Many of the problems confronting citizens with disabilities have been addressed through legislation at the federal level. The Social Security Act of 1935 provided federal grants-in-aid to states for maternal and child health and welfare programs, and for services to children with handicaps. In the Cooperative Research Act of 1957, Congress provided $675,000 to support research concerning the education of children with disabilities. In the next year, Public Law 85-926 recognized that relatively few professionals were involved in research and training and so provided aid to colleges and universities to prepare teachers and leaders to work in the field of mental retardation. Public Law 88-164, passed in 1963, extended Public Law 85-926 to include training of professionals to work with children with all types of disabilities. Public Law 89-313 amended the Elementary and Secondary Education Act and included among the disadvantaged those who were school aged and lived in state residential institutions or state-supported, private schools.

Inaccessible buildings segregate the walking, seeing, and hearing population from those with disabilities. The Architectural Barriers Act of 1968 requires certain buildings and facilities designed, constructed, altered, or leased with federal funds to be accessible to, and usable by, individuals with physical disabilities. Five years later, Congress created the Architectural and Transportation Barriers Compliance Board (ATBCB) under section 502 of the Rehabilitation Act of 1973 to enforce the Architectural Barriers Act of 1968. As long as buildings are architecturally accessible, individuals with disabilities can participate in recreation programs that are available to the general public.

The 1970s have been referred to as the *Decade of the Disabled*, for during those 10 years, historic civil and human rights advances by persons with disabilities were dramatically achieved. The 1973 Rehabilitation Act, as amended in 1974, is one of the most significant landmark pieces of legislation in the struggle of individuals with disabilities. Section 504 of the Rehabilitation Act entitled "Nondiscrimination Under Federal Grants," or the "Civil Rights Act for the Handicapped," states that: "No otherwise qualified handicapped individual in the United States shall, solely on the basis of his handicap, be excluded from participation in, be denied the benefits of, or be subjected to discrimination under any program or activity receiving federal assistance." The Education of All Handicapped Children Act, was signed into law in 1975 by President Ford. The Act provided equal education opportunity to all children with disabilities. "It is the purpose of this Act to assure that all handicapped children have available to them a free and appropriate public education and related services designed to meet their unique needs, to assure that the rights of handicapped children and their parents or guardians are protected, to assist states and localities to provide for the education of all children, and to assess and assure the effectiveness of efforts to educate handicapped children (Sec. 601(3)(c))." This law addresses the use of related services in least restrictive environments. Related services are those additional services necessary for the child to benefit from special education instruction. Related services include transportation, and such developmental, corrective, and other supportive services including speech pathology and audiology, psychological services, physical and occupational therapy, medical and counseling services, and recreation.

Legislative initiatives have facilitated the movement of large numbers of persons with disabilities into community living situations, consequently shifting the responsibility of recreation programming to community agencies. However, providing services in least restrictive environments for persons with (and without) disabilities (e.g., in community recreation settings) requires funding and preparation for recreation professionals.

FUNDING

Those concerned with developing community recreation programming for persons with disabilities must be knowledgeable about funding sources. Vaughan and Winslow (1979) found that the major funding source for community recreation programs for persons with disabilities is the general tax fund. Slightly more than 87% of all community leisure service agencies surveyed used the general tax as a source of funding. Fees and charges were the second largest source, utilized by 44.2% of the agencies. The types of resources utilized in addition to those mentioned above, depended on the size of the community. Communities of under 100,000 tended to fund 30 to 40% of their programs from donations. Government grants were a major source of funding for those communities over 250,000. Other sources of funding were special taxes, private grants, and contractual agreements.

One state has used legislation to establish special taxes to support community recreation programs for persons with disabilities. Park districts and municipalities in Illinois have been successful in establishing community recreation programs because of legislation that allows park districts and other governmental bodies to cooperate by forming special recreation associations and to levy a special tax of up to $.02 for $100 of assessed valuation for special recreation programs.

Fund raising is another means of obtaining funds and may include a number of techniques. Sources of funds that may be tapped through fund-raising initiatives include governmental and foundation grants, memorial giving, capital fund campaigns, direct mail solicitations, house-to-house solicitation, and special events.

Community leisure settings can enter into contractual agreements with schools, sheltered workshops, group homes, and other agencies to provide community recreation programs. Contractual agreements offer an additional source of support, although they are not likely to be a major financial resource.

PERSONNEL

People too often assume that the organizing and carrying out of recreation programs is relatively simple and that anyone can do it without specialized training. This assumption is made because many youth and adults in our society do provide recreation leadership *without* such training. The professional's assignment, however, tends to be far more complex than that of the typical volunteer leader or coach. It typically involves carefully thought out goals and objectives and sophisticated planning techniques. Recreation professionals at all levels should be familiar with a wide range of recreation activities and their potential values and outcomes. They need to possess knowledge of direct leadership and supervision, group dynamics, patient or client assessment, evaluation and research, and skill in oral and written communication. Particularly important is the knowledge of the history and traditions of the field, and the meaning of recreation and leisure in human society and their value in human growth and development. In the case of therapeutic recreation programs that serve individuals with disabilities, the recreation specialist needs to have an extensive knowledge of disabilities and its effects on the individual, medical terminology, anatomy, physiology, and psychopathology.

In the past, many persons entered the field of recreation without professional training, before college and university curricula were established. Today, higher education in recreation is available throughout the United States and Canada. Specialized curricular options are available in areas such as recreation management, resource management, commercial recreation, campus recreation, and therapeutic recreation. One of the most significant efforts to upgrade curricular standards and practices in recreation has been the accreditation process. In the course of this process, clearly defined standards and procedural guidelines regarding courses, administrative support, student selection and services, faculty resources, and similar curriculum components need to be documented. The accreditation process has been immensely supportive to college and university departments and has resulted in a continuing flow of departments seeking initial accreditation, as well as applying for follow-up reviews at the authorized five-year periods. As of the late 1980s, approximately 100 departments had been accredited, and the number continues to grow.

Therapeutic recreation was one of the first professional specializations in recreation to institute a strong, national registration plan. Registration programs for therapeutic recreation specialists were available as early as 1956. In 1981, the term registration was changed to certification, upon the creation of the National Council for Therapeutic Recreation Certification (NCTRC). The nine-member NCTRC has three major responsibilities: setting national evaluative standards for the certification and recertification of therapeutic recreational personnel, granting recognition to those who meet the standards, and monitoring adherence to standards by certified personnel.

Purpose/Intent

RATIONALE

Recreation is an essential component of healthy living and quality of life, along with proper nutrition, shelter, education, employment, and community living. Since many individuals with disabilities continue to remain unemployed, or employed only part time, recreation becomes a major focus of a large part of their daily living. Recreation participation in community settings offers the individual with a disability an opportunity to develop a positive self-concept through the successful experiences and satisfying relationships with peers. Channels for self-expression, opportunities to interact with the environment, and the potential to establish a more personally satisfying way of life are other implications of integrated, community leisure participation by individuals with disabilities.

The rationale for the development of recreation opportunities for persons with disabilities in community settings has been developed from both a theoretical (i.e., normalization) and a practical (i.e., deinstitutionalization) perspective. Integration of children and adults with disabilities into community leisure services and facilities may be viewed as an outgrowth of the normalization principle and the resulting movement toward community placement. Normalization, a concept defined by Nirje (1969), involves making available to persons with disabilities the same patterns and conditions of everyday life, as close as possible to the patterns of society. Normalization involves valuing the life, rights, and dignity of persons with disabilities and believing that they should participate in the activities enjoyed by other members of society.

UTILIZATION CRITERIA

The integration of persons with disabilities into community leisure programs and facilities is essential if the process of normalization is to be completed. Successful integration of community leisure programs requires that those involved in service delivery adopt a philosophy and value system consistent with the principles of normalization. Of particular importance is a recognition that people with disabilities are valuable as individuals and have a right to participate in the same leisure programs in which persons who are not disabled participate. Agencies committed to the principle of normalization must articulate and practice a philosophy of inclusion of individuals with disabilities into existing programs being provided for the general public, rather than just the provision of special, segregated programs. A belief that the creation and provision of only segregated programs is exclusionary and amounts to the removal of a person with a disability from the rest of society is a vital component of this philosophy. Commitment to the integration of programs also requires that agencies actively recruit participants with disabilities to their programs and facilities.

Integration of individuals with disabilities into community recreation environments is supported through an examination of the benefits derived from participation in an integrated environment. The opportunity to learn from, and socialize with, peers who are not disabled has been cited as one benefit for individuals with disabilities participating in integrated programs. For example, teenagers with moderate retardation showed an increase in appropriate playground behavior and increased their frequencies of appropriate social interactions with teenagers who were not disabled who volunteered to teach them playground skills (Donder & Nietupski, 1981). Stainback and Stainback (1985) supported the notion that students who are not disabled provide students with disabilities with models of age-appropriate dress, language, gestures, and leisure behavior. While these findings should not be extended to account for the behavior of all people with disabilities, they do provide support for the belief that integrated activities prove more beneficial than do segregated activities, and in some cases may be preferred by individuals with disabilities.

SPECIAL CASE MANAGEMENT NEEDS

Community leisure service agencies also have a responsibility to ensure that personnel in their agencies are prepared to share the responsibility for integrating participants with disabilities. Education for staff regarding the leisure needs of persons with disabilities and training in how to facilitate the successful integration of programs is vital to the success of efforts to integrate programs. Effective integration will require that general program staff and specialists in therapeutic recreation begin working together. An emphasis must be placed on the utilization of generalists, rather than specialists to supervise integrated programs. The utilization of specialists as support for the generalists will assist integration efforts by de-emphasizing a person with a disability's need for specially trained staff and for special programs. Lord (1983) offers important advice that will be useful for personnel involved in integration efforts. Lord states that instead of asking the question "Is this person ready for integration?," it makes more sense to ask, "What support does this person need to be involved and to participate?"

Client Services

When persons with disabilities enter into recreation programs offered at community recreation settings, they do so with varying levels of ability, knowledge, skill, and interest. The nature of their disabilities could limit successful participation in recreation activities with peers who are not disabled. For example, a young woman who is mobility impaired and uses crutches realizes that she will be unable to keep pace with other participants actively playing kickball. Persons with cognitive impairments are often dependent upon group home staff to locate, plan, and lead outings into the community because they are unaware of the many options. This may be due to a lack of education and awareness, and the lack of opportunities to make independent choices about preferred recreation activities. Other persons often find themselves participating in activities which do not allow them to practice or enhance the skills they do have. An example would be the visually impaired cross-country skier who learns to ski at an out-of-town event, only to find, upon arriving home, that no one there is qualified to guide him on local ski trails. Finally, all persons, regardless of ability, vary in their degree of interest and motivation prior to and during participation in a recreation activity. The person with a hearing impairment may find increased strength, fitness, and self-worth while participating in a volleyball league. However, her teammates may be more interested in the socialization which occurs, the competition among teams, the "escape" from life's pressures, or a simple appreciation of the elements of the game. These examples are not necessarily disability specific as participants who are not disabled enter into recreation programs with varying levels of skill or experience. It is important, therefore, that the community recreation professional be aware that individual differences do exist in the skills, abilities, knowledge, and interests of persons with and without disabilities.

DESCRIPTION OF SERVICES

Because the characteristics of a person's disability can handicap their participation in regular programs, recreation professionals must develop a range, or continuum of services that are accessible to all persons with disabilities. This range of services helps to move those persons requiring large amounts of specialized staff, services, and equipment toward more accessible leisure experiences. Community recreation services for persons with disabilities have essentially three primary levels.

The first level provides for persons participating in programs who typically need a special environment in which to gain a positive and successful leisure experience. Specialized staff (e.g., therapeutic recreation specialist, care provider, teacher) are employed because they have a complete knowledge and understanding of the participant's skills, abilities, and behaviors. They can provide specialized services through appropriate interventions (e.g., speech interpreter, behavioral manager) to help ensure that the program runs smoothly. Special adaptive equipment (e.g., therapy balls, positioning cushions) and facilities (e.g., therapeutic swimming pools in hospitals, activity rooms in institutional settings) are purchased or scheduled to accommodate participants with disabilities. Persons typically utilizing these programs are those who prefer to associate with peers who are similarly disabled.

The second level provides persons with disabilities opportunities to be mainstreamed into regular programs and to participate alongside participants who are not disabled. While specialized staff (e.g., volunteer advocates), services (e.g., care providers' assistance with registration), and equipment/material (e.g., built-up paintbrush for artists with motor limitations in their hands) may still be utilized, little or no assumption is made beforehand that these considerations are appropriate, or even necessary.

The third level should be the ultimate goal of recreation personnel. Participants with disabilities should know that independent access to community leisure settings and programs is possible. Persons with disabilities are considered "participants," not "the disabled." Therefore, they are entitled to the same respect and attention afforded any other member of the community when considering individual involvement in recreation programming.

It is apparent that there is a need for programs at all three levels. Many persons with disabilities need the specialization offered through a special environment in order to participate in community recreation services. However, those persons with disabilities who have the potential to participate alongside peers or who have the skills to independently choose and attend an accessible leisure setting, should be given sufficient opportunities to do so. Decisions on which level to start this process rests not only with the parent or professional, but through collective assessments of the skills and abilities of the potential consumer with disabilities.

References

Donder, D., & Nietupski, J. (1981). Nonhandicapped adolescents teaching playground skills to their mentally handicapped peers: Toward a less restrictive middle school environment. *Education and Training of the Mentally Retarded, 16*, 270-276.

Lord, J. (1983). Reflections on a decade of integration. *Journal of Leisurability, 10*(4), 4-11.

Nirje, B. (1969). The normalization principle and its human development implications. In R. Kugel & W. Wolfensberger (Eds.), *Changing patterns of residential services for the mentally retarded* (pp. 181-195). Washington, DC: President's Committee on Mental Retardation.

Stainback, S., & Stainback, W. (1985). *Integration of students with severe handicaps into regular schools.* Reston: The Council for Exceptional Children.

Vaughan, J., & Winslow, R. (1979). *Guidelines for community based recreation programs for special populations.* Alexandria, VA: National Therapeutic Recreation Society.

Financial Assistance

Donald E. Vaughn, Ph.D., C.P.A.

History/Legislation

Prior to the 1930s, the elderly in the United States did not have a federal retirement system. France and certain other European countries had initiated such programs in the mid-nineteenth century. When FDR took office in 1933, he set about remedying certain ills of the country, including the poverty level for masses of persons beyond the age of 65. On August 14, 1935, the Social Security Act was signed into law. The Social Security Act of 1935 covered employees in nonagricultural industry and commerce only. Since 1935, coverage has been extended to additional employment, so that today the old-age retirement survivors, disability, and health insurance program approaches universal coverage. Over 90% of those who work in paid employment or in self-employment are either covered or eligible for coverage.

In 1939, Social Security became a family program rather than a program for retired workers only, providing monthly benefits for a worker's dependents and survivors. It was not until January 1940 that the first benefit checks were issued. Prior to that date, some states had old-age assistant programs for the elderly, but many such persons had to either live with working children or other relatives, or depend on local municipalities for shelter, food, and other necessities of life.

Beginning in the early 1950s, farm and household employees, as well as self-employed persons, were brought under the program. Benefits were provided for disabled workers in 1956. Beginning in 1960, disability benefits could be paid at any age. For a person fully covered under Social Security, the amount of disabled benefits is equivalent to what would be paid to a retired person at base age (65). A person must be fully disabled from doing any type of work, and disability benefits are begun six months after one becomes fully disabled.

Under the initial program, retirement benefits were not paid until a person reached aged 65. The minimum eligibility age was lowered to 62 for women in 1956, and to 62 for men in 1961. A person may retire and begin to draw benefits at any age 62 or older. One beginning benefits at an earlier age than the base age (65 in 1991) receives reduced benefits of about 6.7% yearly. Those that defer initial benefits to age 66, 67, or older also receive an increase of a similar ratio. Since persons are living longer, and about half the retiring workers at age 62 to 65 continue to work part-time, two years are being added from year 2000 to 2022 in increments of two months each two years during this period in computing base benefits. That is, someone retiring in year 2000 must be 65 years and 2 months to receive base benefits. By the year 2022, he or she must be age 67 (or monthly benefits will be reduced slightly from the base).

Survivors' benefits extend to children under the age of 18 (or to 19 if the person is still a high school student), to the surviving parent that has to care for a child under the age of 16, and to certain dependent parents of deceased bread winners.

In 1990, about 7.2 million people in the U. S. received monthly Social Security benefits as survivors. About 133 million workers earn survivors' insurance protection for their families under the program. Widow (widower) survivor's benefits begin when she or he reaches the age of 60 if he or she has not remarried by the time of reaching that age. The age is 50 for someone that is physically handicapped. Children who are disabled before attaining age 22 qualify for survivors' benefits so long as they remain fully disabled.

Medicare was introduced in 1966 for persons aged 65, and was extended to the disabled in 1972. Persons normally apply for Medicare when reaching age 65. This is a type of health insurance that may be a primary type coverage or a secondary type coverage. Over the years, the amount of monthly payment into the program (as premiums) has escalated about in line with the rising cost of health costs, or roughly 4% above the annual increase in the cost of living index as measured by changes in the Consumer Price Index. Medicaid is provided to financially indigent persons with the level being set by each state, which is dependent somewhat on the level considered to be the poverty level within a given state.

FUNDING

The effective earnings base and actual tax rate assessed each the employer and the employee on Old Age Survivors and Disability Insurance (OASDI) earnings have generally increased from 1937 through 1991 about in line with inflation. In the initial year—1937—1% was charged each the employee and employer on the base earnings of $3,000. The rate was increased to 7.51% on each the employee and employer's upward adjusted taxable base to $48,000 in 1989 with higher base amounts in later years. Beginning in 1957, a small fraction was assessed for disability coverage with an additional amount assessed beginning in 1966 for health insurance (Medicare/Medicaid).

Funds collected through payroll deductions are deposited to a depository bank or other institution, along with withholdings for federal and state income taxes. Beginning in 1990, deposits were sent directly to the Internal Revenue Service. The funds flow into one of several funds, the largest of which is the Social Security account. Funds collected for the health portion are accounted for separately, and funds are sometimes borrowed by one fund from another to make necessary benefit payments.

In general, self-employed persons pay about the same rate for social security coverage as the combined amount of the employee and employer. While a small credit was given against the rate paid by self-employed persons from 1984 to 1989, this credit was eliminated in 1990 and one-half of the amount of self-employment tax was considered to be a business deduction. Prior to 1990, it was not a business deduction, so the actual impact was about equal. Single proprietors, partners, certain professional persons (e.g., ministers), and shareholders of S corporations are considered to be self-employed. Persons who earn more than $400 yearly must generally pay self-employment taxes on the net earnings (after deductible business expenses).

Base benefits are computed on a price adjusted base during the years in which social security taxes are paid. The five years of lowest earnings are excluded. Benefits on some base amount is computed at 90%, another tier is allowed base benefit payments of 32%, and additional amounts are provided benefits at 15%. Thus, low-income earners might draw base social security retirement (or disability) benefits equal to about 50% of working income. It runs about 25% on above average income earners—those that are earning and paying in on about the maximum amount of OASDI earning base. Many of these high-income persons, however, are receiving other retirement income from supplemental programs, covered below. Prior to retirement, a covered person should contact the nearest Social Security office, obtaining an estimate of probable monthly benefits and applying for OASDI benefits (including the application for Medicare at the age of 65). In general, a dependent spouse qualifies for an amount up to 50% of the primary benefits being paid to the spouse. In some instances, a divorced, dependent spouse may draw on the account of the ex-spouse where the marriage contract existed for longer than 10 years.

Purpose/Structure

The primary purpose of Social Security is to bring a certain level of financial security to persons (a) during retirement years, (b) to those disabled and unable to work, (c) to surviving dependents and widows (widowers) of covered wage earners, and (d) health care payments to those covered by Medicare or Medicaid. The program is one of wealth redistribution—taking funds from the workers and redistributing it to those not earning above some preset level. The United States Congress and most U. S. Presidents have voiced their dedication to continuing to make the program a viable one, but steps were taken in the 1980s to reduce benefit payments to certain types of recipients to eliminate the need for more rapid taxation of the OASDI tax-paying workers.

These reductions generally include the elimination of certain types of social security recipients. In the early 1980s, dependent college students were eliminated from obtaining survivors' benefits. Dependent spouses who had retirement benefits from programs (e.g., state or federal retirement programs) not covered by social security were required to offset OASDI benefits with those received from the non-OASDI covered program benefits. Thus, most persons in this category do not receive dependents' retirement or survivors' benefits. Primary social security benefits were likewise reduced somewhat for persons paying into the social security program for less than 30 years when they received benefits from some program not covered by OASDI. Half the benefits received from social security were subjected to taxation for federal income tax purposes, thus further reducing the net payments to recipients. It is likely that other ways to reduce net benefit payments to workers with significant amounts of income will be developed, although the assessed cost of catastrophic health insurance imposed on those above age 65 was revoked in early 1990 as being age discriminatory.

PROGRAMS TO MEET VARYING NEEDS

As stated above, the Old Age Survivors and Disability Health Insurance (OASDHI) program was developed to provide a certain base level of financial security to the aged, the survivors of workers (dependent children and widows reaching the minimum age under the law), disabled workers, and health insurance coverage for those above age 65 (Medicare), and those that are assessed to be financially indigent (at the poverty level) and who qualify for Medicaid. In 1990, about one benefit recipient under the program existed for each 2.7 persons paying into the program. When the heavy births of the late 1940s and early 1950s reach retirement, the viability of the program will be severely tested, inasmuch as each benefit recipient will be supported by less than two current payers. By that time, hopefully, the program will be more substantially funded (i.e., covered with a buildup of investments held in government securities and other assets) than at the present time.

HISTORY OF PRIVATE PENSION LEGISLATION

Some corporate pension plans and plans designed by municipalities and for selected groups of persons (e.g., college teachers) have been in existence for almost a century. More recently, the IRS Section 403(b) plans and the Keogh plan for self-employed persons were designed. Persons who do not have one of these deferred income plans are eligible for an Individual Retirement Annuity (up to $2,000 annually). Each of these plans will be discussed briefly.

Before the advent of Social Security, some corporations provided a pension plan for their workers. Railroads, utilities, banks, and many large industrial corporations established their own retirement plans. With the advent of social security and the push by labor unions for more fringe benefits in the form of deferred compensation, still other firms established corporate 401(k) corporate plans. Under this plan, a worker may defer up to $7,000 of earned income annually. The firm may also contribute to these plans, with not over $30,000 flowing to each account (with joint contribution by firm and employee). In general, the contributions by a person may not exceed 20% of earned income.

Section 403(b) accounts permit teachers, policemen/firemen, hospital workers, and so on, similar retirement deferral accounts, up to $9,500 annually not to exceed 20% of earned income yearly. A catch up is permitted to someone with 15 or more years of employment with a given employer if no deferral has yet been made. Such deferral can carry the total up to $12,500 of income annually.

Self-employed persons (defined above) may, since 1952, defer up to 20% of self-employment income (not to exceed $30,000 yearly in 1990).

Federal government workers have their own retirement plan, placing about 7% of their income in the Federal Employees Retirement System. Since about 1984, new federal workers have been required to split their contributions into a federal retirement plan and into OASDI. They receive some benefits when they retire under each of these plans.

Military service personnel are paid a pension if they serve an appropriate number of years in active duty (or a combination of active and reserve status). In past years, 20 years of active military service would provide a pension, with retirement benefits to begin at retirement, equal to 50% of base pay. The number of years of service required was increased to 22 in the late 1980s. A person with 20 or more years of combined active and reserve service might also qualify for a deferred pension beginning at age 60. Since 1956, servicemen have been paying into social security, so it is possible for an active military person to build more than one type of retirement. Since most take another full-time job upon leaving the military, it is possible for them to build three or four different types of retirement benefits.

FUNDING OF PRIVATE RETIREMENT PLANS

Private pension plans are funded in different ways. Corporate pension plans usually transfer cash or shares of their own securities to a fund to be managed by a bank trust department or by an insurance company. Benefits paid to retiring employees might be in addition to social security, or computed and reduced by primary social security benefits. Some of these may begin at an early age for the individual (e.g., at age 55) or later for one with 30 years or more of service. Some of these plans are contributory, which means that the employees makes some (all or partial) payment to the plan. Others are noncontributory, meaning that the employing firm makes the total contribution. The benefits on them are, thus, taxed in a different way. The tax laws hold the view that return of investment should not be taxed, but return on investment or payment of funds by a contributing firm are taxed. Thus, if a person has contributed about 25% of the total amount in the fund, and the balance comes from earned investment income or untaxed contributions, then 75% of monthly benefits would be taxable.

Many public school systems, including colleges and universities, have developed plans where each the employee and employer contribute from 5 to 8% of earned income into the account. Persons are permitted to retire at various ages, such as age 55 with reduced benefits or age 60 with full benefits. The monthly benefits are usually based on the years covered in the system times the base income (often the average of the highest consecutive 36 or 48 months of service). Retirement at less than the base age of 60 or 62, will often be at about a 6% annual reduction in benefits. In general, the federal employees retirement system is similar to this, permitting retirement at 55 or older with 30 years of covered service. Retirement at age 62 is permitted with fewer years of service.

Self-employed persons establishing a Keogh plan may contribute into qualifying insurance annuities, mutual fund shares, or a wide array of money market accounts. In general, the tax law requires that annuity benefits begin between the ages of 59.5 and 70.5 for persons to avoid taxation on deficiencies of withdrawals.

Persons who do not have another type of deferral of income supplemental retirement plan may establish an IRA (individual retirement annuity) with an insurance company (or other qualifying financial institution), placing up to $2,000 in the account each year. A spousal IRA permits up to $2,250 to be divided between both spouses, so long as one is not credited with more than $2,000 yearly. Again, benefits must begin between the ages of 59.5 and 70.5 to avoid the 10% penalty tax on failure to make timely withdrawals.

PURPOSES OF THE PROGRAMS

As benefits were reduced under the social security program, income earners were encouraged to provide their own supplemental retirement system. Thus, some of the above plans were developed to provide a supplemental retirement (income deferral system) to virtually every wage or salaried person. The major benefit from the plans are that they permit the deferment of income taxes on the contribution until benefits are withdrawn, and place a penalty tax on early withdrawals, which serves to reduce premature withdrawal from the accounts. In the early 1990s, about 90% of retiring persons seemed to qualify for some OASDI benefits. Almost one-half of retiring families had built some type of supplemental retirement benefit.

OTHER FEDERAL ASSISTANCE PROGRAMS

Certain low-income families may qualify for Supplemental Security Income (SSI) or food stamps. The SSI program pays monthly checks to people who are aged, disabled, or blind and who do not own many assets or have a lot of income. Persons who receive SSI benefits often also receive food stamps and Medicaid (which helps to pay doctor and hospital bills). The basic federal SSI check for one person is $386 (in 1990), or $579 a month for a couple. In general, in order for a family to receive SSI benefits, they may own their home, one auto, some personal assets, and up to $2,000 in financial assets. Application for SSI benefits are made through the nearest federal Social Security office.

The food stamp program helps needy people buy the food they need for good health. The federal program is run by local state agencies. The amount of stamps that each family is able to receive depends on the size of the family and the amount of cash income it receives. In order to receive food stamps, an application must be filed. Many food stores take food stamps, but not necessarily for nonfood items. Neither do they qualify for hot foods served on the premises. Any questions about the food stamp program should be referred to the food stamp office or to a regional Social Security office.

PLANNING IS ESSENTIAL

It is in the best interest of wise consumers and the U. S. economy that senior citizens and those unable to work be provided with a humane level of income to cover necessities of life. Thus, the federal OASDHI program was developed, first beginning in the mid-1930s. Coverage has been extended to other groups of persons, as stated above, since its inauguration in 1935.

Since Social Security only pays a fraction of earned income to the recipient as benefits, it is in the best interest of wage earners and salaried persons to build a supplemental retirement benefit by deferring some earned income until years of retirement, when the federal income tax rate will be nil or low. Several types of deferrals have been developed, as described above, to meet the needs of persons working for business firms, government agencies, or the self-employed. For those not qualifying for one of these plan, the IRA was begun in about 1981.

It is probably in the best interest of a working person to set aside from 10 to 20% of gross income into OASDI or other retirement systems to provide an adequate retirement income when the worker and spouse are no longer able to work. The careful budgeting of income and expenses, with good expense control and effective money management, should permit a development of one or more retirement plans. A budget might be helpful in planning and controlling monthly household expense and leaving funds for saving and investment.

Sources

Gitman, L. J. *Personal finance*. Chicago: Dryden.
Health Care Financing Administration. (1990). *The medicare handbook*. Publication No. HCFA 10050.
Mathur, I. (1989). *Personal finance* (2nd ed.). Cincinnati: Southwestern.
Social Security Administration. (1986). *Food stamp program*. SSA Publication No. 05-10100.
Social Security Administration. (1989). *History of Social Security*. SSA Publication No. 05-10011.
Social Security Administration. (1990). *Retirement*. SSA Publication No. 05-20035.
Social Security Administration. (1990). *Supplemental security income*. SSA Publication No. 05-11000.
Social Security: Partnership with tomorrow, 50th Anniversary edition. Sparta, IL.
Stillman, R. J. (1988). *Guide to personal finance* (5th ed.). Englewood Cliffs, NJ: Prentice-Hall.
Vaughan, E. J. (1989). *Fundamentals of risk and insurance* (5th ed.). New York: John Wiley.

Housing and Urban Development

Robert Lee Matkin, Rh.D.

History/Legislation

The Department of Housing and Urban Development (HUD) was established by the Department of Housing and Urban Development Act, approved September 9, 1965. HUD is the principal federal agency responsible for making housing affordable for low- and moderate-income families, enforcing fair housing opportunities, helping end the tragedy of homelessness, and creating jobs and opportunities in distressed urban and rural communities.

In carrying out its responsibilities, the department administers a wide variety of programs, including: Federal Housing Administration mortgage insurance programs that help families become homeowners and facilitate the construction and rehabilitation of rental units; rental assistance programs for lower income families who otherwise could not afford decent housing; the Government National Mortgage Association mortgage-backed securities program that helps ensure an adequate supply of mortgage credit; programs to combat housing discrimination and to affirmatively advance fair housing for all; programs that aid community and neighborhood development and preservation; and programs to help protect the homebuyer during real estate transactions. The department also takes steps to encourage a strong private sector housing industry that can produce affordable housing, as well as stimulate private sector initiatives, public/private sector partnerships, and public entrepreneurship.

The Department of Housing and Urban Development has a five-part mission:
- Administer the principal programs that provide assistance for housing and for the development of the nation's communities;
- Assist the President in achieving maximum coordination of the various federal activities that have a major effect upon community preservation and development;

- Encourage the solution of problems of housing and community development through states and localities;
- Encourage the maximum contributions that may be made to vigorous private homebuilding and mortgage lending industries, both primary and secondary, to housing, community development, and the national economy; and
- Provide for full and appropriate consideration, at the national level, of the needs and interests of the nation's communities and of the people who live and work in them.

Priorities of HUD under President George Bush and Secretary Jack Kemp are to expand home ownership and affordable housing opportunities, create jobs and economic development through *Enterprise Zones*, empower the poor through resident management and homesteading, enforce fair housing for all, help make public housing drug free, and help end homelessness.

Purpose/Intent

OFFICE OF THE SECRETARY

HUD is administered under the supervision and direction of the secretary, a cabinet-level position. The secretary is responsible for the administration of all programs, functions, and authorities of the department, including secondary mortgage market operations of the Government National Mortgage Association, also known as *Ginnie Mae*. The secretary advises the President on federal policy, programs, and activities relating to housing and community development. The secretary formulates recommendations for basic housing and community development policies for purposes such as the department's legislative program, the State of the Union message, and the President's budget.

The secretary's job includes (a) working with the Executive Office of the President and other federal agencies to ensure that economic and fiscal policies in housing and community development are consistent with other economic and fiscal policies of the government; (b) encouraging private enterprise to serve as large a part of the nation's total housing and community development needs as possible; (c) promoting the growth of cities and states and the efficient and effective use of housing, and community and economic development resources, by stimulating private sector initiatives, public/private sector partnerships, and public entrepreneurship; (d) taking steps to ensure equal access to housing for all, and to affirmatively prevent discrimination in housing; and (e) developing enterprise in achieving the objectives of the department. The secretary provides general oversight (as required by law) of the Federal National Mortgage Association, also known as *Fannie Mae* and the Federal Home Loan Mortgage Corporation. The secretary serves as a member of the Resolution Trust Corporation's oversight board.

The Office of the Secretary also contains staff offices having department-wide responsibility in specialized functional areas such as coordination of field activities, Indian and Alaskan Native programs, small and disadvantaged business utilization, intergovernmental relations, labor relations, international affairs, administrative judicial proceedings, and contract appeals. External organizations chaired by the secretary include the Interagency Council on the Homeless, the Martin Luther King, Jr. Federal Holiday Commission, and the Federal Housing Finance Board.

REGIONAL ADMINISTRATOR-REGIONAL HOUSING COMMISSIONERS

The field operations of the department are carried out through a series of regional and field offices. The regional offices of the department have boundaries prescribed by the secretary. Each regional office is headed by a Regional Administrator-Regional Housing Commissioner, who is responsible to the secretary for the overall satisfaction of the department's goals and objectives and for the management of the offices within the region.

While program and staff assistant secretaries exercise technical supervision over their field counterparts, the Regional Administrator (RA) is the responsible line official for all HUD programs in his or her region. The RA is responsible for (a) ensuring that program goals are met and that programs function in accordance with headquarters' guidance; (b) directing and evaluating performance of field offices in the region; and (c) allocating funds and staffing within the region. In addition to their regional management responsibilities, regional offices manage HUD's programs in their immediate geographic area. The 71 Field Office Managers supervise and direct programs within their jurisdictional areas. They are accountable to the Regional Administrators.

Program Areas and Legislation

ASSISTANT SECRETARY FOR HOUSING-FEDERAL HOUSING COMMISSIONER

The Assistant Secretary for Housing-Federal Housing Commissioner directs the housing programs and functions of the department, supporting the production, financing, and management of new and substantially rehabilitated housing, and the conservation and preservation of the existing housing stock.

The Office of the Assistant Secretary provides federal mortgage insurance to facilitate homeownership and construction or improvement of housing through approximately 40 mortgage insurance and loan programs. These insurance programs include mortgage for single family, multifamily, property improvement, manufactured homes, hospitals, and nursing home loans. This office administers special purpose programs designed specifically for the elderly, the handicapped, and the chronically mentally ill. It provides affordable housing for low- and moderate-income families through assisted housing programs. This office also protects consumers against fraudulent practices of land developers and promoters.

The assistant secretary is responsible for the following programs: mortgage insurance and other financial and related assistance authorized by the National Housing Act; the assisted-housing program (section 8) under the United States Housing Act of 1937; the rent supplement program under title I of the Housing and Urban Development Act of 1965; the repair, construction, improvement, removal, demolition or alteration, management, rehabilitation, rental, maintenance, operation, and disposition of real and related personal property managed by the Secretary; the elderly and handicapped housing loan program under section 202 of the Housing Act of 1959; technical and financial assistance to nonprofit sponsors under section 106 of the Housing and Urban Development Act of 1968; administration and enforcement of regulatory programs aimed at consumer protection; and the housing development grant program under section 17 of the United States Housing Act of 1937. The assistant secretary also serves as the chairman of the Mortgage Review Board and is authorized to withdraw mortgage approvals.

Insurance

Mortgage insurance is provided under the terms of the National Housing Act for the purchase, refinancing, construction, or rehabilitation of single-family housing, rental housing, cooperative housing, condominiums, and manufactured homes. Mortgage insurance also is provided for property improvement loans, housing for the elderly, nursing homes and intermediate care facilities, and nonprofit hospitals and group practice medical facilities. Special programs are provided for loan and mortgage insurance for land development, manufactured home parks, experimental housing, housing in urban renewal areas, armed services housing, and single-family housing for home ownership subsidized by interest assistance payments.

Applicants who wish to participate in the single-family mortgage insurance program must apply to a HUD-approved mortgage lender, who then applies to HUD. For multifamily projects, an applicant may elect to apply for a site appraisal and market analysis or, together with an approved mortgage, apply for a conditional or firm commitment depending upon the completeness of the drawing's specifications, and other required exhibits.

Loans and Rental Assistance

The department is authorized to provide loans to private, nonprofit borrowers to develop sound housing projects for the elderly or handicapped. In addition, interest-free loans are authorized under section 106 to cover up to 80% of the preconstruction costs incurred by nonprofit sponsors in planning a federally assisted section 202 housing project.

The section 8 housing assistance payments program authorized by the Housing and Community Development Act of 1974, provides housing assistance payments to participating private owners and public housing agencies to provide decent, safe, and sanitary, rehabilitated or existing housing for low-income families and elderly persons with affordable rents.

Housing Development Grants

Under the housing development grant program, HUD provides grants to cities, urban counties, and states acting on behalf of local governments to support the development of rental housing in areas with severe rental housing shortages. Grantees use the HUD funds to provide capital grants or loans, interest-reduction payments, rental subsidies, or other construction or substantial rehabilitation of rental projects by private owners.

Loan Management

HUD-insured and government-held mortgages are managed and serviced for all mortgage insurance programs under the National Housing Act, as amended, including nursing homes and manufactured home parks, hospitals and group practice facilities, and land development. Management and administration of assistance is offered for contracts for interest-reduction payments and rent supplements, home ownership for low- and middle-income families, operation and forbearance agreements, and assistance of mortgages. Loans are serviced and managed for housing assisted by department lending and grant programs.

Property Disposition

Real and related property conveyed to or in the custody of the secretary is managed, rehabilitated, rented, and disposed of by the department.

Real Estate Settlement Procedures

The Real Estate Settlement Procedures Act of 1974, as amended, was enacted by Congress to minimize abuses and to protect home buyers. The program requires lenders to provide loan applicants "good-faith estimates" of settlement costs that are incurred, and an information booklet describing the settlement process. The home buyer and seller each receive a Uniform Settlement Statement at the time of settlement, detailing services paid for the purchase of the house. The act also prohibits kickbacks and places limits on the amount of funds held in escrow by lenders.

ASSISTANT SECRETARY FOR PUBLIC AND INDIAN HOUSING

The Assistant Secretary for Public and Indian Housing is responsible for administering all public and Indian housing programs administered under the United States Housing Act of 1937, as amended. The assistant secretary advises the secretary regarding the production, financing, and management of public and Indian housing programs, as well as the preservation, improvement, and upgrading of the management and operation of the existing housing stock.

The office of the assistant secretary administers Public and Indian Housing Programs, including rental and homeownership programs, and provides technical and professional assistance in planning, developing, and managing low-income projects. This office administers an operating subsidy program for Public Housing Agencies (PHAs) and Indian Housing Authorities (IHAs), including operation/management of low-income housing projects. It also administers the Comprehensive Improvement Assistance Program for modernization of low-income housing projects to upgrade living conditions, correct physical deficiencies, and achieve operating efficiency and economy. The office of the assistant secretary administers the Resident Initiatives Program for resident participation, resident management, homeownership, drug prevention control, economic development and supportive services programs. This office also protects tenants from the hazards of lead-based paint poisoning by requiring PHAs and IHAs to comply with HUD regulations for the removal of lead-based paint from low-income housing units.

Low-income Public Housing

Local Public Housing Agencies (PHAs) are provided with technical and financial assistance in planning, developing, and managing housing for low-income families. Financial assistance is provided for planning, paying off bonds and notes issued to finance project development, and operating subsidies to ensure the low-income nature of the projects, and to enable PHAs to maintain adequate operating and maintenance services and reserve funds. Special provisions allow for purchase of such housing by low-income families. Modernization funds are provided for project upgrading.

Indian Housing

The department's Indian mutual-help home ownership opportunity program and low-income rental housing program utilize delivery systems that are responsible to the special housing requirements of Indian and Alaska Native communities. These programs are administered by Indian Housing Authorities (IHAs). Modernization funds are also provided for upgrading existing housing stock.

ASSISTANT SECRETARY FOR COMMUNITY PLANNING AND DEVELOPMENT

The office of the Assistant Secretary for Community Planning and Development administers Community Development Block Grants (CDBG) which provide communities with funds to carry out a wide range of community development activities. It provides section 108 Loan Guarantees under which HUD guarantees loans to communities to finance the acquisition and rehabilitation of real property. This office administers the Urban Development Action Grant (UDAG) program which encourages private investment in cities and urban counties experiencing severe economic distress, and stimulates development which aids in economic recovery. (Currently this program has not been refunded and, therefore, no new grants are being awarded.) It administers the Urban Homesteading Program which provides home ownership opportunities for individuals and families, using existing housing stock. It provides Rehabilitation Loans (312 Loans) which are low-interest loans for rehabilitation of property, primarily for low- and moderate-income persons. It administers the Rental Rehabilitation Program which provides funds to states and local governments to support rehabilitation of existing residential housing units and to provide rental assistance to low-income families. This office administers title V of the McKinney Act which establishes a procedure for the identification and use of unutilized and underutilized federal real property for facilities to assist the homeless.

The Assistant Secretary for Community Planning and Development is responsible for the following programs and activities:

Community Development Block Grants

The Community Development Block Grant (CDBG) program was established by title I of the Housing and Community Development Act of 1974 to meet a wide variety of community development needs in the *entitlement* and *nonentitlement* communities. Its primary objective is to develop viable urban communities by providing decent housing and a suitable living environment and expanding economic opportunities principally for persons of low- and moderate-income. Entitlement communities, generally cities with more than 50,000 population, central cities, and counties with more than 200,000 population, receive an annual amount of CDBG funds (their entitlement) based on a formula contained in the statute. Thirty percent of the funds appropriated for the CDBG also are allocated among states, using a formula, for use by nonentitlement communities.

Grants are awarded to entitlement communities to carry out a wide range of community development activities directed at neighborhood revitalization, economic development, and the provision of improved community facilities and services.

Entitlement communities develop their own programs and funding priorities. However, grantees must meet one of the following program objectives: benefit low- and moderate-income persons, or aid in the prevention or elimination of slums and blight. In addition, activities may be carried out that the community certifies are designed to meet other community development needs having a particular urgency because existing conditions pose a serious and immediate threat to the health or welfare of the community where other financial resources are not available to meet such needs. Grantees must also certify that during a period of not more than three years, not less than 51% of their CDBG funds will be used for activities that benefit low- and moderate-income persons. Activities that do not meet one of these three broad national objectives may not be undertaken with CDBG funds.

Nonentitlement communities are places that are not entitled to an annual grant. States may administer the nonentitlement CDBG funds, as a result of amendments to the act in 1981. In states that do not choose to administer the nonentitlement funds, HUD administers the Small Cities Program, which was established by amendments to the act in 1977.

The HUD-administered Small Cities Program is competitive; HUD ranks each community's application according to its percentage and absolute poverty, its program's impact, its community needs, and its performance in fair housing and equal opportunity. The most highly ranked applications are then funded to the extent funds are available.

The state-administered Small Cities Program application requirements, and the methods in which funds are distributed to nonentitlement communities, are established by the state. Eligible activities are the same as those for the entitlement communities, and programs must address the same program objectives. In electing to administer the program, the governor must certify that the state has or will:

Plan for community development activities;

Provide technical assistance in connection with community development programs;

Provide from state resources, funds equal to 10% of its CDBG allocation for community development activities; and

Consult with local elected officials in designing the method of funds distribution it will use.

Other applicable laws and requirements may be found in the Housing and Community Development Act of 1974, as amended.

Some of the specific activities that can be carried out with block grant funds include the acquisition of real property, relocation and demolition, rehabilitation of residential and nonresidential structures, provisions for public facilities and improvements (e.g., water and sewer facilities, streets, neighborhood centers), and the conversion of schools for eligible purposes. In addition, block grant funds are available to pay for public services within certain limits, activities relating to energy conservation and renewable energy resources, planning activities, assistance to profit-motivated businesses to carry out economic development activities, and assistance to nonprofit entities for community development activities.

Section 108 Loan Guarantees

Under section 108, HUD guarantees loans to communities to finance the acquisition of real property and the rehabilitation of publicly owned real property, plus certain related activities. CDBG entitlement cities, such as metropolitan cities and urban counties, are eligible to apply for loan guarantee assistance under section 108. To secure the loan guarantee, the community is required to pledge any grant approved or any grant that the community becomes eligible for under title I of the Housing and Community Development Act of 1974, as amended. Obligations guaranteed under section 108 are sold to an underwriting group of investment bankers for resale through periodic public offerings.

Secretary's Discretionary Fund

Under title I of the act, a fund is reserved for secretarial discretion in making community development grants to insular areas and Indian tribes for special project grants in unique and urgent circumstances, and for technical assistance to improve the planning, development, and administration of title I programs.

Urban Development Action Grants

These funds are authorized by title I of the Housing and Community Development Act of 1974, as amended. The Urban Development Action Grant (UDAG) program is designated to encourage new or increased private investment in cities and urban counties that are experiencing severe economic distress. The availability of Action Grant funds permits local officials to capitalize on opportunities to stimulate economic development activity such as new, permanent jobs and increased tax revenues needed to aid in economic recovery. Action Grant funds are available to carry out projects in support of a wide variety of economic recovery activities that involve partnerships with the private sector. As a requirement for funding, a firm private sector financial commitment must be in place. The program demonstrates the federal government's commitment to fostering private investment in cities.

Relocation and Acquisition

The Uniform Relocation Assistance and Real Property Acquisition Policies Act of 1970 (Uniform Act) establishes policies and requirements to ensure fair and equitable treatment of owners of property acquired for a federally assisted project, and persons displaced as a result of such acquisitions. The Office of Community Planning and Development develops HUD policies, standards, procedures, and advisory materials implementing the act and monitors HUD-assisted activities to ensure compliance with the law. Under the law, displaced persons receive relocation assistance, including reimbursement for moving expenses. Eligible occupants displaced from a dwelling unit also receive a replacement housing payment. Property owners are offered fair value for their property and are reimbursed for any incidental sales costs. By regulation, the department has adopted requirements designed to ensure that adequate relocation assistance is provided to tenants displaced by certain HUD-assisted programs that are not governed by the Uniform Act.

Environment

The assistant secretary has responsibility for implementing policies and procedures for the protection and enhancement of environmental quality pursuant to the National Environmental Policy Act of 1969 and related laws and authorities, and the Housing and Community Development Act of 1974 as amended. Environmental activities encompass the development of standards, policies, and procedures for environmental assessments and impact statements, and compliance with laws and executive orders on archaeology, historic preservation, floodplains, wetlands, aquifers, endangered species, and other resources. Activities include the development and administration of strategies for the amelioration of environmental problems and the establishment of standards, such as those for minimum distances between housing and sources of noise or hazardous storage facilities. Emphasis is placed on technical assistance and helping communities in environmental and land-use planning and environmental management practices, including urban environmental design and the quality of the built environment.

Energy

The 1980 and 1981 amendments to title I of the Housing and Community Development Act of 1974 added to the findings and purposes of the act. Recognizing that increasing energy costs have seriously undermined local community development and housing activities, these amendments called for concerted action with state and local governments to address the resulting economic and social hardships and added as new objectives conservation, energy efficiency, and renewable sources of supply. HUD-supported activities include building energy retrofit and installation of solar equipment, production (emphasizing renewable resources), aid for the assessment and design of district heating and cooling systems and resource recovery projects, provision of technical assistance to state and local governments, and the preparation of comprehensive energy-use strategies. The Assistant Secretary for Community Planning and Development functions as energy conservation officer for the department and in liaison with other agencies.

Section 312 Rehabilitation Loans

Under section 312 of the Housing Act of 1964, as amended, low-interest loans for rehabilitation of residential and nonresidential properties are made in conjunction with other federal programs that aid neighborhood revitalization, such as the Community Development Block Grant Program and Urban Homesteading.

Funds are allocated for the rehabilitation of single family and multifamily properties in HUD-approved urban homesteading areas and in communities that receive Community Development Block Grant Assistance. In making section 312 loans, priority is given to applications submitted by low- and moderate-income persons who own property and will occupy it upon the completion of rehabilitation. The interest rate for single-family, owner-occupied properties (1 to 4 units) is 3% if the borrower's family income for the area, adjusted for family size, is within 80% of the median income for the area. For all other applications, the rate of interest will be indexed to the weekly Federal Reserve statistical release for comparable or near terms of the U. S. Government securities. Applicants should contact the local city or county government in their area to determine what local public agency administers the program. An applicant who needs assistance should contact the HUD Field Office in his or her area for more information. The agency will provide advice and assist the applicant with the loan application.

Urban Homesteading

Under title VIII, section 810 of the Housing and Community Development Act of 1974, as amended, HUD is authorized to transfer, without payment, to states, units of local government or their designated public agencies, secretary-owned, unoccupied, unrepaired, one-to-four-family residences for use in a HUD-approved urban homesteading program. The legislation also authorized the appropriation of funds to reimburse the department for any properties transferred under section 810.

An urban homesteading program must provide for the conditional conveyance of property to homesteaders who agree to repair it, maintain it, and live in it as their principal residence for a minimum of five years in exchange for full, legal title. The local program must develop a coordinated plan for improving the neighborhood's services and facilities. The appropriations for the urban homesteading program are used to reimburse the HUD housing loan and mortgage insurance fund for any properties transferred to localities for use in an approved local urban homesteading program.

Section 106 of the Housing and Community Development Amendments of 1979 and section 102(a) of the Housing and Community Development Amendments of 1978 authorized HUD to reimburse the Secretary of Veterans Affairs and the Secretary of Agriculture for properties conveyed for use in a HUD-approved urban homesteading program.

Rental Rehabilitation Grant Program

Under section 17 of the United States Housing Act of 1937, as amended, formula grant allocations are made to state and local governments to make the rehabilitation of rental properties feasible. Direct allocations go to states, cities with populations over 50,000, and urban counties that will receive at least a minimum allocation amount established by HUD. State programs cover areas under 50,000 in population (except for FmHA title V areas) and cities over 50,000 in populations that do not receive the minimum allocation.

Program grant funds may be used only to finance the rehabilitation of privately owned, primarily residential rental properties. In order to leverage the maximum amount of private capital, rehabilitation subsidies are generally limited to 50% of the cost of rehabilitation, not to exceed $5,000 per unit adjusted for high-cost areas.

To ensure maximum benefit to lower income tenants in this program, 70 to 100% of each grantee's funds must be spent on rehabilitated properties initially occupied by lower income tenants. In addition, grantees must target all of the assistance to lower income neighborhoods (median income at or below 80% of median for area) where the rents can be expected to remain affordable to lower income families over time.

Neighborhood Development Demonstration Program

Section 123 of the Housing and Urban-Rural Recovery Act of 1983 authorized a demonstration program to determine the feasibility of supporting eligible neighborhood development activities by providing federal matching funds to eligible neighborhood development organizations. The matching funds are determined on the basis of the monetary support such organizations have received from individuals, businesses, and nonprofit or other organizations in their neighborhoods prior to receiving federal assistance. The legislation seeks to foster the long-term self-sufficiency of such organizations, and improve the business, job creation, and housing availability programs within these neighborhoods.

ASSISTANT SECRETARY FOR FAIR HOUSING AND EQUAL OPPORTUNITY

The Assistant Secretary for Fair Housing and Equal Opportunity advises the secretary and departmental staff on issues and policies affecting civil rights and equal opportunity in housing and related facilities, community development, and employment. The assistant secretary is responsible for developing and implementing fair housing and equal opportunity policies and programs pursuant to various civil rights laws, executive orders, and federal regulations intended to protect affected persons from discrimination based on race, color, sex, national origin, religion, handicap, or age.

This office administers:

Fair Housing Laws and Regulations: Federal law prohibits discrimination in public and private housing on the basis of race, color, religion, sex, age, handicap, familial status, and national origin;

Equal Opportunity Laws and Regulations: Federal law prohibits discrimination in HUD-assisted community development programs on the basis of race, color, religion, sex, and national origin; and

Equal Employment Opportunity Laws and Regulations: Federal law prohibits discrimination on the basis of race, color, religion, sex, national origin, handicap, and age in HUD employment.

ASSISTANT SECRETARY FOR POLICY DEVELOPMENT AND RESEARCH

The office of the Assistant Secretary for Policy Development and Research advises the secretary on policy, program evaluation, and research. The office evaluates and analyzes existing and proposed programs and policies. Under the Housing and Urban Development Act of 1970 and other statutes, the assistant secretary undertakes programs of research, studies, testing, and demonstrations related to HUD's mission. These functions are carried out by its staff and through grants, cooperative agreements, contracts with industry, nonprofit research organizations, educational institutions, private foundations, and agreements with state and local governments, the private sector, and other federal agencies.

To provide the secretary and program administrators with the most complete information possible in the formulation of policy, this office not only assesses alternative policies but also gauges their impact. An important step in that process is linking the findings of long- and short-term research with the policy issues and problems facing the department, making maximum use of the ongoing research, evaluation, and economic analysis conducted by the divisions within this office. This office sets the research agendas of the divisions so they reflect the overall policy needs of the department. This office also participates in the formulation of the department's budget and legislative development process, and reviews all departmental regulations, notices, handbooks, and forms.

The evaluation process is inseparable from policy development. Along with preparing option and quick-response papers on a wide variety of issues, this office also conducts field studies and evaluations of all major programs to provide information on their impact, effectiveness, and administration and to analyze their costs and benefits. The purpose in every case is to generate the comprehensive understanding that leads to new programs and policies in tune with administration goals and a high level of efficiency.

In helping to carry out its mission to improve the nation's communities and housing, HUD's research efforts have been narrowed and intensified to focus on such priority subjects as: improvements in housing finance issues; the impact of proposed tax changes on low-income housing; improving the quality of life in public housing; evaluation of programs authorized by the Housing and Urban-Rural Recovery Act of 1983; affordable housing; evaluation of current fair housing activities and development of the department's Fair Housing Initiatives Program; and the administration's federalism policy.

Sources

National Archives and Records Administration. (1987). *The United States Government Manual* (1987/ 88 ed.). Washington, DC: U. S. Government Printing Office.

U. S. Department of Housing and Urban Development. (1990). *The Secretary's Semiannual Report to the Congress, Number 2 (May 31, 1990)*. Washington, DC: U. S. Department of Housing and Urban Development.

Community Service Organizations

M. J. Schmidt, M.A.

In recent years, the number of persons with special needs has grown immensely. Political activism and overall awareness of civil rights for the disabled has expanded. The array of human services available has improved, and the amount of information and technology specific to special populations has increased dramatically. Funding for human services, however, has become less available. As a result, the job of human-service personnel has become increasingly complex. No longer do human-service counselors and practitioners rely solely on traditional sources of information and individual knowledge of available services. Instead, human-service providers have learned to be more creative in their search for potential client resources. Counselors often must rely on alternative service providers, seek supplemental sources of information, and better access the community.

Traditionally oriented and trained counselors frequently overlook community service organizations as viable resources. Community service organizations are agencies which typically provide services—both directly and indirectly—to special groups of people or to the community at large (Lewis & Lewis, 1989). Some community service agencies exist primarily to serve a specific population or disability group. Others are interested more globally in serving persons with special needs or in addressing related political, economic, and financial concerns. Finally, some community service organizations are simply local groups (e.g., religious or fraternal organizations) who are willing to help those in need in their community. The American Cancer Society, the American Red Cross, and the Lion's Club are all examples of community service organizations.

Community service agencies recognize the need for direct, individualized services and often provide them. They also frequently facilitate self-help groups or mutual support networks. As important as direct services are, however, their primary impact is in supplementing or supporting extant community efforts for the people they serve. Advocacy, information dissemination and research, referral, fund raising, and political action are among their most common activities.

Community service organizations tend to fall into three general categories:

- Specialized agencies—or those organized to address specific needs of a group or a specific cause
- Multiple service agencies—or those organizations concerned with a variety of special groups and concerns
- Fraternal, religious, and other local community service agencies—or those agencies primarily concerned with providing service to those in need within a given community.

Specialized and multiple-service agencies are generally organized on the national, state, and local levels. Frequently, national offices exist in large metropolitan areas, and state and local affiliates develop as needed. While national offices most often have access to information regarding global issues including facts about the disability or area of concern, the organization itself, federal law, and the like, state and local offices are commonly the source of direct services and community education efforts.

Specialized and multiple service organizations often consist of small paid staffs and large numbers of volunteer members. Membership is rarely limited to professionals, consumers, or family members. Instead, members tend to represent all of these parties and interested others. Typically, membership dues are requested of those who can pay. Many times, dues are waived or smaller donations are accepted from those who cannot afford the requested amount. Generally, membership entitles one to a regular newsletter or publication, as well as occasional discounts for upcoming seminars and events. Fraternal, religious, and other local agencies may also be organized nationally, yet, again, services are primarily rendered on a local level. Membership for these organizations also consists of volunteers.

History/Legislation

Community service organizations have existed for a number of years in the United States. As early as 1880, for example, the National Association for the Deaf and the Salvation Army were in operation. However, the number of community service organizations in this country has increased dramatically within the past 50 years. This increase can be attributed to a number of factors including the continually improving survival rates of persons with disabilities, the expanded prevalence of persons with special needs in our society, the civil rights and disability rights movements, and the corresponding increase in potential human services.

The history of the development of various community service organizations is quite diverse. Many community services have originated in response to legislation; the Disability Rights Center, for one, was founded in 1976 to protect and enforce the rights of citizens with disabilities. The agency has been concerned with and continues to focus on the enforcement of section 501 of the Rehabilitation Act of 1973. Other organizations have developed to advocate for or against political action or legislation. The National Association of Developmental Disabilities Councils, for example, was created, in part, to work with legislators to ensure adequate representation of the special concerns of persons with developmental disabilities.

Community service organizations are also established by professionals, consumers, and family members. Namely, the American Criminal Justice Association and the National Rehabilitation Counseling Association were established by professionals in order to create better information sharing and professional networking. Similarly, the National Amputation Association was founded by veterans with service-related amputations. The Alzheimer's Association was established by families of persons with Alzheimer's disease in response to the general lack of available support and information.

Finally, the origin of many of the existing community service organizations today has been facilitated by members of specific disability groups or consumers. However, the origin of most community service organizations has been facilitated by a group of persons including consumers, professionals, family members, and other advocates.

FUNDING

Community service organizations can be funded in any number of ways. Often, they rely on multiple methods of financing. The great majority of community service organizations are funded at least in part by private donations. The American Heart Association, for example, is financed entirely in this manner. Many receive monies from federal and state government in the form of grants for special projects. The Retired Senior Volunteer Program, which manages Meals on Wheels programs, is funded by ACTION, the federal domestic volunteer agency. Membership dues also serve to support operations. In fact, most professional and special interest service agencies request annual dues from their members. Fund-raising efforts are not uncommon. The Muscular Dystrophy Association's annual telethon is a well-known example. Additionally, some community service organizations charge for printed materials provided to others in order to minimize cost. Others, such as Goodwill Industries and the Salvation Army, rely on the resale of goods in thrift shops to generate funds. Some are completely government supported and operated. The National AIDS Information Clearinghouse, for instance, is operated by the Center for Disease Control.

Regardless of the primary funding for community service agencies, information and referral services are typically available at no cost. Support services, such as the National Amputation Association's Amp to Amp program and the National Burn Victim Association's 24-hour crisis counseling program, are also provided without cost to the consumer. Often, allowances for those unable to pay can be arranged through even the direct service providers in this genre, such as Goodwill Industries and the United Way.

STAFFING

Community service organizations are staffed by both paid personnel and volunteers. Many organizations (e.g., United Way, Association for Retarded Citizens, Volunteers of America) operate with relatively small paid staffs and large numbers of volunteers. Fraternal and religious organizations such as the Kiwanis Club and B'nai B'rith Women, consist of voluntary members of widely differing education, experience, and professions. Many special interest agencies rely on donations of time from affiliated professionals, consumers, and family members. Others, like the Salvation Army, are staffed almost entirely by persons specifically dedicated to that agency.

The qualifications of agency personnel varies greatly. At the national level, some of the best known doctors, advocates, and professionals may be on the staff of a specialized community service organization. Consumers, family members, and volunteers with less formal education may also be present. Despite the difference in area of expertise, staff members of specialized agencies are typically quite familiar with the population of concern or interest. When they lack knowledge directly, they often have the resources to gain information. Hence, they make invaluable resources in terms of networking and referral.

Purpose/Intent

Community service organizations exist to serve individuals in the community. Specialized agencies work primarily with specific disability groups or populations or to address related concerns. Fraternal, religious, and locally based service organizations primarily work to serve the local community and to facilitate projects of interest. Nonetheless, each community service organization develops in order to meet certain goals. Although some agencies are quite focused in their mission, most organizations offer a combination of services to achieve two or three objectives. Often, the mission of specialized agencies is centralization or unification of consumers, family members, and professionals interested in a specific disability. Through unification, there is increased networking and information sharing. There is also strength in numbers in terms of political advocacy and fund raising. The objectives of unified disability-specific organizations often include increasing community awareness, advocacy for the rights of the group, improvement in the status of treatment or quality of life, and the provision of support for consumers and their families.

Conversely, some community service organizations develop which are not specifically interested in a particular group, but rather in all persons with special needs. Objectives of these organizations range from service provision, to increased community awareness, to political advocacy. The American Red Cross, the United

Way, and Goodwill Industries are examples of organizations primarily concerned with service provision to those in need. Other community service organizations develop to specifically advocate for, and protect the rights of, all persons with disabilities. Their objectives primarily reflect education of policymakers, enforcement of current legislation, and the continued advocacy for legislation which will protect the rights of persons with disabilities. Finally, many local community service organizations develop primarily as social groups which are also dedicated to furthering efforts of goodwill in local communities.

Regardless of the specific purpose of these agencies, community service is generally part of the mission. Although direct services may not be available to all who request them, information and referral are typically available. Specialized organizations are often excellent starting places in terms of learning more about a specific population, piece of legislation, or related concern. Local service agencies are also an excellent, yet frequently overlooked, resource for counselors in terms of volunteer services and money or fund raising.

Services

In order to achieve their objectives, community service organizations offer a wide range of services—both directly and indirectly to consumers and the community. These services are often offered in varying degrees by the different divisions of community service organizations.

DIRECT CONSUMER SERVICES

Many state and local offices of community service organizations offer direct services to consumers. The type and quality of these services vary greatly. Individualized services are occasionally available. Agencies like Goodwill Industries offer a wide range of direct consumer services including evaluation, training, counseling, and placement for vocationally disabled persons. Similarly, the National Easter Seal Society offers physical, occupational, and speech and language therapies, vocational evaluation and training, recreational opportunities, and even equipment, on loan, to persons of all disabilities. The United Cerebral Palsy Association's direct services include similar therapies, as well as supported and supervised housing. The National Burn Victim Association operates a Medical Disaster Response System which provides emergency services to large numbers of burn victims, as well as offers free blood to those victims in need.

Individual counseling is also frequently offered directly to individual consumers and their families. Special counseling is also commonly available. For instance, the American Heart Association sponsors *Heart to Heart*, a one-to-one visitation program for persons with coronary problems. Similarly, the National Amputation and Spinal Cord Injury Associations offer individualized peer counseling.

Other direct individualized services include meal provision and companionship programs; these are primarily available through local organizations and are most frequently offered to senior citizens and the homebound. Community service organizations like the Children's Defense Fund and the National Coalition for the Homeless also provide legal counseling and assistance. Medical services are provided by various agencies, especially those concerned with prevention, disaster relief, or specific medical conditions. Shriner's Hospitals provide free care to children with burns and disabilities. Financial counseling and assistance is also commonly available. The American Kidney Fund provides financial assistance to those suffering fiscal problems as a result of their condition. Special education, outreach programs for those with special needs, and prosthesis/equipment maintenance and repair services are additional services commonly available through many of these organizations.

Specialized community service organizations frequently offer group services as well as individual care. Self-help and support groups are commonly offered by state and local affiliates of community service organizations. Persons with disabilities and their families often experience gaps in their natural support networks. They may benefit from developing mutually supportive relationships with others in similar situations. Self-help and support groups often provide this opportunity. There are any number of such groups sponsored by community service agencies. They include, but certainly are not limited to:

- Alcoholics Anonymous
- American Schizophrenic Association
- Association for Children with Learning Disabilities
- Burns Recovered
- Epilepsy Foundation
- Gay Men's Health Crisis
- Juvenile Diabetes Foundation
- Muscular Dystrophy Association
- National Alliance for the Mentally Ill
- National Association for Retarded Citizens
- National Federation for the Blind
- National Spinal Cord Injury Foundation
- United Cerebral Palsy Association

Community service agencies also sponsor camps, especially for children with special needs. A great many of these camps are free or of minimal cost. They are almost always staffed by professionals, and can prove to be a great resource to those counselors working with children. The National Head Injury Foundation, the Muscular Dystrophy Association, the American Diabetes Association, and many other community service organizations are involved in these efforts. Similarly, the Children's Wish Foundation International provides terminally ill children with opportunities to engage in desired activities.

INDIRECT CONSUMER SERVICES

Perhaps the greatest component of community service organization work involves indirect services to consumers. Indirect services include information and referral, research, political action and advocacy, research and training, and fund raising. By and large, the vast majority of community service organizations develop and distribute some form of information specific to their population or area of interest. Pamphlets, articles written for laypersons, scholarly publications, and even audio and video tapes are widely available from community service organizations. Many publish newsletters or similar publications routinely. Many even maintain libraries of all types of information specific to their interest. For the most part, written information is available for free or for a minimal fee to cover reprint and postage costs.

Information regarding available services—or referral—is also normally available. Quite often, community service organizations are excellent sources of information regarding locally available services for a particular population. In fact, some organizations specialize in information and referral. The Information Center for Individuals with Disabilities, for example, gathers and stores information in 16 subject categories including accessibility, employment, housing, transportation, and personal care. The National Homelessness Information Exchange is designed specifically to supply local service providers with information relevant to the needs of those without homes. Agencies may also be able to refer counselors and consumers to practitioners with experience in a particular disability or condition, identify related support or self-help groups, or provide similar linkages to other agencies or service providers. Organizations such as the National Multiple Sclerosis Society, maintain large databases of information to facilitate research and referral. Community service agencies may also provide information regarding potential funding for services.

Another important function of many community service organizations involves political action and advocacy. Occasionally, these agencies advocate for consumers on an individual basis. However, for the most part, advocacy efforts pertain to the group as a whole or to persons with disabilities collectively. The Disability Rights Center and the Disabled Rights Education and Defense Fund are primarily concerned with the protection of the rights of persons with disabilities. They work to educate policymakers as to the needs of these persons, as well as to ensure compliance with existing legislation. The Disabled Rights Education and Defense Fund also trains judges on disability rights compliance standards and maintains the Disability Law National Support Center to identify key disability issues.

Disability-specific community service agencies are also quite active in political advocacy. The National Association for the Deaf promotes legislation and programs to benefit persons with hearing impairments. The American Council for the Blind provides information and advisory services on federal legislation, administrative action, and rule making on both national and state levels. Similarly, the National Alliance for the Mentally Ill and the National Association for Developmental Disabilities Councils work to improve the lives of their populations by informing legislators of their special needs.

Additionally, the National Multiple Sclerosis Society, the Arthritis Foundation, the American Diabetes Foundation, and many other community service agencies sponsor tremendous amounts of research regarding the cure and prevention of disabling conditions. Similarly, many organizations offer funding to researchers, as well as specialized training in state-of-the-art diagnostic and treatment techniques. The Arthritis Foundation, for instance, provides training to doctors in the diagnosis and care of rheumatoid arthritis.

Advocacy efforts regarding accessibility issues or other discriminatory policies affecting target population are yet another illustration of services provided by these agencies with both direct and indirect consumer benefits. The National Disability Action Council, the National Coalition for the Homeless, and the National Rehabilitation Association are among the many groups involved in comparable endeavors. Some community service agencies are instrumental in identifying other aspects of the environment which affect the prevalence or severity of the disability or condition. Efforts then to ameliorate or prevent the problem are made. The National Head Injury Foundation, in this manner, has campaigned heavily for seatbelt and carseat legislation, as well as for motorcycle and bicycle helmet use.

Finally, community service organizations are commonly involved in fund raising. The Muscular Dystrophy Association, the American Lung Association, the National Multiple Sclerosis Society, and the National Easter Seal Society, for example, raise millions of dollars each year. These efforts often involve community participation and donations. Telethons, walk- or bike-a-thons, raffles and lotteries, and simple solicitation of donations are not uncommon. Occasionally, large businesses become involved, such as the National Football League's involvement with the United Way. In any case, much of the money raised through these efforts serves to support direct client services and the operation of these agencies.

COMMUNITY SERVICES

Community service organizations are also involved in providing direct services to the community at large. These services often take the form of courses or workshops that provide knowledge or skills that the particular populations they serve have identified as important. Women's centers often provide courses on assertiveness, career development, or women's health concerns. The American Cancer Society and the American Heart Association operate national education and awareness campaigns. Agencies concerned with the elderly may provide education related to retirement planning or social security benefits.

Prevention is a common theme of community education. Many community service organizations provide public workshops on healthy lifestyling and even offer screening for certain conditions. The National AIDS Network, for example, provides community workshops and seminars on AIDS prevention issues, and even financially assists other organizations sponsoring AIDS education. Finally, many organizations work directly with allied health professionals to ensure that practitioners are offering state-of-the-art services to the community.

Community service agencies also frequently bestow awards to deserving care-providers, researchers, consumers, advocates, and educators.

HOW TO ACCESS

Community service organizations are not difficult to access. They generally can be found in the Yellow Pages of local telephone books under such headings as "Community Service Organizations," "Social Service Organizations," "Fraternal Organizations," and even under churches, synagogues, and other religious affiliations. The *Encyclopedia of Associations* (Burek, 1991) is also an excellent source for basic information and addresses and phone numbers of national organizations. Similarly, the United Way regularly publishes a resource book which lists basic information, addresses and phone numbers of community service agencies.

As in any other referral or request for information or services, it is recommended that counselors check with fellow professionals regarding their contacts and resources. It is also recommended that, when possible, counselors refer directly to known individuals in an agency rather than to the agency itself. This process, of course, involves the continual development of professional contacts. In order to facilitate this process, counselors should consider the following:

- Human service professionals should become aware of those agencies in their community involved with service efforts. This includes, but is not limited to, fraternal organizations, local chapters of specialized agencies, religious service organizations, senior citizen organizations, women's centers, university-affiliated services and groups, and government-supported programs and services. Counselors should identify and develop personal contacts at those agencies likely to be used.
- Counselors and practitioners involved with a specific disability group should become aware of the associated specialized organizations and become a member of at least one such association. This is an excellent way of making contacts, keeping up-to-date with pertinent information, finding out about relevant conferences and seminars, and building a professional network.

References

Burek, D. M. (Ed.). (1991). *Encyclopedia of associations* (25th ed.). New York: Gale Research, Inc.

Lewis, J. A., & Lewis, M. D. (1989). *Community counseling*. Pacific Grove, CA: Brooks/Cole.

Index